Glossary of Anaesthetics

For Nurses, Paramedics, and Operating Department Practitioners

John England

Disclaimer

The author has made every effort to ensure that the contents of this book are correct, error free, and a reasonable representation of the design goal, which is to inform and describe some of the relevant concepts and terminology concerning the subject of Anaesthesia, and related topics. This body of work should be regarded as a text book for learning purposes, and not a clinical or operations manual.

The author accepts no responsibility or liability for damages caused by any erroneous contents of this book and, in all situations, recommends that professional guidelines, national policies, and direction from suitably qualified medical staff, take precedence over the information contained herein.

☆ ☆ ☆ ☆ ☆ ☆ ☆ ☆ ☆

Preface

Perioperative patients depend on doctors (anaesthetists and surgeons) to maintain or improve their conditions, and these same doctors rely on a team of allied professionals to support them. Within the field of anaesthetics, the support role is fulfilled by anaesthetic trained nurses, Operating Department Practitioners (ODPs), and Anaesthetic Technicians.

Anaesthetic training, for the above practitioners, is non-standard and practical, where a student learns their role by mimicking their mentor, which means focusing on the manual aspects of working in anaesthetics, such as equipment and drug preparation, protocol compliance, and setting up for intravenous fluid administration.

For these personnel, the science of anaesthetic practice is not, on the whole, part of training. An anaesthetic practitioner (with exceptions) will, for example, prepare a syringe containing a drug of a specific concentration, without understanding how the concentration is calculated, or what the dosage information means. With respect to the application of an inhalational gas, such as Isoflurane, anaesthetic practitioners are not taught how a patient's physiology is affected by that gas, or the significance of the properties of individual gases. The same situation occurs with basic scientific concepts, such as diffusion, gas pressures, osmosis, and molar measurements.

There is, quite clearly, a gap between the practical side of working in anaesthetics, and the basic science and theoretical aspects which underpin practice. The purpose of this book is to help fill that gap, by providing definitions and explanations of selected perioperative terminology, basic science, and principles of anaesthetics.

After mastering the *Glossary of Anaesthetics*, the reader will have gained a greater understanding of some of the more significant principles of anaesthesia, and be more informed as to how the patient is affected by the imposition of an anaesthetic regime. As a consequence, the reader will become a safer and more confident professional, be more qualified to be a patient advocate, and be better equipped to take the path to more advanced roles.

☆ ☆ ☆ ☆ ☆ ☆ ☆ ☆ ☆

Introduction

This book has been designed, principally, to be a handy anaesthetic reference for nurses, Operating Department Practitioners, and Paramedics, and a guide as to what areas of Perioperative science such practitioners might have to develop, if they wish to progress to more senior and advanced roles.

Part one is a glossary of terminology, short definitions, and explanations of a compendium of theoretical and practical issues, which are central to an understanding of anaesthetics.

Part two is the Appendix, which contains more detailed discussions and explanations of some of the items in part two. For students, there are examples of case preparation, such as setting up for Epidural blocks, and Central Venous Pressure monitoring.

Audience

Students

For the student anaesthetics assistant, the glossary and appendices provide a comprehensive introduction to the fundamental science and day to day language of anaesthetics.

Experienced practitioners

For established practitioners, the explanations of more specific issues, for example, *Flow Rate* factors, *Blood:Gas* and *Oil:Gas Partition Coefficients*, will help to expand their understanding of those matters which are well understood by anaesthetists, but not so well understood by supporting practitioners.

Advancement

For anyone with the ambition to progress to a more advanced role, such as Practice Educator, Physician Associate, or Anaesthesia Associate, having a thorough comprehension of the basic science and related subjects, in this book, might indicate an aptitude for the type of study which these more advanced roles require. As a marker for those ambitious individuals, some glossary entries have been emboldened, because they represent topics, an understanding of which, indicate the aptitude for the above mentioned advanced roles.

OdpQandA@Twitter.com

For readers who want to test their knowledge, test questions, based on this book, are presented at the above Twitter handle, which is a non "Follow back" account, so that there is minimal clutter from other tweets.

☆ ☆ ☆ ☆ ☆ ☆ ☆ ☆ ☆

Glossary

~ (Tilde)

The tilde symbol signifies "approximately".

[ ]

Square brackets are a symbol to show that the entity within the brackets is referred to in the context of concentration. For example, 4 mmol/L Na (sodium) concentration: [Na] = 4 mmol/L.

A-a Gradient (PAO_2 - PaO_2)

The oxygen partial pressure gradient (difference) between the calculated alveolar (pAO_2) and measured (blood gas) arterial (paO_2) pressures. Normal A-a is between 4 and 8 mmHg (0.53-1.06 kPa), but a rough calculation can be used, specifically: (age + 10) / 4. For example, a healthy 20 year old patient has an expected gradient of (10 + 20) / 4 = 7.5 mmHg. So, if this patient has an alveolar oxygen pressure of 104 mmHg (13.8 kPa), then the arterial oxygen pressure (paO_2) is expected to be 104– 7.5 = 96.5 mmHg (12.8 kPa). The gradient can help differentiate causes of hypoxaemia to be either intrapulmonary or extrapulmonary; if the patient has a larger than expected gradient, the cause might be right to left shunt, diffusion problems, or poor ventilation-perfusion (V/Q) ratio. But, if a hypoxaemic patient does not have a wide A-a gradient, the hypoxic condition might be caused by hypoventilation, because both alveolar (pAO_2) and arterial (paO_2) values will be lower than normal, so the difference (gradient) between the two may also be normal. **Note**: Every decade of life increases the gradient by ~1 mmHg.

Abdominal Aortic Aneurysm (AAA)

Dilation of part of the aorta to 50% + above normal diameter, and which requires urgent surgical intervention. For the anaesthetic team, **equipment** needed might include: ECG, Pulse oximeter, BP, Capnography, Arterial and Central Venous monitoring; Rapid fluid infuser; Urine output monitoring; Transoesophageal echocardiography; LIDCO cardiac output monitoring; Warmed blood products; Cell-saver; Body Warming; Temperature monitoring; Arterial blood gases. See Appendix A1 (pg 339).

Absorber

A component of an anaesthetic machine, forming a *circle* breathing circuit, and whose functional part is a chemical crystalline structure that absorbs the patient's expired CO_2 (carbon dioxide), and produces heat and moisture as a side-effect. A CO_2 absorber allows a low flow circle breathing system to be used, otherwise, a higher fresh gas flow would have to be continuously added to the circuit, so that CO_2 can be flushed out to the atmosphere. In most cases, the chemical element, known as “soda lime”, has calcium hydroxide as the absorbent ingredient, plus potassium hydroxide and sodium hydroxide. Other chemical absorbents, such as lithium hydroxide, are available. When the soda lime has reached its saturation point (colour change), it can no longer absorb CO_2, and must be replaced. If a CO_2 absorber is integrated into a Mapleson C circuit, it becomes a “Water's” circuit. CO_2 absorbers are also found in submarines, decompression chambers, and spacecraft, where they are more commonly referred to as "CO_2 scrubbers".

Absorption

Biology: Assimilation of substances into cells, by diffusion or osmosis. For example, an inhalational anaesthetic, such as isoflurane, some of which is absorbed by plasma proteins, and where the amount being absorbed is governed by the agent's *Blood:Gas Partition Coefficient.* See *Drug Absorption.*

Acetylcholine (ACh)

The primary neurotransmitter (has no antagonist) for nerves of the parasympathetic nervous system, stored in synaptic vesicles within nerve terminals at the neuromuscular junction, released by exocytosis (nerve impulses) *{Acetylcholine is also found in the brain, autonomic ganglia, and heart}*. ACh binds with cholinergic (nicotinic) receptors on nerve neurons in the motor end plate of the neuromuscular junction, producing depolarisation and muscle contraction. ACh is also released by the heart's cardiomyocytes, where it binds with muscarinic receptors, producing muscarinic effects, including bradycardia, decreased force of heart contractions, salivation, and secretions, which may be countered by antimuscarinic drugs such as Glycopyrrolate. When a patient is paralysed with a competitive neuromuscular blocker, such as Atracurium, it binds with the cholinergic receptors in competition with ACh, so locks out enough ACh to prevent depolarisation (muscle contraction). Thus, the patient is "paralysed". Note: ACh can be thought of as having the opposite effect of noradrenaline.

Acetylcholinesterase (AChE)

Cholinesterase enzyme that breaks down Acetylcholine (ACh) into choline and acetate, in the central nervous system and at motor end plates, for recycling. By decomposing ACh, muscle contraction is reduced. Acetylcholinesterase is essential because, without it, muscle contraction would be continuous.

ACGO

See Auxiliary Common Gas Outlet.

Acid

A substance that releases hydrogen ions (H+) when it dissociates in a solution, such as water. Hydrogen atoms leave their electrons behind, with the substance they detached from, which is why they are sometimes referred to as protons, because that is all that is left of the hydrogen atoms. An acid has more H+ ions than hydroxide ions (OH-). The "opposite" of acid is base, or alkali if it can be absorbed in water. Note that an H+ ion combines with a hydroxide ion to produce H_2O (water). See also *pH*.

Acid-Base Balance

The balance between acid and base values is managed, normally, by homoeostatic systems, and deviation from these normal values can have sudden and severe consequences to health. For the anaesthetist, the fundamental guide to acid-base balance is by pH – the measurement of [H+] (hydrogen ion concentration). The three main methods of achieving proper acid-base balance are:

◇ **Expiration** - the respiratory control system adjusts the rate and depth of breathing so that an appropriate amount of carbon dioxide, which is acidic, is removed, via the lungs.

◇ **Kidneys** - help regulate acid-base balance by excreting H+ ions into the urine, and reabsorbing bicarbonate from urine.

◇ **Buffer systems** - the body's acids and bases regulate their own levels by resisting changes to [H+], and utilising the neutralising effect which a buffer has on H+ ions. See *Buffer*.

Acid-Base Compensation

The body's attempt to bring pH into the normal range, by regulating CO_2 levels with breathing rate/depth, and the kidneys reabsorbing or excreting H+ ions, or recycling bicarbonate, during metabolic and respiratory acid-base disturbances.

Acid-Base – Mixed Cases

Conditions that mixed cases might be accompanied by...

- Mixed *respiratory/metabolic acidosis*: cardiac arrest, multi organ failure.

- Mixed *respiratory/metabolic alkalosis*: cirrhosis with diuretics, vomiting in pregnancy, COPD.

- Mixed *respiratory acidosis + metabolic alkalosis*: severe hypokalaemia, NG suctioning, COPD with vomiting or diuretics.

- Mixed *respiratory alkalosis + metabolic acidosis*: sepsis, kidney failure, liver disease, aspirin overdose.

- Mixed *metabolic acidosis/alkalosis*: (pH and HCO_3^- normal values) ketoacidosis with vomiting, NG suctioning, or diuretics.

Acid Reflux

Stomach acid, moving into the oesophagus, through a faulty or relaxed *lower oesophageal sphincter* (muscle). If stomach acids pollute the lungs, the consequences, such as aspiration pneumonia, can be severe. If reflux is a persistent condition, this is known as *Gastro-oesophageal reflux disease – GORD*. Patients undergoing emergency surgery are at greatest risk of acid reflux.

Intubation protects the patient from reflux, but there is a risk before and after intubation, hence the need for *Rapid Sequence Induction*, and pharyngeal suctioning. See Appendix A2 (pg 340).

Acidaemia

A state of excess H+ (hydrogen) ions in the blood, signified by low blood pH. Effect is to cause peripheral vasoconstriction, negative inotropic cardiac contractility, and the Bohr Effect. Acidaemia is caused by either the kidneys (metabolic acidosis) not eliminating H+, the lungs (respiratory acidosis) not eliminating CO_2, or because there is a loss of bicarbonate from the GI tract.

Acidity

A solution having a pH lower than 7, the neutral level at which the concentration of H+ ions is equal to the concentration of OH- (hydroxide) ions. In the body, acidity refers to a blood pH lower than what is normal for optimum physiological function, 7.4.

Acidosis

The process that creates acidaemia. Note: a patient may have an "acidosis" process in progress, but compensation may push pH into the normal range, thereby hiding the acidosis. Acidosis causes a right shift on the Oxygen-Hb Dissociation Curve, producing a lower O_2 saturation for a particular paO_2 (arterial O_2 pressure).

Acquired Aortic Valve Disease

Abnormalities of the aortic valve, which develop with age. The valve is too narrow (stenosis) or does not open enough, to allow sufficient blood into the aorta, or does not close (regurgitation) properly, so allows some blood to leak back into the left ventricle.

Action Potential

A brief decrease and rise of electrical potential (voltage) acting on a muscle cell membrane - the realisation of a nerve impulse - and propagated to adjacent cells, like a Mexican wave, until the "action" (such as contraction of muscle fibres) occurs. To contract a skeletal muscle, the neurotransmitter ACh is released, at the neuromuscular junction, to initiate an action potential.

Actrapid

A soluble replacement human insulin product, from *Novo Nordisk*, for hyperglycaemic diabetic mellitus patients. A typical ampoule will be 10 ml (cc), containing 1,000 IU, and the usual dosage is 0.3 – 1 IU/kg/day. The anaesthetic practitioner (nurse, technician, ODP etc) may be required to draw up an Actrapid solution for an anaesthetised patient, which might be 50 IU (0.5 ml) and 49.5 ml of normal saline, into a 50 ml syringe. It might take thirty minutes before the blood sugar level falls.

Acute Coronary Syndrome (ACS)

Any condition with a sudden reduction of blood flow to the heart, and which can lead to, for example, myocardial infarction (MI: heart attack). The three types are **unstable angina**, **STEMI** (ST Elevation MI), and **NSTEMI** (Non ST Elevation MI), where ST refers to the ECG ST segment. See also *Myocardial Infarction*.

Acute Respiratory Distress Syndrome (ARDS)

"Acute Lung Injury" (< 1 week) life threatening inflammatory pulmonary injury, where the lungs can't supply enough oxygen (O_2) for the tissues, due to excess vascular permeability, reduction in lung compliance and aerated lung tissue, and increased venous admixture and physiologic dead space. The condition "must not be explained by cardiac failure or fluid overload". Severity measured by Berlin ARDS Rating scheme.

Causes: Sepsis, pneumonia, aspiration, smoke, producing lung inflammation, resulting in fluid leaking into alveoli.

Symptoms: Hypoxia refractory to O_2 therapy (low P/F ratio); Bilateral opacities; Shallow and rapid breathing; Fatigue; Confusion; Shortness of breath.

Treatment: Sit up; O_2, proning; diuretics, intubation, ECMO.

Addison's Disease

An immune system problem with the adrenal glands – one cause of normal anion gap metabolic acidosis.

Adenitis

Inflammation of a gland or lymph node. Ensure difficult intubation aids are at hand.

Adenosine

A 15 second half-life anti-arrhythmic (supraventricular tachycardia) agent, slows impulses to normal sinus rhythm - **not** for patients with: asthma, AV block, COPD, or severe hypotension.

Adhesive Arachnoiditis

Chronic adhesion and inflammation of the arachnoid and dura maters, impedance of CSF flow in the subarachnoid space, and associated entrapment of nerve roots, causing pain and dysfunction of various organs. Can be caused by trauma, spinal injection, or by pushing an epidural needle too far, to pierce the dura mater, and injecting anaesthetic into the subarachnoid space.

Adipose Tissue

Connective tissue containing fat, used as an energy store.

Adjunct

Some item or process which is used to supplement the main item or process. Examples: (1) a guedel airway, is used to help the ventilation process; (2) Hyaluronidase is used, in ophthalmology, to increase the onset speed of eye blocks; (3) a volatile agent supplements anaesthesia. In general, a pharmacological adjunct allows a lower dose of the main agent to be given.

Adjustable Pressure Limiting (APL) Valve

Expiratory relief valve - calibrated between 0 and 75 cmH2O - on an anaesthetic machine or portable breathing circuit. Governs PEEP in spontaneous breathing, and can protect against barotrauma, but not volutrauma. During non-spontaneous ventilation, the APL valve has no effect. The integrity of an APL valve should be checked, prior to every list, both for maintaining circuit pressure, and for quick release of pressure.

Adrenaline (USA: Epinephrine)

Positive inotropic hormone and neurotransmitter, affecting *alpha [arteries]* and *beta* [heart, lungs, skeletal muscle arteries] receptors, secreted by the adrenal glands, and stimulates the sympathetic nervous system to increases the force of cardiac contractions. Potency requires administration by infusion, not bolus. A low dose infusion mostly affects *beta* receptors, producing increased heart rate, output, and contractility. A high dose has more of an affect on *alpha* receptors, producing vasoconstriction and increased blood pressure. Adrenaline is added to local anaesthetics when vasoconstriction is desirable, such as during ENT cases - to reduce blood in the surgical field, with the added benefit of less anaesthetic being flushed away with blood, and lower absorption, to reduce risk of toxic affects. In a **shockable** cardiac arrest rhythm, 1 mg adrenaline is given (or 10 microgram/kg paediatric dose), intravenously, after alternate shocks, starting after giving the third shock, until the return of spontaneous circulation. In a **non-shockable** rhythm, give 1 mg as soon as venous access is made. Also used in severe asthmatic and bronchospasm attacks, and anaphylaxis (iv 50-100 microgram bolus from 1 in 10,000).

Adrenergic

Synonym for *Sympathomimetic.*

Aerobic Respiration

Transfer of oxygen and glucose into mitochondria (in cells), where a chemical reaction releases energy. Byproduct is CO_2 and water.

Afferent

From the periphery to the centre. An *afferent reservoir* circuit, such as Mapleson A/B/C, has the reservoir bag on the limb that carries fresh gas flow towards the patient. Mapleson C does not have an **efferent** limb. Afferent nerves are sensory – they send impulses to the brain. See also *Efferent.*

Affinity

Pharmacological phenomenon that describes how well drug molecules bind with target receptors. A drug with high affinity will displace another drug, of lower affinity, from those receptors.

Afterload/SVR (Systemic Vascular Resistance)

SVR is the resistance the heart must overcome to open the aortic valve, before propelling blood into the systemic circulation. An increased afterload reduces the volume of blood pumped per beat.

Agon

An ancient Greek term for a struggle or contest.

Agonal Breathing

An abnormal and uncomfortable pattern of breathing, produced by spasm of the diaphragm and facial muscles. Agonal breathing may occur in stroke and cardiac arrest events, where anoxia causes the respiratory control centre into a desperate effort to breathe. The agonal breathing patient is NOT ventilating, so should be regarded as not breathing at all.

Agonal Rhythm

A slow ventricular rhythm, and type of asystole, with a wide QRS complex (> 120 millisecond) and few, if any, P waves. The wide QRS complex suggests a slow spread of the polarisation of the ventricles, perhaps due to damaged Bundle of His, Purkinje fibres, or other heart muscle problems. Considered a cardiac emergency, the resuscitation pathway for asystole should be followed, and 1 mg of 1 in 10,000 adrenaline should be administered.

Agonist

A substance which initiates a response, such as when acetylcholine binds with a cholinergic receptor, leading to muscle contraction.

Aintree Intubation Catheter

An adaption of the Cook Airway Exchange Catheter, used for intubating through a laryngeal mask airway, and oxygenation through a central lumen. See Appendix A3 (pg 341).

Air

Not strictly a gas, but the naturally occurring mixture of gases which form the atmosphere. The main constituents of air include:

Gas	*Fraction (%)*
Nitrogen	78.1
Oxygen	20.95
Argon	0.93
Carbon Dioxide	0.04

Air pressure varies with temperature, altitude, and local meteorological conditions. During general anaesthesia, a patient is given air, in addition to oxygen, to titrate the fraction of inspired oxygen to a pressure which does not prove to be toxic.

Air Leak Syndrome

A class of respiratory disorder, where air, or other inspired gas, escapes from ruptured alveoli, and collects in tissues around the lungs or heart, resulting in a tamping of those organs. Syndrome examples include pneumothorax, subcutaneous emphysema, pneumopericardium, and pulmonary interstitial emphysema.

Air Oxygen Mixtures

An anaesthetised patient will be given O2 (oxygen), diluted with medical air, to a required O2 fraction, and with a total gas volume or flow rate. To set the O2 and air flows so that they provide the target FiO2 (Fraction of inspired Oxygen), fractions of O2 and air must be calculated. For common range of FiO2 values, the particular flow rate fractions, are as follows:

Target FiO2	Oxygen flow rate	Air flow rate
0.3	12.5%	87.5%

0.4	25%	75%
0.5	37.5%	62.5%
0.6	50%	50%
0.7	62.5%	37.50%

For example, if the patient is to receive a total gas flow of 1 litre, with an FiO2 of 40% (0.4), then the oxygen flow rate should be set to 0.25 (25%) of a litre, and the air flow to 0.75 (75%) of a litre.

Air Trapping

The accumulation of air in the lungs (alveoli), possibly causing hyperinflation. Caused by COPD, airway obstruction, breath stacking, or PEEP.

Airtraq

Proprietary name for difficult intubation aids, produced by VYGON, which provide periscopic views of the larynx, without needing to align the patient's oral, pharyngeal and tracheal axes.

Airway

The generic term to describe the route for air, or anaesthetic breathing gases, from the mouth/throat cavity, pharynx larynx, trachea, left and right mainstem bronchi, secondary and tertiary bronchi, segmental and respiratory bronchioles, alveolar duct, and alveoli. In anaesthesia, reference to the “airway” can mean the upper respiratory tract. or a nasal or Guedel pattern airway device.

Airway Obstruction

Partial or total impedance of gas flow between lungs and atmosphere (or circuit) is a potential emergency.

Causes include: CNS depression, anaphylaxis, blood, vomit, trauma, inflammation, secretions, tumour, nerve damage, active muscle relaxants (anaesthetic), foreign objects, food, laryngospasm.

Signs: Visible swelling, stridor, coughing, breathing and swallowing difficulty, speech problems, hunched over.

Symptoms: Hypoxia, assisted ventilation difficulty, hypotension, central cyanosis.

Treatment: 100% oxygen, jaw thrust, guedel airway, BVM, remove obstruction with Magill Forceps, intubation, cricothyrotomy.

Airway Pressure (PAW)

[Flow * Resistance] + alveolar pressure. Airway pressure during IPPV, at different phases of the respiratory cycle, reflecting efficacy of ventilation. A high pressure may be due to a blocked circuit or ET tube, high BMI, bronchospasm, ARDS, or pulmonary oedema. See also *Peak Inspiratory, Plateau,* and *Mean Pressures*.

Akinesis/Akinesia

The inability to make movements; paralysis due to central nervous system disease, or by anaesthetic paralysing drugs.

Aladin Cassette

Newer type of volatile agent plenum vapouriser – slides into place. Agent concentration is governed by the amount of gas flowing through the cassette.

Albumin

Made by the liver; the most abundant protein in plasma. Albumin gives viscocity to blood, and prevents blood from leaking (oncotic pressure) into the extravascular space e.g., lungs and abdomen, and to transport vitamins, hormones, and enzymes around the body. If albumin level is low, it may be due to shock or significant inflammation, or due to a liver or kidney (nephrotic syndrome) problem. With respect to blood gas reports, albumin forms the largest source of unmeasured anions, so accurate measurement is needed for HAGMA evaluation; a low albumin level can make a HAGMA look like a NAGMA, because each 1 g/litre loss of albumin decreases the AG by ~ 2.5 mmol/litre. If albumin is high, it may be due to dehydration, infection, post-surgery, or MI. Normal range is 3.4 – 5.4 g/100 ml. {ABO not needed}

Aldosterone

A hormone, produced by the adrenal glands (cortex), that governs sodium reabsorption and secretion of potassium, in the kidneys. High levels of aldosterone cause extra secretion of H+ (hydrogen ions), producing an alkalotic condition. Low levels of aldosterone do the opposite, and produce an acidotic condition.

Aldrete Score

A system of grading a patient's physiological status, with the aim of deciding whether or not it is safe to transfer the patient to a ward or second stage recovery/PACU unit. Different versions of Aldrete's system are used, but the common parameters include:

- Δ Respiration ability
- Δ BP difference from pre-anaesthesia
- Δ Acceptable pain level
- Δ Minimal nausea/vomiting
- Δ Level of consciousness
- Δ Oxygen saturation level
- Δ Temperature
- Δ Blood sugar
- Δ Haemoglobin
- Δ Number of limbs patient can move

Alfentanil

Very quick acting opioid (because of high lipophilicity, so crosses blood-CSF barrier quickly), similar to fentanyl, but less potent and with less than half the duration. Dose 10 microgram/kg from 500 microgram/ml concentration. See *Opioids*.

Aliquot

An exact fractional part of something eg, divide a 20 ml syringe of metaraminol into 4 syringes gives 4 aliquots of 5 ml each.

Alkali

A base that is soluble in a solvent, such as water, and produces dissociation of hydroxide ions (OH^-). Alkalis neutralise acids. An alkali has more hydroxide ions (OH^-) than hydrogen ions (H^+).

Alkalosis/Alkalaemia

Alkalaemia (pH > 7.45) means an excessive base of the blood. **Alkalosis** refers to the process that creates the alkalaemia.

Allen's Test

A technique to determine patency of arterial blood flow to a hand, by using finger pressure to occlude the ulnar and radial arteries. If blood supply appears normal, the test is said to be Negative.

Technique:

- Elevate the patient's hand above his/her heart.
- Ask the patient to make a fist.
- Use finger pressure to occlude the radial and ulnar arteries.
- Maintain pressure until blood flow stops (pale palm).
- Release pressure on one artery; blood supply should be returned by the other artery within a few seconds.

Alligation

Method of calculating how to produce a concentration of a solution from the combination of two other concentrations, using a 3*3 grid. The higher % concentration is placed in the top left box; the lower concentration in the bottom left box; the required concentration in the centre; the difference between the required and higher concentrations in the bottom right box, and the positive difference between the lower and required concentrations in the top right box. The high:low ratio is given by the top right and bottom right values.

Example: Produce 20 ml of a 30% w/v concentration from a supply of a 20% and 60% concentrations.

60		30-20=**10**
	30	
20		60-30=**30**

The ratio of the higher (60%) to the lower (20%) concentrations is given by the top right and bottom right boxes: 10:30 or 1:3.

The 1:3 ratio means that ¼ of the 20 ml solution (5 ml) should be from the 60% solution. The smaller concentration (20%) makes up the remaining 15 ml. The result is 20 ml of a 30% concentration.

Allosteric

A part of a receptor, other than the agonist (active) part, that a molecule can bind to and prevent receptor activation.

Alteplase

A thrombolytic (dissolves blood clots) agent, given to ischaemic stroke victims, as soon as possible after the event.

Alveolar Dead Space

V/Q mismatch condition where alveoli are ventilated, but are not perfused (no blood flow), so no gas exchange takes place.

Alveolar Oxygen Diffusion

The concentration gradient from alveoli causes oxygen to diffuse through surfactant, alveolar epithelium (lining), basement membrane, and finally through capillary epithelium.

Alveolar Hypoventilation

Insufficient ventilation – leading to hypercapnia.

Alveolar Gas Equation

The method for estimating the partial pressure of oxygen (pAO_2) in the alveolar space, to enable calculation of the alveolar-arterial oxygen (A-a) gradient:

$$pAO_2 = (FiO_2 (P_{atm} - PH_2O)) - (PaCO_2 / RQ) \text{ mmHg}$$

$$pAO_2 = (FiO_2 (760-47)) - (PaCO_2 / 0.8) \text{ mmHg}$$

FiO_2 = Fraction Inspired oxygen

P_{atm} = Atmospheric pressure (mean=760 [mmHg])

PH_2O = Alveolar water vapour pressure (47)

RQ = Respiratory Quotient (0.82)

At mean sea level, (healthy adult) pAO_2 is ~104 mmHg.

Alveolar Pressure (Palv)

Relative alveolar pressure (in cmH_2O) during different phases of the breathing cycle. A normal maximum (relative to ambient) pressure is 30 cmH_2O (22 mmHg, 2.94 kPa), and 0 at inspiratory and expiratory pauses. High pressure may be due to high PEEP, incorrect ventilator settings, or poor lung compliance.

Alveolar Recruitment Manouevre (ARM)

Techniques, such as PEEP, to open collapsed alveoli, by increasing intra-pulmonary pressure.

Alveolar Shunt

See Intra Pulmonary Shunt.

Alveolar Ventilation (V_A)

Volume of gas exchanged between the environment and alveoli, in ml/minute; found by subtracting *dead-space ventilation* from *minute ventilation*.

Alveolus

Plural, *alveoli*. An air sac, in the lungs, which facilitates gas exchange, due to pressure gradients, where oxygen diffuses from alveoli to the blood (during inspiration AND expiration), and carbon dioxide diffuses from the blood to the alveoli. Also, an *alveolus* is a jaw socket for the root of a tooth.

Ambu Bag

Proprietary name for a *bag-valve-mask*.

American Society of Anesthesiologists (ASA) Rating

Rating scheme for the physical state of a patient.

Rating	Significance
I	Normally healthy individual
II	A patient with mild systemic disease
III	A patient with severe systemic disease which is not incapacitating
IV	A patient with incapacitating systemic disease which is a constant threat to life
V	A moribund patient who is not expected to survive 24 hours with, or without, an operation.

VI	A brain-dead patient whose organs are being removed, with the intention of transplanting them into another patient.
E	Added as a suffix for emergency cases.

Ametop Cream

A topical local anaesthetic (tetracaine) cream, used for patients who are sensitive to the pain of injection, especially children. Should be kept clear of open sounds, eyes, and lips. Should not be used with babies or pregnant or breastfeeding women, and might not be suitable for epileptics. Takes 30-45 minutes to effect.

Amikacin

Aminoglycoside antibiotic for significant bacterial infections.

Aminophylline

Bronchodilator for bronchospasm or severe asthma attacks: 5 mg/kg to max dose of 500 mg, IV, followed by infusion.

Amiodarone

An emergency anti-arrhythmia drug, when vasopressors and defibrillation are ineffective. In shockable adult **cardiac arrest**, 300 mg Amiodarone in 20 ml 5% glucose is given, intravenously, after the third shock, and may be repeated another two times. Amiodarone may be contraindicated in the presence of thyroid and some cardiac problems, and side-effects may include nausea, allergic reaction, respiratory impairment, and bronchospasm.

Anaemia

Reduced level of oxygen supply to the tissues, due to low haematocrit or low haemoglobin (Hb) count, resulting in hypoxia.

Anaerobic Respiration

Anaerobic respiration is when cells break down glucose, and produce energy, without using oxygen.

Anaesthesia

Loss of sensation, to relieve the patient from awareness, pain, or muscle control. See Appendix A4 (pg 343).

Anaesthesia Side-Effects

Anaesthetic staff have to be alert to allergic reactions to anaesthetic agents, but some reactions are side-effects only, usually post-surgery, rather than allergic reactions, so should not be confused. Common postoperative side-effects: aching muscles, PONV, shivering, headache, confusion, and itching.

Anaesthetic Drugs

Anaesthetic induction is achieved by a standard set of agents, based on the triad of anaesthesia, and prophylactic agents, such as anti-emetics and antibiotics. See Appendix A5 (pg 344).

Anaesthetic Gas Analyser

Part of an anaesthetic machine's suite of monitoring tools; measures inspired and expired partial pressures (concentrations) of oxygen, carbon dioxide, and volatile agents.

Anaesthetic Induction

Inducing a patient into a state of anaesthesia, where the primary consideration is ensuring adequate ventilation, which is monitored, primarily, by end tidal carbon dioxide ($EtCO_2$) capnography. For the anaesthetic assistant, a response to an apparent ventilation failure is to verify that the capnometer equipment is functional, and properly connected to the breathing circuit. See Appendix A6 (pg 347).

Anaesthetic Machine Checks

Before connecting a patient, the anaesthetist must ensure the anaesthetic machine conforms with relevant regulations and guidelines. Separately, an anaesthetic practitioner, or nurse, must perform the same checks. See Appendix A7 (pg 349).

Analeptic

A drug, such as Doxapram, which stimulates the central nervous system to initiate breathing.

Analgesic Ladder

World Health Organisation approach to pain relief, realised by three stages, until relief occurs:

Step	*Description*	*Examples*
1	Non-opioids	Aspirin, Paracetamol, NSAIDs
2	Weak opioid, with or without non-opioids	Lidocaine, Codeine, Oxycodone, Tramadol
3	Strong opioids	Morphine, Fentanyl

Anaphylactic Shock

Severe reaction to drugs or allergens, with hypotension → cardiovascular collapse, and cardiac arrest. Appendix A8 (pg 354).

Anaphylaxis

Acute onset of an allergic reaction to something which the sufferer is sensitive to, such as bee stings, pollen, or a food item. **Symptoms**: tachycardia, anxiety, lightheaded, unconsciousness, shallow breathing, wheezing, clammy skin, plus **allergy symptoms**: angioedema (swelling), raised rash (hives), nausea, and stomach pain. Immediate **action** is to call for help, remove the trigger (leaf, sting etc), lie the patient flat, with legs raised, and give intramuscular adrenaline (widens airways): dose for 12 years and older is 500 microgram (0.5 ml) of a 1 in 1,000 weight to volume concentration; Child, 6-12 years is 300 microgram; Younger child is 150 microgram. See Appendix A8 (pg 354).

Anatomic Dead Space

The volume (~150 ml, adult) of the conducting airways (mouth, nose, pharynx, larynx, trachea, bronchi, terminal bronchioles) which do not take part in gas exchange, but convect gases between the atmosphere/gas supply and terminal bronchioles.

Aneurysm

An abnormality of a blood vessel, where the vessel wall is weakened, and expands or balloons into a blood filled sac.

Angina

Tight sensation of strangling, heaviness, or pain in the chest, usually caused by the narrowing of arteries by *atherosclerosis*. Typically treated with GTN (glycerine trinitrate). **Angina Pectoris**: Cardiac pain, caused by insufficient blood supply to the heart. **Unstable Angina** is a less predictable and less controllable from of angina, and is classed as a least serious Acute Coronary Syndrome, because the restricted blood supply to the heart is not low enough to cause permanent damage to the heart muscle.

Angioedema

Swelling of the deeper layers of the skin, caused by a build-up of fluid. Swelling can occur on any part of the body, but usually on the eyes, lips, genitals, hands, or feet. This condition is often accompanied by urticaria (hives).

Angiogram

A technique to inspect the integrity of blood vessels. The test incorporates an X-ray and camera to capture images of a dye, previously injected into the patient's bloodstream. Angiograms are the gold standard for determining the occlusion of an artery.

Angioplasty

The widening of a narrowed artery by inflating a balloon at the narrow point of the artery. Often also includes insertion of a permanent stent (tube of wire mesh).

Angiospasm

A spasm which constricts blood vessels.

Anion

A negatively charged ion (atom, molecule, compound) - more electrons than protons. **Chloride** and bicarbonate constitute 85% of the body's anions. In blood, the anions are acidic. See cation.

Anion Gap (AG)

In blood, total cations = total anions, and AG is the difference between unmeasured (UM) anions and cations (UM anions-UM cations), helping to confirm the type of metabolic acidosis, either High Anion Gap (HAGMA) or Normal Anion Gap (NAGMA). AG is derived from the calculation: *sodium + potassium – chloride – bicarbonate* but, by convention, potassium is excluded from the calculation, giving *AG = sodium – chloride – bicarbonate* (142-105-25). If AG is > 30 mmol/L, it is most likely a HAGMA; if 20-29, there will be a 70% chance of HAGMA. The usual AG range is

4-12 mmol/L. See Appendix 9 (pg 357).

Anodyne

A pain relieving drug.

Anoxia

Absence of oxygen supply to the organs/tissues.

Antagonist

A substance (drug, ligand) which opposes (blocks) the normal action of a system, or action of a drug. Typically, antagonists bind to receptors, thereby blocking those receptors from agonists.

Antiarrhythmic

Agents which normalise an irregular cardiac rhythm. Example agents: Amiodarone, Flecainide.

Antibiotic

A substance which destroys or prevents growth of bacteria.

Antibody (Immunoglobulin)

A Y shaped protein, on the surface of B cells (B-lymphocyte, white blood cell, produces the antibodies), in response to the presence of antigens. Antibodies attach to antigens on infectious organisms then, either destroy them, or render them harmless.

Anticholinergic

Antagonist of acetylcholine (ACh) receptors, particularly muscarinic, in the central and peripheral nervous systems, preventing ACh from binding with those receptors, inhibiting parasympathetic nerve (autonomic system) signals responsible for cardiac and smooth muscle activity. Anticholinergic drug **side-**

effects include: dry mouth and eyes, constipation, urinary retention, arrhythmias, postural hypotension.

Antimuscarinic agents, such as Atropine, Glycopyrrolate, and Hyoscine (Buscopan), block (bind with) muscarinic receptors.

Antinicotinic agents, such as Atracurium and Mivacurium, used for non-depolarising neuromuscular (peripheral muscle) blockade, bind with nicotinic receptors.

Anticholinesterase

Drugs (e.g., Neostigmine, Distigmine, Pyridostigmine) to inhibit acetylcholinesterase from metabolising (breaking down) ACh (acetylcholine, parasympathetic neurotransmitter). As the amount of ACh starts to outnumber the blocking agent (eg, Atracurium), paralysis wears off, and normal muscle control is resumed. Contraindications: intestinal or urinary obstruction.

Anticoagulation

Using a drug to reduce the chance of a blood clot forming, such as when helping to prevent a stroke, by interrupting the process involved in the formation of the blood clots. Commonly used anticoagulant drugs are Heparin and Warfarin.

Anticonvulsant

Substance which relieves convulsions e.g., Phenytoin.

Antiembolism Device (Flowtron)

A mechanical "cuff" that wraps around the patient's calf, and is intermittently inflated, by machine, so that blood flow is maintained in the lower limbs, and reduces the chance that a blood clot will develop. See also *Deep Vein Thrombosis*.

Antidiuretic Hormone (ADH)

Aka *Vasopressin*: Peptide hormone secreted by the posterior lobe of the pituitary gland. ADH causes reabsorption of water in the renal tubules, with consequent reduction in urine output. In larger doses, ADH causes constriction of plain muscle, which increases peripheral vascular resistance, resulting in increased arterial blood pressure. Used in the treatment of *diabetes insipidus*.

Antiemetic

Drug to relieve nausea/vomiting (often caused by opioids and nitrous oxide). Examples are: Ondansetron, Metoclopramide, Promethazine, Cyclizine. See Appendix A10 (pg 358).

Antifibrinolytic

A substance that inhibits fibrinolysis (natural process of breaking down blood clots, by halting the deconstruction of fibrin), and so promotes blood clotting.

Antigen (antibody generator)

A substance which evokes the production of antibodies.

Anti-hypoxia Device

See Hypoxic Guard.

Antimuscarinic (Anticholinergic)

Antimuscarinic drugs, such as Atropine, Glycopyrrolate, and Hyoscine (Buscopan), inhibit some of the parasympathetic effects (bronchoconstriction, bronchospasm, bradycardia) caused by acetylcholine binding with muscarinic receptors (M3). In anaesthesia, the antimuscarinic (muscarinic receptor antagonist) drug Glycopyrrolate is used to reduce the muscarinic effects of Neostigmine, by countering bradycardia and bronchoconstriction, relaxing smooth muscle, decreasing secretion of saliva, and reducing the production of sweat and digestive fluids.

Anti-platelet Agents

Drugs which care used to suppress platelet action, with the aim of preventing myocardial infarction (heart attack), by stopping formation of blood clots. Example agents include NSAIDs (non-steroidal anti-inflammatory drugs), aspirin, and clopidogrel.

Antipyretic

Agents to reduce fever: eg, aspirin, paracetamol, and ibuprofen.

Antispasmodic

Drugs, such as Buscopan (Hyoscine), which relieve/prevent urinary tract or intestinal muscle spasms.

Antitussive

Something which prevents coughing, eg, honey.

Anton Helman's Triple 15 Rule

A guide to optimising preoxygenation: Use **nasal prongs** with 15 L/min O_2, and give 15 L/min by **non-rebreather mask**. If O_2 sats is < 95%, then apply 15 cmH_2O of **CPAP** (APL valve).

Anuria

The failure of the kidneys to produce urine.

Anxiolytic

Substances to relieve anxiety e.g., Benzodiazepines.

Aorta

The largest artery in the body, carrying oxygenated blood from the heart, to the systemic circulation. During cardiac arrest, chest compressions are meant to force blood into the aorta.

Aortic Stenosis

A narrowing of the aortic valve orifice, restricting blood flow from the left ventricle to the aorta.

Aortocaval Compression

The gravid (pregnant) uterus compressing the mother's abdominal aorta and inferior vena cava: reason for C-Section left lateral tilt.

APGAR score

Method to assess health of neonates. See Appendix A11 (pg 359).

Apheresis

Extraction of specific components of whole blood - plasma, white blood cells, red blood cells, or platelets.

APL

See Adjustable Pressure Limiting Valve.

Apnoea

Suspension of breathing, caused by:

- Residual effects of a narcotic premedication
- Residual effects of induction, or maintenance agent
- Hypocapnia - no stimulus for breathing
- Hypercapnia - can be caused by a faulty anaesthetic circuit
- Severe hypotension
- Suxamethonium apnoea
- Pszeudo cholinesterase - caused by liver disease
- Tracheal Stenosis

Apnoea-Hypopnoea Index (AHI)

The number of apnoea and hypopnoea events per hour, which gives a measurement of the degree of sleep apnoea.

Apnoeic Oxygenation

In the patient is apnoeic, and not receiving assisted ventilation, safe apnoea time, beyond pre-oxygenation, may be extended by feeding the patient with oxygen through the use of nasal specula, with the aim of allowing pressure gradients to ventilate the lungs, without lung expansion. This occurs because more oxygen diffuses **to** the bloodstream than CO_2 diffuses **from** the bloodstream, causing a reduced alveolar pressure that draws in oxygen from the upper airway, thereby allowing continued diffusion to the blood. The modern term for this process is *aventilatory mass flow*.

Aqueous Solution

A solution with water as the solvent, where the dissolved solute is hydrophilic (affinity for water).

Arachnoid Mater

The middle meninx of the three spinal meninges, and the main barrier for drugs from the epidural space reaching spinal nerves.

ARDS

See Acute Respiratory Distress Syndrome.

Arm-Brain Circulation Time

The time it takes an intravenously administered drug to travel from the hand/arm to the brain. Typically, 20-60 seconds.

Armoured Endotracheal tube

An ET (endotracheal) tube, embedded with a metallic helix strip, to prevent kinking and crushing, commonly used in head and neck surgery, where acute flexion of the neck may occur.

Arnold's Nerve Cough Reflex

Reflexive coughing, by 2% of people, induced by activation of the Arnold Nerve, such as when putting something in the ear, due to stimulation of the external auditory meatus. The Arnold is the auricular section of the vagus nerve.

Arrhythmia

An irregular or abnormal beating of the heart. Examples: atrial fibrillation, heart block, supraventricular tachycardia.

Artefact

Something introduced or made by man, and which may create misleading results - a common feature of monitoring systems, such as an ECG artefact resulting from diathermy equipment.

Arterial Blood Gases (ABG)

Blood analysis to determine levels of dissolved O_2 and CO_2, acid-base balance, compensation, and electrolyte values. ABG machines will measure, for example:

- Acidity (pH)
- Lactate
- Bicarbonate (HCO_3^-)
- Electrolytes
- Base Excess
- O_2 partial pressure (paO_2)
- Carbon dioxide partial pressure (pCO_2)

When pH and $paCO_2$ move in opposite directions, the acid-base imbalance is respiratory; the same direction is metabolic. Note: Full compensation is indicated by pH returning to the normal range. See *Appendix A12* (pg 360), *Anion Gap, Delta Ratio, Metabolic Acidosis/Alkalosis, Winters' Formula*. Note: for more on acid-base balance, refer to ***Blood Gases: The Basics – And a Little More*** (John England, Amazon Publishing).

Arterial Line Monitoring

A catheter placed in a peripheral artery, such as the radial, axillary, femoral, brachial, or pedal, to display real-time arterial blood pressure. See Appendix A13 (pg 362).

Arterial Line Square Wave Test

Fast Flush or *Dynamic Response Test*. When an arterial line's fast flush toggle is briefly opened, the transducer is exposed to the higher pressure of the saline solution, and produces a square shaped wave on the monitor. At the end of the down stroke there should be 2 oscillation spikes, with the second being 1/3 the size of the first. If there are more than 2 oscillations, plus larger than usual *dicrotic notches* on the downward slope of the non-square waves, the **under-damping** could mean there are too many stopcocks in the apparatus, long tubing, tachycardia, or high cardiac output. With under-damping, the systolic value is displayed higher than the real value, and the diastolic value is displayed lower than it actually is. Conversely, an **over-damped** condition shows only 1 oscillation spike, plus small or absent dicrotic notches, and a systolic value that is displayed lower than the real value; a diastolic value might be displayed higher than it actually is. Over-damping causes: tubing kinked or too small, air bubbles in the tubing, obstructions between the transducer and catheter, blood clots, spasms. See Appendix A13b (pg 367).

Arterial Thrombosis

A blood clot which develops in an artery, and usually associated with atherosclerosis (hardening and narrowing of the arteries). A heart attack can occur when a blood clot blocks the arteries leading to the heart, inhibiting the blood supply. A stroke occurs when a blood clot blocks an artery in the brain. Risk factors include: smoking, saturated fat, salt, and a sedentary lifestyle.

Artery

A blood vessel which takes blood away from the heart. The arteries are smaller, in cross section, than veins, and have relatively smaller lumens, but the wall of an artery is stronger than that of a vein, because it has to contain blood at a higher pressure. Most arteries carry oxygenated blood, which supply arterioles which, in turn, feed the capillaries, whence, gas exchange takes place. Some of the main arteries, and the parts of the body they serve, include:

Aorta	Trunk
Brachial	Upper arm, Radial and Ulnar arteries
Carotid	Brain, Face, and Neck
Femoral	Upper leg, feeds Popliteal and Tibial
Iliac	Pelvis, feeds Femoral
Subclavian	Arms and head
Vertebral	Supplies the brain

ASA

See *American Society of Anesthesiologists* Rating.

Ascites

Accumulation of ascitic (contains protein) fluid in the abdomen, typically caused by hepatic venal hypertension, due to cirrhosis. The fluid causes breathing difficulty and hypoxia and, if the fluid becomes infected, could result in bacterial peritonitis. The ascitic patient's airway might be better protected by intubation (upright position?), as opposed to using a supra-glottic device.

Aspiration

Drawing off fluid from a cavity, or inhalation of gastric contents (pulmonary aspiration). In anaesthesia, aspiration is the most common cause of death. See Appendix A14 (pg 368).

Aspiration Pneumonia

Lung infection due to aspiration. See also *Pulmonary Aspiration*.

Aspirin (Acetylsalicylic Acid)

A non-steroidal anti-inflammatory drug, used to treat minor aches and pains, but with a more notable function of reducing the formation of blood clots, particularly for patients with cardiovascular disease, or who are susceptible to ischaemic stroke. Aspirin works by blocking the effects of cyclooxygenase (enzyme), which would otherwise produce prostanoids, which are the hormones that take part in blood clotting, by enabling platelets to stick together. For safety, surgical patients will usually be asked to stop taking aspirin seven to ten days before their surgery.

Asthma

An obstructive airway disease, with chronic bronchial wall inflammation, causing smooth muscle to constrict bronchioles, reducing their diameter, with resulting increased resistance to airflow, reduced volume, and expiration difficulties. [**Intrinsic** (non-allergic) asthma is triggered by stress, weather, or infection. **Extrinsic** asthma is triggered by allergies] **Symptoms**: coughing, wheezing, and breathlessness. Ideally, intubation should be avoided for asthmatics, because positive pressure ventilation may cause complications, such as bronchospasm, and atelectasis. Also, some drugs, such as Morphine, Mivacurium, and Atracurium, are best avoided for asthmatics, because they cause histamine release.

{Inhaled Salbutamol (beta agonist) should be available}

Asystole

Absence of electrical and mechanical activity in the heart - a non-shockable cardiac arrest event. See Appendix A15 (pg 369).

Atelectasis

Greek for "incomplete expansion". Partially collapsed alveoli, resulting in acute respiratory failure, signified by tachypnoea and low O_2 sats. Atelectasis is common after surgery, due to respiratory splinting. See Appendix A16 (pg 370).

Atheroma (Plaque)

The deposition of cholesterol, fat, and other substances, which adhere to and clog up the arteries, resulting in *atherosclerosis*.

Atherosclerosis

State where fatty deposits, called *atheroma* or *plaque,* accumulate on the interior walls of the arteries, causing a reduction in their effective internal diameter, with consequent reduction in their blood carrying capacity. If untreated, can lead to cardiovascular diseases, such as stroke or myocardial infarction (heart attack).

Atmospheric Pressure

The air pressure, which fluctuates with altitude and weather. Mean atmospheric pressure, at mean sea level, and 0° Celsius, with units:

- Φ 1 atmosphere (atm)
- Φ 1.01325 bar
- Φ 101.325 kPa
- Φ 1,033.23 cmH_2O
- Φ 760 mmHg
- Φ Molar Volume: 22.4 litre

Vapourisers must be calibrated to ambient pressure. The modern definition for atmospheric pressure is given by *Standard Temperature and Pressure (STP).*

Atony

Muscular weakness, typically the ability of an organ to contract, such as the uterus failing to contract after delivery of the baby.

Atracurium

A non-depolarising neuromuscular blocking drug (NMBD), which antagonizes (inhibits) the action of acetylcholine by competitively binding with post-synaptic nicotinic (cholinergic) receptor sites on the motor end-plate. As acetylcholine is blocked from binding with receptors, which have been "occupied" by the NMBD, no skeletal muscle activity can occur, thus paralysis is achieved. Intubation dose 0.5 mg/kg from 10 mg/ml (refrigerated).

Atrial Fibrillation (AF)

An arrhythmia. Rapid and asynchronous contractions of the atrium, causing irregular contraction of the ventricles. Pulse rate and strength will be irregular, wrist and apex pulse rates will be asymmetrical, and P waves will be absent. Once Atrial Fibrillation is under control, aspirin might be administered, to reduce the risk of emboli. For higher risk patients, long term Warfarin may be appropriate. See Appendix A17 (pg 371).

Atrial Flutter

Rapid contractions of the Atria, 240-350 beats/minute, often accompanied by atrioventricular block.

Atrial Tachycardia

Abnormally fast heart rhythm where electrical impulses originate in the atria, rather than from the more normal sinus node. The rhythm is usually regular, and exceeds 100 beats/minute. A common sign is a narrow complex saw-tooth ECG.

Symptoms

- Exertion
- Syncope
- Chest discomfort
- Palpitations
- Fatigue
- Dyspnoea at rest
- Dizziness

Causes

- Anxiety
- Fatigue
- Caffeine
- Alcohol
- Smoking

Treatments

- Pacemaker
- Anti-arrhythmic drugs
- Cardioversion

Atrioventricular Block (AV Block)

Electrical signals are interrupted between the Sinus Node and Atrioventricular Node. It is the most common type of heart block.

Type of AV Block	**Effect on impulses**
First degree	Slowed (least serious block type)
Second degree (Mobitz types 1/2)	Becoming progressively slower
3rd degree (complete block)	Impulses do not reach ventricles (most serious block type)

Atropine

An antimuscarinic, which antagonises the effects of acetylcholine (parasympathetic neurotransmitter) at muscarine receptors. Atropine blocks vagal action on the sinus node that causes tachycardia, thereby, making it useful in treating bradycardia, with dose of 20 microgram/kg.

Side-effects

- Constipation
- Arrhythmia
- Vomiting
- Dizziness
- Palpitations

Contra-indications

- Prostate enlargement
- Ulcerative colitis
- GI obstruction
- Urinary retention
- Intestinal weakness

Auscultation

Listening to internal organs with a stethoscope.

Autologous

Something that a patient receives from themselves. For example, transplant of their own tissue, from one body part to another; or autologous red blood cell transfusion by *cell-saver* system.

Automated External Defibrillator (AED)

A portable, non-invasive, and durable device to deliver an electrical charge to the heart, to stop an arrhythmia, which will be Ventricular Fibrillation or pulseless Ventricular Tachycardia. {The AED detects these arrhythmia, via chest pads}

Automaticity

The attribute of behaving automatically, and without external stimulus. Some heart cells, particularly of the sinus node, will normally instantiate action potentials (impulses), without external stimuli. In abnormal cases, other cardiac cells may initiate action potentials, with the possible consequence that atrial or ventricular arrhythmias may occur. In such abnormal cases, anti-arrhythmic drugs may not be as effective as they otherwise might be.

Auxiliary Common Gas Outlet (ACGO)

An anaesthetic machine's second common (all gases) gas outlet (bypasses the APL and reservoir bag), which allows an extra circuit to be connected to the anaesthetic machine, supplementary to the main circuit, so that the anaesthetist can switch from one to the other, without having to disconnect and reconnect. An example situation is when a paediatric patient is induced from a Mapleson F (Jackson-Rees T-piece) circuit, connected to the ACGO, but is then switched to the main circuit, which is connected to the main Common Gas Outlet (CGO). A prominently located lever will allow switching between the ACGO and CGO – **ALWAYS CHECK**!

AVPU

Alert/Voice/Pain/Unresponsive: A method of estimating a patient's level of consciousness, with four levels of discrimination:

Level	*Response type*
Alert	Awake, has motor control, responds to voice and eye movement
Voice	Only responds to voice
Pain	Only responds to painful stimuli
Unresponsive	No voice, eye, or motor response

Avulsion

Tearing something away, such as in varicose vein procedures.

Awake Intubation

Technique to intubate an awake patient having a “difficult” airway, so that the airway can be protected for longer than with a normal intubation. The upper airway should be anaesthetised, using local anaesthetic (4% or 10% lidocaine), and “vasoconstricted” with adrenaline, to reduce bleeding from nasal mucosa. Nasal or oral intubation may be performed. The oral route is more stimulating and requires a cooperative patient. See Appendix A18 (pg 372).

Axilla

The armpit – a location for taking body temperature.

Ayre's T-Piece

A Mapleson E valveless circuit, with corrugated reservoir tubing, minimal dead space and resistance. Exhaled CO_2 flows through the efferent (expiratory) limb, and flushed out of the circuit by gas flow. For safety, there should be a minimum oxygen flow rate of 6 litre/minute, but 10 litre is probably better, as low flow rates can result in dangerous levels of CO_2 being rebreathed. See also *Mapleson F.*

Back Bar

The platform on which vapourisers are connected.

Background Infusion

Continuous infusion; may be supplemented by boluses eg, by PCA.

Backup Cylinder

Size J molybdenum gas cylinder, used when a main supply fails.

Backward Heart Failure

One of the ventricles fails to pump out all of the blood that comes into it, so causing blood to pool behind the ventricle, and producing pulmonary and systemic oedema.

Backward Upward Right Pressure (BURP)

Pressure, by the anaesthetic assistant, on the thyroid cartilage, to help visualise the vocal cords when intubating. The assistant moves the larynx backward, upward, and to the patient's right, whilst the tongue is displaced to the left by the laryngoscope blade.

Bacteriostatic Water

A *Water For Injections* diluent, which has bacteria removed, and added antimicrobial 0.9% benzyl alcohol, as an excipient.

Bag Valve Mask (BVM)

A portable Mapleson C, hand-held, self-inflating reservoir bag, for emergency positive pressure ventilation to a patient who is not breathing adequately. Sizes range from 250 ml (low tidal volume, rarely used) to 2 litre, and the bag can deliver about half of its volume. A 1-way valve prevents re-breathing, so can be used with low flows. A pop-up relief valve limits pressure to 4 kPa. Beware: the applied positive pressure increases the risk of aspiration of gastric contents. Note: a patient end "fish tail" valve means gas only flows when pressure is applied to the bag. See *Ambu Bag*.

Bagging The Patient

Manually ventilating a patient, with reservoir bag to push breathing gases into the patient's lungs; typically used between the phases of spontaneous and ventilator controlled breathing. Bagging helps the "bagger" determine where the cause of a ventilation problem might be: if the patient is **easy** to bag, the problem is probably with the anaesthetic circuitry and settings; if bagging is **difficult**, the problem is probably with the patient, eg, compliance, obstructions etc.

Bailey Manoeuvre

Deep extubation, where the endotracheal (ET) tube is replaced by a laryngeal mask airway (LMA): the LMA is railroaded over the ET tube, the cuff is then inflated, then the ET tube cuff is deflated, before carefully removing the ET tube.

Bain Circuit

Functionally, a coaxial Mapleson D efferent reservoir (bag in expiratory limb) circuit, typically used in anaesthetic rooms, connected to a Nuffield Penlon 200 ventilator. Fresh gas flows down the inner tube; exhaust gases flow through the outer tube. Needs fresh gas flow of 2-4 * minute volume to prevent re-breathing. If the circuit is attached to a block assembly, connected to the gas outlet of the anaesthetic machine, and incorporates an expiratory valve, gas scavenging and intermittent positive pressure ventilation may be facilitated. Bain circuits are better for assisted than spontaneous ventilation.

Balanced Anaesthesia

Combination of drugs that produce the optimum balance of hypnosis, sedation, analgesia, and relaxation, whilst minimising side effects and toxicity.

Balanced Salt Solutions

Any solution having a pH and tone matching normal body values, and usually used for washing eyes and other sensitive tissues. Examples: calcium, chloride, magnesium, potassium, and sodium.

Barbiturates

Sedative and hypnotic (induction) drugs, derived from barbituric acid. Examples: *Thiopentone* and *Methohexitone*. Dependency is a drawback of barbiturates (Marilyn Monroe died of barbiturate OD).

Baricity

In anaesthesia, baricity describes the density of a substance, compared with CSF, and is used to determine the spread of the substance, when injected into the CSF. "Heavy" marcain has a higher density than CSF and, therefore has higher baricity (hyperbaric), making it flow through the CSF, following gravity.

Baroreceptors

Nerve endings, particularly in the neck (carotid sinus, aortic arch), which detect, by negative feedback, flow and pressure changes in the arterial system, and send messages to the central nervous system to correct any imbalances in blood pressure, by instructing vascular smooth muscle to alter vessel diameter: increase to lower BP, decrease to increase BP.

Baroreflex

The name given to the baroreceptor negative feedback system.

Barotrauma

Lung (pulmonary barotrauma) or ear (otic barotrauma) injury, due to excess pressure. For example, if an oxygen flush is made during the ventilator inspiratory phase, the excess gas in the circuit (including lungs) cannot be vented, because the ventilator relief valve is closed, the result of which could be a "burst lung".

Basal Flow

On older anaesthetic machines, minimum O_2 flow of 300 ml/min.

Base

A substance that either donates an electron, accepts a proton (+hydrogen ions), or releases a hydroxide ion (OH^-) if it is dissolved in water. An aqueous base reacts with an aqueous acid, forming water and a salt, by accepting protons from the acid. In the blood, the bicarbonate (anion) base is the body's most important buffer that mops up H^+ ions, forming H_2CO_3, thus reducing acidity. A base has pH > 7. Most bases are not soluble in water; those that are soluble are termed *alkalis*.

Base Deficit (BD)

Base Deficit (BD) is the complementary of Base Excess (BE); when BD is positive, BE is negative, and vice versa.

Base Excess (BE)

A value derived from pH and pCO2, where a positive value means alkalosis, describing how much acid (mmol) would have to be added to a litre of the patient's blood (at 37°C, and pCO2 of 40 mmHg), if pH is to be reduced to 7.4. A negative value (Base Deficit) that indicates acidosis, and describes how much base must be added to the blood if pH is to be raised to 7.4. If BE is greater than +2 mmol/L level, the abnormal excess of base in the blood will be caused by metabolic alkalosis. Conversely, if BE is less than -2 mmol/L, the low level will be caused by metabolic acidosis.

BD Connecta

Proprietary name for a 3-way tap and 4 inch (10 cm) extension line, for intravenous line access.

Benzodiazepines

Drugs used for sedation, anxiety relief, muscle relaxation, anti-convulsive, by boosting the effects of the Gabba Amino Butyric Acid neurotransmitter, in the brain. Examples: Midazolam, Oxazepam, Diazepam, Lorazepam. Overdose can cause respiratory depression, loss of consciousness, and hypotension. Benzodiazepines are antagonised (reversed) by Flumazenil.

Berlin ARDS Rating Scheme

Rating system for Acute Respiratory Distress Syndrome, created by the European Society of Intensive Care Medicine (2011), which uses the P/F Ratio to define severity as: **Mild** = 200-300 (27% mortality), **Moderate** = 100-199 (32% mortality), **Severe** = < 100 (45% mortality), with 5 cmH2O of PEEP. Note: An ability to calculate the Berlin score is an attribute that differentiates between knowledgeable and average anaesthetic assistants.

Berman Intubating Airway

Similar to the Guedel pattern Airway, but with a plastic hinge down the left side, a lateral opening down the right side, and used as an aid to blind or fibre-optic intubation.

Beta (β) Blockers

Beta-adrenoceptor blocking agents: Negative inotropics that block effects of adrenaline on the heart and blood vessels, by weakening Sympathetic Nervous System affects on heart conductivity, and reducing blood pressure (vasodilates) and heart rate. Used to treat hypertension, angina, atrial fibrillation. Examples are Esmolol, Atenolol, Metoprolol. See Appendix A19 (pg 374).

Beta Lactam Antibiotics

A family of antibiotics which includes:

- ☺ Carbapenems
- ☺ Cephalosporins
- ☺ Penicillins
- ☺ Monobactams
- ☺ Cephamycins
- ☺ Beta-lactamase inhibitors

Beta-lactam antibiotics inhibit growth of bacteria, by inactivating a set of enzymes located in the bacterial cell membrane, which are involved in the third stage of cell wall synthesis.

Bicarbonate (HCO_3^-)

Aka *Hydrogen Carbonate*: A negative electrolyte and conjugate base of carbonic acid (H_2CO_3). Generated, excreted and reabsorbed by the kidneys, in response to pH levels. When CO_2 combines with water, carbonic acid is formed, and this separates into H+ (positive ions) and negative bicarbonate (HCO_3^-) ions. Bicarbonate levels are raised during respiratory acidosis, to counter (compensate) the acid state by mopping up (**buffering**) H+ ions, thereby lowering pH. The body lowers bicarbonate levels during respiratory alkalosis. Diarrhoea can cause enough loss of bicarbonate to produce metabolic acidosis; the decrease is normally replaced by chloride ions. The range is calculated (blood gases), from pH and CO_2 as 22–26 mmol/litre. Note: bicarbonate values in mEq/L have a 1:1 mapping with mmol/L, so the units are inter-changeable.

Bier Block

Intravenous regional anaesthesia, where an extremity, such as a leg, is made numb for surgery, by injecting a local anaesthetic into a vein, after a tourniquet has been placed distal to the surgical site, and the blood squeezed out of the extremity. The tourniquet prevents the local anaesthetic from leaving the extremity, and blood from entering it, giving the surgeon a bloodless field in which to work. The tourniquet should be inflated to a pressure at least 50 mmHg above the patient's systolic blood pressure.

There is a 1-2 hour time limit on the application of a tourniquet, due to the oxygen starvation which occurs in the region. If the tourniquet is released whilst a large amount of the anaesthetic is yet to be metabolized, blood toxicity may result. Common anaesthetics used are 0.5% Prilocaine or 0.5% Lignocaine. A typical adult dose for a leg is 50-60 ml, and 40 ml for an arm.

Bifurcation

The junction where a vessel divides into two branches.

Bigeminy

Twinned heart beats, which disrupt a normal rhythm.

Bilevel Positive Airway Pressure (BiPAP)

A non-invasive ventilatory pressure support mask, providing higher positive pressure (8 cmH2O) for inspiration than the pressure on expiration (4 cmH2O), so breathing out is easier than with CPAP, where the delivered gas pressure remains constant. Synchronises with the patient when spontaneous breaths are made. The BiPAP machine allows programming for an easier breathing pattern than CPAP. Used for COPD, Pneumonia, and Obstructive Sleep Apnoea.

Bioavailability

The fraction of an administered drug (A) which reaches the systemic circulation (S) unaltered: Bioavailability = S/A. For intravenous drugs, bioavailability is 1, because there is NO first pass metabolism.

Bioconnector/Bionector

Needle free intravenous access device (7 days), from Vygon, providing a sealed access port (less chance of CRBI), and requires a Luer lock device for connecting to a fluid source. May not be suitable for large bore cannulae - flow rate is only 105 ml/min.

Bi Spectral Index (BIS)

Depth of anaesthesia monitor, using electroencephalogram (EEG) activity, via a forehead electrode strip, to calculate depth of sedation and, in GA (general anaesthesia), level of awareness. A hypnotic state measurement scale of 0 (no electrical activity) to 100 (awake) is used. In GA, a reading between 40 and 60 is expected.

Blood

The body's communication/transport system. See Appendix A20 (pg 375).

Blood Brain Barrier

The membrane which separates the bloodstream from the brain, across which, anaesthetic agents diffuse.

Blood:Gas Partition Coefficient (BGPC) λ

Ostwald Coefficient: is the ratio between the concentration of an inhalational agent in the blood phase, and that in the gas phase, when pressures are equal. A higher value (eg, isoflurane=1.4) means higher solubility, lower MAC, and slower anaesthetic onset, because more of the agent must be dissolved (bound to plasma proteins) in the blood, before equilibrium with the alveolar concentration occurs, and commencement of anaesthesia. A low coefficient (eg, desflurane=0.45) means low solubility, higher MAC, faster onset of, and recovery from, anaesthesia.

Blood Groups

Classification system that determines blood type (ABO). See *Group and Save* and Appendix A21 (pg 378).

Blood Pressure (BP)

Pressure exerted by the blood on arterial walls - typical value for a healthy young adult is 120/80 mmHg. The higher reading is the **systolic** pressure, the pressure when the heart is ejecting blood into the arteries; the lower reading is the **diastolic** pressure, which measures the blood vessel's resistance to flow, and occurs when the aortic and pulmonary valves are closed, and the heart is relaxed (between beats). Normal mean arterial pressure is 75-105 mmHg. Factors that affect BP: Cardiac Output, Blood Volume, Blood Vessel Resistance and Compliance (elasticity), Blood Viscosity. BP is derived by Cardiac Output * Peripheral Resistance.

Blood Products

For transfusion: Cryoprecipitate, FFP, Fibrinogen, Platelets, RBCs, Whole Blood, Immunoglobulins, Human Albumin Solution.

Blood Sugar (Glucose)

Extracted from food, glucose is the body's main energy source, with serum glucose concentration measured by BM machine. In some countries, concentration is expressed in millimoles/litre; elsewhere, the levels are measured in mg/dL (to convert from mmol/litre to mg/dL, multiply mmol by 18). Glucose is not an electrolyte, and does not dissolve in water. When glucose is **low** (hypoglycaemia), the liver makes ketones, which break down amino acids and fat (ketogenesis) to use as fuel. **Symptoms**: hunger, sweating, confusion, anxiety, shaking. Intravenous glucose may be required for Diabetics. When **high** (hyperglycaemia), symptoms are: thirst, excessive peeing, fatigue, blurred vision, fruity breath - insulin may be needed. The system for testing blood sugar was developed by Boehringer Mannheim (now Roche) hence the name – *BM* test. See also Appendix A39.

Blood Testing - bottle colours

Bottle cap colours, cardiac arrest: Full Blood Count (lavender), Glucose (grey), U&Es (gold). See Appendix A24 (pg 381).

Blood Transfusion

Infusion of a donated product: RBCs, platelets, FFP, cryoprecipitate. In a standard “blood transfusion”, it is RBCs that are given, not whole blood. See Appendix A25 (pg 382).

Blood Viscocity

Viscosity is "thickness" and how resistant a fluid is to flow, and change in shape. Water has low viscosity, it flows easily, but blood has relatively high viscosity, it oozes more slowly. The more viscous blood is, the more resistance it has, and the slower it will flow. To speed up a blood infusion, warming the blood will reduce its viscosity, with the result that it will flow more easily.

Bodok Seal (Bonded Disk)

A neoprene type of O-ring, with aluminium rim, providing a gas tight seal between gas cylinder and the connecting indexed pin fitting on an anaesthetic machine.

Body Mass Index (BMI)

Weight (kg) divided by the square of the height (m). A BMI of 30 is considered obese. Patients with high BMI will desaturate more quickly than those with low BMI.

Body Surface Area

Square root of [weight (kg) * height (cm) / 3,600]. Sometimes used in drug dose calculations for paediatric patients.

Bohr Effect

Describes how oxygen's binding ability with haemoglobin is reduced as CO_2 concentration increases. See *Oxyhaemoglobin Dissociation Curve, Haldane Effect.*

Bolus (USA, Push)

An injection of an agent, given in one continuous injection.

Bone Cement Implantation Syndrome

Hypoxia, hypotension, and alter mental state, when bone is being cemented, prosthetic insertion, joint reduction, or tourniquet deflation, in a patient having cemented bone/joint surgery.

Bonfils

Rigid retromolar intubation fibreoptic scope, with a straight shaft, and 40 degree curved tip, which facilitates targeted intubation in difficult airway cases, such as Retrognathia. The slim profile makes it useful in patients with limited mouth opening, or cervical spine movement. Unlike fibreoptic scopes, the rigidity of a Bonfils allows it to move past obstructions.

Bougie

French for "candle": A gum-elastic semi-rigid device, with a 30° anterior pointing proximal coude (elbow) "J" tip, to introduce an endotracheal (ET) tube into the trachea. The bougie is carefully advanced through the larynx. Whilst the anaesthetist maintains the laryngoscope and bougie in position, the assistant railroads the ET tube over the end of the bougie, and into the larynx; the bougie is withdrawn, whilst stabilising the ET tube.

Boyle's Law

$\mathbf{P_1 * V_1 = P_2 * V_2}$: At a constant absolute temperature (kelvin), the pressure (P) of a given amount of an ideal gas is inversely proportional to its volume (V). This is why, when the lungs inflate (increase in volume), pressure drops below ambient pressure, resulting in an inward flow of air. **P * V = *constant*.**

Brady-

Slow or slowing.

Bradycardia

Slow heart rate < 60 beats/min (average adult), which can be caused by problems with the sinus node or other heart electrical conduction problem, or by various conditions, such as thyroid problems. Drugs, also, can induce bradycardia. **Symptoms** include: fatigue, chest pain, breathlessness, confusion, syncope. In the perioperative setting, antimuscarinics, such as **Atropine** and **Glycopyrrolate**, are often used to counter bradycardia. If bradycardia is caused by Neostigmine, when reversing neuromuscular blockade, it is countered with Glycopyrrolate. Bradycardia can adversely effect coagulation, so must be managed properly. See also *Reflex Bradycardia*.

Bradypnoea

A regular but abnormally low breathing rate (< 12 breaths/min).

Breath Stacking

Breathing in several small breaths, and a short pause between each mini-breath, then holding a small pause before expiration.

Breathing

See Pulmonary Ventilation.

British Thoracic Society Oxygen Delivery and Device Codes

Codes for NEWS2 obs charts. See Appendix A114 (pg 539).

Bromage Scale

Multi-version assessment system for motor nerve blocks.

Grade	*Assessment*
I	Legs and feet move freely
II	Ability to flex at the knee, and move feet
III	Unable to flex knee, but can move feet

IV Unable to move legs or feet

Bronchial Intubation

Intubation when the endotracheal tube is placed too far, and into a primary bronchus (usually right), and ventilation of only one lung.

Signs include:

- Unusually high airway pressure (peak), e.g., 35+ cmH_2O.
- Unilateral chest expansion.
- Mismatched breathing sounds.
- Reduced or increased end tidal carbon dioxide.
- Low oxygen saturation: < 90%.
- Mediastinal shift.

The ventilated lung may receive the full tidal volume meant for two lungs, and suffer barotrauma (such as pneumothorax). The unventilated lung could suffer collapse (atelectasis).

Bronchiestasis

Widened airways (bronchi), with resultant build-up of mucus, which increases the risk of infection. Signs are breathlessness, persistent cough, and bringing up phlegm.

Bronchiole

From a bronchus, air passages branch out and become progressively smaller, and with decreasing amount of supportive hyaline cartilage as the passages get closer to the alveolar ducts. *Terminal* and *Respiratory* are the smallest bronchioles.

Bronchiolitis

Lower respiratory tract inflammation, in children under two years; caused by RSV, spread from droplets in sneezes and coughs.

Similar to bronchitis, but affects bronchioles, not the bronchi.

Bronchitis

Inflammation of the main bronchi lining, the tubes (airways) which carry oxygen from the atmosphere to the lungs. The inflammation increases mucus production in the airways, producing phlegm, and a cough reflex. **Acute** bronchitis is temporary, often following a common cold or flu. **Chronic** bronchitis, along with emphysema, is classed as a *Chronic Obstructive Pulmonary Disease*, and lasts for several months at a time, with an annual recurrence. Symptoms include headaches, aching, fatigue, sore throat, nasal congestion.

Bronchodilator

An agent that relaxes and dilates the smooth muscle of the bronchial passages, reducing resistance to gas flow, and making it easier to breathe, particularly for asthmatics and COPD sufferers. Bronchodilating agents include beta-2 agonists, such as salbutamol, and anticholinergics, such as glycopyrrolate. Sevoflurane and desflurane have bronchodilating properties.

Bronchopneumonia

An acute inflammation of bronchiole walls, which become clogged with mucus; inflammation spreads to alveoli and alveolar ducts. Signs include: fever, chest pain, coughing up mucus, aches, fatigue, sweating, confusion, and tachypnoea.

Bronchopulmonary Segment

A functionally independent region of a lung (10 right, 8 left), supplied by a tertiary (segmental) bronchus, and which can be surgically removed, without effecting the rest of the lung.

Bronchoscopy

Viewing of the airways and lungs, by camera, using a flexible endoscope. The patient may be awake and sedated, or intubated.

Bronchospasm

Breathing difficulty due to constriction of smooth muscle in bronchiole walls (not protected by cartilage, unlike bronchi). **Signs**: longer expiration time, audible wheeze (except in complete constriction), increased $EtCO_2$ and peak airway pressure, shark fin trace, reduced volume. **Treatment**: inform surgeon, call for help, give 100% O_2, deepen anaesthesia (propofol, ketamine, sevoflurane), give salbutamol (via ETT), adrenaline 10 mikes, hydrocortisone 100 mg, ECMO (last resort). Bronchospasm can lead to hypoxaemia, hypotension, and cardiac arrest. Unless there is good reason for intubation, bronchospasm risk is reduced with spontaneous breathing and LMA use, and using drugs that do not trigger histamine release. See Appendix A26 (pg 385).

Bronchus

Plural *bronchi*, Latin for "throat": One of the larger passages of the respiratory tree, below the trachea, which transports inspired gases to the lungs, and expires waste gases. A bronchus differs, structurally, from a bronchiole, by being supported by hyaline cartilage, so that it cannot constrict, whereas a bronchiole is surrounded by smooth muscle, which allows it to have a dynamically changing diameter. See Appendix A27 (pg 389).

Broviac line

Skin tunnelled cuffed central venous catheter, to provide long term intravenous access. Typically used for paediatric patients.

Buccal

The cheek, or mouth cavity.

Buffer

An aqueous solution that helps keep blood pH within the normal range, by reversibly binding with hydrogen ions ($H+$), when pH is low (acidic), and releasing them when pH is high. The main extracellular buffer systems are bicarbonate (HCO_3-) and plasma proteins. In the cells, buffering is by Hb, phosphate, and proteins.

Bundle Branch Block

Heart Block, an *intraventricular conduction defect*, where electrical impulses are partially or wholly blocked from reaching the ventricles. Left Bundle Branch Block suggests an underlying cardiac issue. A Right Bundle Branch Block may or may not mean an underlying condition.

Bundle of His (Atrioventricular Bundle)

Cardiac muscle fibres, between atria and ventricle, conducting atrioventricular node impulses to the interventricular septum, then divide to connect with Purkinje Fibres.

Bupivacaine Hydrochloride

Local anaesthetic with slower onset (20+ mins) and longer duration (2-6 hours) than Licodaine. Available in ~ 0.25% and 0.5% w/v solutions. Marketed under the name *Marcaine*. Also available with Adrenaline. Note: 0.5% is not to be used for paediatric caudal anaesthesia.

Burette

A paediatric microdrip giving set which administers 60 drops/ml.

Butrylcholinesterase

Aka *plasma cholinesterase*, or *pseudocholinesterase*. A butryl enzyme, made by the liver, and present in the bloodstream, which breaks down Suxamethonium. A deficiency results in Suxamethonium apnoea.

BVM

Bag Valve Mask.

Caesarean Section

The surgical delivery of a baby, by cutting through the abdomen and womb. See Appendices A28 (pg 391) and A29 (pg 393).

Calcium (Ca)

An extracellular electrolyte, to facilitate muscle contraction, skeletal validity, blood clotting, heart rhythm, and enzyme function. Blood calcium levels (2.2–2.6 mmol/L) are regulated by calcitonin (thyroid hormone) and parathyroid hormone. If not enough calcium is in the diet, it drains from the bones, weakening them. Calcium deficiency may be countered with calcium (gluconate or chloride), which is also given for magnesium toxicity. 10 ml of 10% w/v calcium is given in PEA (pulseless elec activity), when caused by hyperkalaemia, hypocalcaemia, or calcium channel blocker overdose.

Calcium Chloride, Gluconate

To treat hypocalcaemia, hyperkalaemia, and magnesium toxicity. Calcium chloride is an irritant, so extravasation can cause soft tissue damage (best use a larger cannula). Calcium gluconate is not so irritating, so is preferred to calcium gluconate, but has to be metabolised by the liver before it exerts its action, so may not be an option if the patient has liver dysfunction.

Calculus

An aggregation of an insoluble crystallised matter which forms, for example, within the gallbladder, urinary bladder, and kidneys. In simple terms, a solid growth or "stone".

Cannula

Latin "small reed": A flexible hollow needle, inserted into a vein, to facilitate intravenous fluid administration and blood extraction. Generally, smaller than a catheter. See Appendix A30 (pg 395).

Can't Intubate, Can't Oxygenate/Ventilate

The algorithm, produced by the Difficult Airway Society, on how to proceed with failed intubation and oxygenation, culminating in **Plan D**, which involves emergency front of neck access, by Scalpel Cricothyroidotomy. The algorithm can be downloaded from: *https://www.das.uk.com/guidelines/cvci.html*

Capillary

A blood vessel, one cell thick, which allows diffusion of gas, nutrients, waste, and fluid, between the blood and tissue cells. The capillary is connected, upstream, to a supplying arteriole, and downstream, to a venule. The capillary wall only allows particles below a particular size to escape (like a fishing net - only smaller fish escape through the net). Larger substances, such as colloids, continue their journey through the capillary, without "escaping".

Capillary Refill Time (CRT)

Guide to tissue perfusion: refilling of a capillary after exsanguination by externally applied pressure, typically to the nail bed (or sternum), until it blanches (turns white), the patient should then raise their hand above their heart, and the time taken for colouring to return is recorded - normally 2 seconds, or 4 seconds on the chest; longer might indicate shock or hypovolaemia.

Capnogram

Series of capnographs. See Appendix A31 (pg 397).

Capnograph

Two dimensional graph that gives information about expired CO_2, with time plotted on the X axis, and CO_2 concentration on the Y axis. In theatres, *time capnographs* are usually used, but *volume capnographs* are also available. In some conditions, such as lung disease or some congenital heart diseases, the difference between arterial ($paCO_2$) and E_TCO_2 can exceed 1 kPa, but usually the difference is small. Fever and shivering increase CO_2 production. Capnography can warn of: hypoventilation, oesophageal intubation (flat trace), cardiac oscillations (serrated alveolar plateau), patient attempt to breathe during IPPV (*curare cleft* in alveolar plateau), emphysema (reversed alveolar slope), bronchospasm or asthma (*shark fin* trace), circulatory failure, leaking circuit/ETT (*dunce hat* trace). A peak at the end of the alveolar phase, known as *pig-tail*, suggests poor lung compliance, and might also be seen in pregnancy or obesity. E_TCO_2 is considered the gold standard for ensuring ventilation, particularly to confirm endotracheal intubation (*top hat* trace). Mantra: NO TRACE = WRONG PLACE. See Appendices A31 (pg 397), A31b.

Capnography

Depiction of capnographs. See Appendix A31b (pg 398).

Capnometer

The numerical presentation of expired carbon dioxide. Typical (adult) range values are 35 - 45 mmHg, or 4.6 – 6 kPa.

Carbaminohaemoglobin

Haemoglobin molecules bound with carbon monoxide.

Carbon Dioxide (CO_2)

A respiratory acid, and metabolic waste product of oxidisation of sugar in the mitochondria (in cells). CO_2 (20 times more soluble in blood and alveolar fluid than oxygen) is a heavy, colourless, odourless, incombustible, corrosive, and volatile compound of carbon and oxygen, also formed as a waste product of combustion, and organic decomposition. ~200 ml of CO_2 is produced per minute, diffuses very quickly from the blood to the alveoli. Of the CO_2 produced, ~5% is dissolved in plasma, 10% binds to Hb, and the rest combines with water to form carbonic acid, which quickly dissociates into hydrogen (H^+) and bicarbonate (HCO_3^-) ions which, in turn, move from blood cells into the plasma. If cardiac output is reduced, end tidal CO_2 ($EtCO_2$) may also be reduced. CO_2 is an indicator of respiratory function, and a normal $EtCO_2$ reading is a sign of valid endotracheal tube placement and airway "sealing". When bicarbonate and H^+ ions reach the lungs, they recombine to form CO_2, and are exhaled. Normal $paCO_2$ (arterial CO_2 pressure) is 4.6-6 kPa (35-45 mmHg). Normal $pACO_2$ (alveolar CO_2 pressure) is ~0.66 kPa (5 mmHg) lower than $paCO_2$.

Carbon Dioxide Narcosis

A potentially serious, but reversible, state of confusion and convulsions caused by excessive CO_2 levels, of ~50 mmHg or more, rather than the normal 40 mmHg. When arterial CO_2 climbs to a level where the respiratory control centre loses its ability to respond to CO_2, respiratory control is transferred from the *respiratory* drive to the *hypoxic* drive, which relies on oxygen levels, detected by peripheral chemoreceptors, to stimulate breathing. If the affected patient is given a high concentration of oxygen, the hypoxic drive stimulus to breathe is reduced, and CO_2 levels climb further still, and CO_2 narcosis occurs. COPD patients are most susceptible to carbon dioxide narcosis.

Carbon Monoxide (CO)

CO is a by-product of incomplete combustion, a toxic gas that has no colour or smell, and kills by preferentially occupying the Hb (haemoglobin) molecules (carboxyhaemoglobin) that would otherwise be available for binding with oxygen (CO has 200 times more affinity for Hb than oxygen). CO gives the same red colour to arterial blood as oxygen does. **In CO poisoning, arterial O_2 partial pressure (paO_2) is unaffected, but O_2 saturation by CO-oximetry is low**. A CO blood level greater than 10% causes arrhythmias and respiratory problems. Many pulse oximeters do not detect CO poisoning – only CO-oximeters do that. In severe CO poisoning, hyperbaric oxygen treatment is needed, so the high oxygen pressure can dislodge the CO from Hb. [In 1994, tennis player Vitas Gerulaitis died of CO poisoning, from a leaking gas heating system] See *CO-Oximetry, Haemoglobin Electrophoresis*.

Carbonic Acid (H_2CO_3)

A weak acid, created when carbon dioxide is dissolved in water, and which then dissociates into hydrogen (H^+) and bicarbonate (HCO_3^-) ions. Carbonic acid is a volatile respiratory acid, because it is the only acid excreted as a gas (as CO_2) by the lungs.

Carboxyhaemoglobin (COHb)

Haemoglobin (Hb) molecules that have been occupied by carbon monoxide (CO) and cannot, therefore, be used to transport oxygen, because Hb has a stronger affinity for carbon monoxide than it does for oxygen. A normal COHb fraction (FCOHb) from total Hb is 1-2%, but smoking and pollutants can increase the level until the sufferer experiences hypoxia. Only *CO-oximetry* oximeters differentiate Hb bound with CO with oxygen from Hb bound with CO; non CO-oximeters count Carboxyhaemoglobin along with Oxyhaemoglobin, giving a false high sats value.

Cardiac Arrest

The heart stops pumping, due to a problem with electrical activity. Not to be confused with a "heart attack". Primary characteristics of cardiac arrest are: **Unresponsiveness, Unconsciousness**, and cessation of **Breathing** (resulting in respiratory acidosis). Successful treatment is governed by compliance with the *Chain of Survival*. The most common cause of sudden cardiac arrest is an arrhythmia. See Appendix A92 (pg 506).

Cardiac Cycle

Heart electrical activity: the four phases of the Cardiac Cycle:

① **Atrial diastole**: Vena cava blood passively flows into the right atrium, and pulmonary vein blood flows into the left atrium.

② **Atrial systole**: Both atria contract, and push blood into the ventricles.

③ **Ventricular diastole**: Both ventricles relax; and receive blood from the atria.

④ **Ventricular systole**: Both ventricles contract; right vent pushes blood into the pulmonary arteries, and the left vent pushes blood into the aorta.

Cardiac Index

Provides a more patient specific description of cardiac output, by dividing the cardiac output by body surface area, with the answer given in litres per minute per square metre. A "normal" range of values is 2.5 to 4 L/min/m^2.

Cardiac Output (COP)

Amount of blood ejected from the left ventricle per minute. The product of *stroke volume* and *heart rate*. The significance to anaesthesia of a **high COP** is that it stimulates diffusion of inhalation agents from the alveoli, to the blood, and this results in a prolonged period that the concentration gradient exists. Consequently, the anaesthetic effect is delayed, because there is no partial pressure equilibrium between the alveoli and blood (hence, alveoli and brain). COP can be increased by stimulation of the sympathetic nervous system, or an increase in calcium. A **low COP** shortens time to anaesthesia, because the body prioritises blood flow to the brain, thereby delivering a greater concentration of induction agent. COP can be reduced by parasympathetic stimulation, low calcium levels, hypoxia, or acidosis. At rest, a normal adult COP is 4-6 litre/minute. Notably, low COP is linked to a reduced $EtCO_2$, and high COP with higher $EtCO_2$.

Cardiac Resynchronisation Therapy (CRT)

Aka *biventricular pacemaker*: A **CRT-P** device is a pacemaker, with leads to connect to the ventricles, and send signals to synchronise their contractions. Another implanted device is the **CRT-D**, which is a CRT-P plus defibrillator (aka biventricular ICD).

Cardiac Shunt

Cardiac blood that does not follow a normal circulatory pattern but, instead, follows abnormal connections. Abnormal flow may be from left to right or right to left sides of the heart, or between the pulmonary and systemic (aorta) circulations, resulting in deoxygenated blood being fed into the systemic circulation.

Cardiac Sphincter

See Lower Oesophageal Sphincter.

Cardiac Tamponade

Pericardial effusion that has reached the point where the excess fluid in the pericardium puts pressure on the heart, stopping the atria and ventricles from filling and pumping, and stopping the pulse. Determine with ultrasound; fluid drainage is either by ultrasound guided pericardiocentesis, VATS, or thoracotomy. Cardiac tamponade can lead to obstructive shock. Indicators of cardiac tamponade include *pulsus paradoxus* and *Beck's Triad.*

Beck's Triad of Cardiac Tamponade Signs

Symptom	*Cause*
Hypotension	Decreased stroke volume
Jugular-venous distension	Increased superior vena cava pressure, with impaired venous return to the heart
Muffled heart sounds	Fluid in the pericardium

All 3 symptoms are rarely found together, except during surgery.

Cardiogenic (Cardiac) Shock

Hypoperfusion to organs and tissues. Compensation is increased SVR and vasoconstriction. Typically, caused by myocardial infarction or thrombus, such as pulmonary embolism. Main signs are (1) Prolonged hypotension (2) Cool peripheries (3) Hypoxia. **Symptoms**: confusion, tachycardia, tachypnoea, breathing problems, hypoxia, pale skin. Treatment: inotropic or vasopressor agents, followed by percutaneous coronary intervention, or coronary artery bypass graft (CABG).

Cardiomyopathy

The heart muscle is thickened (hypertrophic), stretched (dilated), or stiff (restrictive), and does not pump as well as it should.

CardioQ Doppler Monitor

A minimally invasive real-time monitoring device, for higher risk surgery, using ultrasound to create the "doppler" effect in measuring blood cell velocity. The CardioQ system is very sensitive to changes in central circulation flow, and provides immediate and accurate measurement of stroke volume and cardiac output. A lubricated probe is inserted (nasal/oral) 14-16 inch (35-40 cm) into the oesophagus, to T5/6 vertebra, where the oesophagus and descending aorta lie at their closest point, to monitor blood flow leaving the descending aorta; this allows the anaesthetist to detect a reduction in circulating blood volume, guiding the anaesthetist to improve cardiac output with fluid challenges. Optimising a patient's haemodynamic status in this way, by giving the right amount of the right fluid at the right time, is known as individualized Doppler Guided Fluid Management.

Cardiovascular Disease

A condition which adversely affects the heart and blood vessels.

Type	*Condition*
Angina	Chest pain
Coronary Heart Disease	Heart arteries clogged with plaque
Myocardial Infarction	Blood supply to part of heart stops
Peripheral Arterial Disease	Inadequate blood supply to the legs, causing pain
Stroke	Reduced blood supply to brain

Transient Ischaemic Attacks	Temporary stroke symptoms

Cardioversion

Conversion of an arrhythmia, such as atrial fibrillation or tachycardia, to sinus rhythm, using an electrical defibrillator, or by pharmacological means. See Appendix A32 (pg 401).

Carina

Where the trachea divides into the right and left main bronchi.

Carrico Index (P/F Ratio)

The ratio (fraction) of the partial pressure of oxygen in the arteries (paO_2), against the Fraction of Inspired Oxygen (FiO_2). A useful measurement of pulmonary condition, and how well the patient's blood is being oxygenated from the alveoli and, hence, whether underlying causes, such as *intra pulmonary shunt*, might be present. The value is determined by dividing paO_2 (mmHg) by FiO_2 (decimal). Example, if paO_2 is 100 mmHg, and FiO_2 is 0.21, the index is 100/0.21 = 476. A value (index) > 400 (at Standard Temperature and Pressure) is considered “normal”; anything lower than 300 might indicate hypoxaemia or lung damage. See *ARDS*.

Carrier Gas

Non-anaesthetic component of the gases that are delivered in the breathing circuit, to allow delivery of an inhalational agent, such as sevoflurane, to the patient. The carrier gas mix always contains oxygen and/or air, and may also include nitrous oxide.

Catheter

A hollow flexible tube for insertion into a body cavity, duct, or vessel, to allow the drainage of fluids, eg, a Foley catheter drains urine from the bladder.

Catheter Mount

Single-use flexible tube between an angle piece, on a mask, and HME filter. Some catheter mounts have angle piece attached, some separate. Some have a port for tracheal suction.

Catheter Related Bloodstream Infection (CRBI)

Catheter Related Sepsis: The presence of bacteria in the blood, introduced by a catheter tip. CRBI is the biggest cause of hospital acquired infection, particularly when centrally placed.

Cation

A positively charged ion, atom, or molecule, because it has more protons than electrons. See also *Anion*.

Caudad

Adverb: Towards the tail or posterior.

Caudal Analgesia

Epidural blockade, for procedures below the level of the umbilicus, that need sacro-lumbar and mid-thoracic blockades. Commonly used in paediatric patients, analgesia is realised by injection of local anaesthetic, such as 0.25% (not 0.5%) bupivacaine, into the caudal canal, with resultant block of the sacral and lumbar nerves.

Cell Salvage

Also known as autologous blood salvage; a medical procedure involving the recovery of blood lost during surgery, cleaning, and re-infusing it into the patient. See Appendix A33 (pg 402).

Cellular Respiration

The processes that cell's use to convert energy from oxygen and nutrients into adenosine triphosphate.

-centesis

Puncturing a cavity or organ, such as when aspirating fluids.

Centimeter of Water (cmH2O)

A manometric unit of airway pressure, equivalent to 98 pascals.

Central Nervous System

The brain and spinal cord, which receives sensory (afferent) information, processes it, and sends out (efferent) control signals.

Central Venous Catheter (CVC)

A catheter inserted into a neck vein (rt internal jugular, subclavian), chest (subclavian, axillary), or groin (common femoral), and threaded to the vena cava, at the entrance to the right atrium, from where administration of agents, monitoring blood pressure (CVP), and drawing blood may occur. Two main types are tunnelled (lying under the skin, then into a vein), for longer term use, and non-tunnelled (straight into a vein), for short term use eg, during surgery. See Appendices A34 (pg 408), A80 (pg 488).

Central Venous Pressure (CVP)

Vena cava mean pressure, using a CVC, at the entrance to the right atrium, typically, 4-11 cmH2O (3-8 mmHg). CVP is equivalent to the filling pressure of the right atrium, and is an indicator of the heart's effectiveness as a pump. If the pressure is less than 4 cmH2O, the patient may be hypovolaemic. (Appendix A34).

Cephal-

Orientation towards the head.

Cerebral/Somatic Monitoring

Real-time monitoring of regional blood oxygen saturation (rSO_2), of the brain or other regions lying beneath the sensor.

Cerebrospinal Fluid (CSF)

Clear and colourless fluid, created from arterial blood in the choroid plexus of the brain. CSF exists in the subarachnoid space and in the ventricular system around/inside the brain and spinal cord, providing nutrients to the spinal cord, and cushions the spine and brain against shock. A test can measure spinal fluid pressure. Normal CSF glucose level is 50 - 80 mg/100 mL, or > 2/3 blood sugar level.

Chain of Infection

Three stages: 1: Agent leaves the host or reservoir via a portal of exit. 2: Agent is transported by a mode of transmission. 3: Agent enters a host's portal of entry.

Chain of Survival

The sequence of steps, developed by the *International Liaison Committee on Resuscitation* (ILCOR), which cooperates on research and processes to save lives through the development of an *International Resuscitation Consensus on Science and Treatment Recommendations* for treating victims of cardiac arrest. The main steps are: Early recognition and call for help Early CPR Early defibrillation Post resuscitation care.

Chalasia

Relaxation of the cardiac sphincter (ring of oesophageal muscle), allowing regurgitation of gastric contents - could pollute the lungs.

Challenge

Giving a drug, under strict observation, to determine whether or not the patient has a reaction to it, starting with a very small dose, then higher doses over several hours.

Charles Law

$V_1/T_1=V_2/T_2$. The **V**olume of an ideal gas, at constant pressure, is directly proportional to its **T**emperature (Kelvin).

Chemoreceptor

A sensory organ, or group of cells, that respond to chemical stimulation, by translating chemical reactions into nervous system signals. In the respiratory system, **peripheral** (carotid and aorta bodies) chemoreceptors cause respiratory rate and tidal volume changes by responding to changes in the partial pressures of CO_2 (actually, carbonic acid and hydrogen ions) and oxygen. **Central** chemoreceptors in the brain (pons, medulla oblongata) respond to changes in the pH of cerebrospinal fluid, by decreasing ventilation when low CO_2 is low, and increasing ventilation when CO_2 is high.

Chest drain

A tube inserted into the pleural space to remove air (pneumothorax), fluids (pleural effusion), or pus (empyema), and attached to a bottle containing water, which acts as a seal to prevent air from leaking back into the pleural space.

Cheyne-Stokes Breathing

An irregular pattern of breathing, alternating between fast and slow, and breaths that are deep and shallow, lasting for seconds, or minutes. Cheyne-Stokes breathing can be seen in patients with congestive heart failure, or anyone very near the end of life.

Chirocaine

Trade (AstraZeneca) name for *levobupivacaine*.

Chlorhexidine

A chemical antiseptic, effective against Gram-positive and most Gram-negative bacteria.

Chloride (Cl-)

An abundant blood electrolyte (anion of chlorine), with levels controlled by the kidneys, which serves to maintain: fluid balance between cells and extracellular space, osmotic pressure, hydration, blood pressure, volume, and pH. A **low** level might be due to low sodium, and caused by: congestive heart failure, metabolic alkalosis, COPD, vomiting, diarrhoea, diuretics, bicarbonate administration, laxatives, steroids, chemotherapy. A **high** level can be due to high blood sodium (perhaps from too much normal saline, or salt ingestion), kidney disease, or dehydration. Symptoms include dry mucous membranes, weakness, thirst, and hypertension. Normal serum range is 95 – 108 mmol/litre.

Chlorphenamine

Sedating antihistamine.

Chlorpromazine

An antipsychotic agent, used to treat schizophrenia patients.

Chole-

Referring to bile/gallbladder.

Cholecystectomy

Open or laparoscopic removal of the gallbladder.

Cholinergic

The neurons, synapses, and receptors that use acetylcholine (ACh), the main neurotransmitter for nerve impulses of the parasympathetic nervous system. Cholinergic neurons release ACh, which bind with cholinergic receptors (in cell membrane) - either of the nicotinic (also found in the sympathetic system) or muscarinic type. Peripheral muscle contraction occurs when ACh binds with nicotinic receptors on skeletal muscles. Cholinergic drugs mimic, enhance, or block the action of ACh. When ACh binds with muscarinic receptors, heart rate and force of contraction decreases, causing increased exocrine gland secretions of gastric acid, saliva, and airway mucosa.

Cholinesterase

Two types of nervous system enzyme - acetylcholinesterase (AChE) and butrylcholinesterase (BchE) - that break down acetylcholine at the neuromuscular junction.

Chronic

A long lasting disease state.

Chronic Obstructive Pulmonary Disease (COPD)

Chronic bronchitis or emphysema – lung diseases where the airways become obstructed or narrowed, causing reduced flow of air to and from the lungs, bringing shortness of breath, and getting progressively worse. Caused by noxious particles or gas - most commonly from smoking - which trigger an inflammatory response in the lung. **Symptoms**: coughing up phlegm, chest infection, wheezing, shortness of breath, aches, fatigue, nasal congestion, sore throat. If the COPD patient has clubbed fingers, they may be suffering from more severe issues, such as lung cancer. COPD patients retain carbon dioxide, which they have lost the ability to detect, which means reduced respiratory drive. Instead, they rely (in theory) on low oxygen levels (hypoxic drive) to regulate their breathing. Note that, sometimes, a finger/toe oxygen saturation probe is unreliable, so an ear probe should be used instead. Target oxygen saturation is 88-92%.

Chronotrope

A substance that changes heart rate. Positive chronotropes (eg atropine) increase heart rate, negative chronotropes (eg metoprolol) decrease the rate.

Chvostek's Sign

Spasm of the facial muscles, due to calcium deficiency.

Chyme

Semi-liquid mix of food and gastric juice, formed in the stomach.

Circle Circuit

Developed by Brian Sword (1926); uses low gas flows, and removes CO_2 by chemical reaction (soda lime).

Cl

Chemical symbol for chloride.

Clark's Rule

In the absence of drug dose instructions, a paediatric (up to 2 years) dose will be: adult dose * weight (in pounds) / 150

Clearance Rate

Estimated volume (**V**) of drug that is removed from the plasma per unit of time. The elimination rate (**E**) divided by the mean plasma (**P**) concentration of the drug. If **E** is 100 mg/min, and **P** is 5 mg/ml, then clearance rate is 100/5 = 20 ml per minute.

ClearSight Arterial Line

A non invasive device for real-time measurement of arterial blood pressure, using a photoplethysmographic (optical) method to measure blood volumes, using a finger cuff.

Cleido-

Referring to the clavicle.

Clonidine (Catapres)

A drug to, primarily, treat hypertension, but also drug withdrawal, diarrhoea, and menopausal flushes. Side-effects include: hallucinations, anxiety, depression, and sleep disturbances.

Clopidogrel

Anti-platelet drug (tablet), to stop platelet aggregation, and prescribed to prevent blood clots, by interfering with the behaviour of platelets. Used by those at risk of heart attack, along with aspirin (300 mg) when heart attack occurs.

Clostridium Difficile (C Diff)

A very contagious bacteria that can seriously affect the bowel, and often affects those who have recently taken antibiotics. Other vulnerable people include those with weakened immune systems (from cancer, kidney problems, diabetes, chemotherapy), had bowel surgery, over 65s, or have prolonged care home or hospital stays.

Surgical patients should be subject to isolation and barrier protocols and, in most cases, will bypass the anaesthetic room, to be anaesthetised in theatre. Anaesthetic assistants should keep copies of Infection Control policies with them, because doctors are unlikely to be up to date with their details. Staff and patients should comply with hand washing guidelines, rigourously.

Clothes Line Injury

Trauma to the neck, usually occurring in children, caused by high force collision with a taut line (rope, cord, wire), resulting in injury to the oesophagus, larynx, trachea, cricoid or thyroid structures. Incidences are rare, but mortality is high.

C-MAC

Proprietary name of Karl Storz set of video intubation devices, including the use of Macintosh, Miller and hyperangular "D" laryngoscope type blades.

CNS

See Central Nervous System.

Co-Oximetry

A CO-oximeter uses a spectophotometric analyser to measure oxygen saturation, and recognises both dyshaemoglobins and Hb molecules that are loaded with oxygen (O_2Hb). The fraction of total Hb that is O_2Hb gives the value for oxygen saturation. A blood gas machine or pulse oximeter that use CO-oximetry gives more accurate oxygen saturation values than without CO-oximetry. See also *Oximetry, SaO_2*.

Coagulation Cascade

The series of steps where clotting factors initiate each other to form a fibrin clot: (1) *Vasoconstriction*: Platelets release serotonin and other substances that cause the vessel to constrict. (2) *Platelet plugging*: Plateletes plug the breach. (3) *Clotting*: The coagulation cascade reinforces the breach in the vessel. (4) *Thrombolysis*: Removal of the clot, and commencement of wound healing.

Coagulopathy

An abnormality in the blood clotting process.

Co-axial Breathing Circuit

Single limb circuit with an inner tube to separate FGF and expired gas flows.

Co-codamol

A potentiating combination of codeine and paracetamol, used for mild to moderate pain relief.

Cocaine Hydrochloride

Solution (10% w/v) to provide local anaesthesia and vasoconstriction (reduces bleeding) in nasal/throat procedures.

Codeine

An opioid, metabolised to morphine, for mild-moderate pain.

Coeliac

Referring to the abdomen.

Colloid

The mixing of a particle, with a diameter between 1 and 1,000 nanometre, into another fluid or solid, to form an evenly distributed substance, and which has less tendency to settle than a suspension. Intravenous colloids help support blood volume, and will not cross semi-permeable membranes (unlike crystalloids), such as capillaries, but will remain within the cardiovascular system. **Examples**:

☺ Volulyte ☺ Dextrans70 ☺ Dextrans40

☺ Gelatin ☺ Volulyte ☺ Hydroxyethyl Starch

Note: Crystalloids are better at correcting electrolyte imbalances.

Coma

Unconsciousness; the patient cannot be aroused, has no normal eye movements, and does not respond to stimuli, such as pain.

Combined Gas Law

Explains the relationship between Pressure (P), Volume (V), and absolute Temperature (T, kelvin), for an ideal gas:

$$\mathbf{P_1 * V_1 / T_1 = P_2 * V_2 / T_2}$$

For one mole of gas, PV/T equals R (universal gas constant). Rearranging gives **PV = nRT**, where n is the number of moles.

Knowing any two factors of pressure, volume, and temperature, the third factor can be calculated. The above equation is essential knowledge for designing hospital gas supply systems, otherwise it would not be possible to predict whether or not the pipe work is strong enough to contain a gas whose pressure has increased, for example, due to an increase in ambient temperature.

Combined Spinal/Epidural

Offers the fast onset of a Spinal anaesthetic (sub-arachnoid block), with topping up of anaesthetic offered by an Epidural. A Tuohy needle enters the epidural space, a spinal needle (25g) passed through the Tuohy, to pierce the dura mater (pop felt), to the subarachnoid space, where CSF leaks through the spinal needle, proving that the needle is in the right space, so a local anaesthetic can be injected. The spinal needle is then withdrawn, and an epidural catheter placed in the epidural space.

Combitube

Twin lumen combined oesophageal and endotracheal tube, used in emergency and difficult airway situations, which is blindly passed into either the trachea or oesophagus, without laryngoscope visualisation. The tube has a small distal cuff (white), and a larger blue cuff (50-75 ml), about 2/3 the length of the tube, from the proximal end. If the tube enters the **trachea**, then the combitube functions as a normal endotracheal tube. Alternatively, if the tube has entered the **oesophagus**, ventilation is by means of apertures in the side of the tube, between the two cuffs. Insertion is midline, along the tongue, until depth markers are reached. Tip location can be proved by *Positube* (checks air flow resistance) or auscultation. See Appendix A35 (pg 414).

Common Gas Outlet (CGO)

The outlet from the anaesthetic machine to the main breathing circuit, where oxygen, air, nitrous oxide, and vapourised gases are delivered. Checking the function of the CGO downstream (inhalation) and upstream (exhalation) one-way valves is part of machine checking. On some anaesthetic machines, the CGO is connected to the machine by a Cardiff Swivel, which allows it to revolve on ts axis. See also *Auxiliary Common Gas Outlet*.

Common Volume

The part of an infusion set that brings together two or more infusions, via a multi-way connector. Ideally, this shared tube space should be as short as possible, near the cannula, as per “B”, in image: Appendix A30 (pg 396).

Comorbidity

A health problem (morbidity) that is additional to another condition. An anaesthetist must know about a patient's comorbidities, such as asthma, allergies, restricted head movements etc., so they can optimise the anaesthetic regime.

Compartment Syndrome

Increased level of pressure within an enclosed (confined) bundle of muscles – known as a muscle "compartment"; caused by bleeding or swelling (typically) in fascial compartments. The resultant pressure restricts blood flow to the affected area. Affected compartments can be in the hand, arm, buttocks, leg (especially below the knee), foot, and abdomen. Emergency treatment is by fasciotomy - where the fascia is cut to relieve pressure. Symptoms include: tightness, cramping, tingling, and burning pain.

Compensation

When one body system fails to function normally, other systems might compensate for the failure. Eg, if a kidney problem causes metabolic acidosis, the respiratory system can compensate by reducing the contribution that CO_2 makes to acidity, by breathing out more CO_2 than normal. Note: If a disease condition is compensated, the sufferer might not experience any symptoms or deficiencies but, if the patient does have symptoms and dysfunction, their condition is deemed to be decompensated.

Compensated Shock

The body's mechanism to reduce the effects of low blood volume by constricting blood vessels, and increasing heart and respiratory rate, thereby helping to maintain blood pressure and perfusion.

Competitive Antagonist

A substance that binds to its target receptor (does not activate it), so blocking an agonist from binding with the receptor (think of sitting in a car's driver seat, blocking the driver from driving).

Compliance (elasticity)

The more compliant (stretchable) a vessel is, the more able it is to absorb increases in volume of blood flow. In **cardiovascular** physiology, general effect of good compliance is to put less strain on the heart and blood vessels. In **respiratory** physiology, compliance refers to lung elasticity. See *Lung Compliance.*

Compound

Substance composed of different chemically bonded elements. If a compound's name ends with "ide", it comprises 2 elements. If the name ends with "ate", the molecule is composed of 3 or more elements, one of which is usually oxygen.

Computerised Axial Tomography (CAT) Scanner

Aka CT: A machine that uses X-rays to produce a detailed image of a slice of the body, shown in 2-D or 3-D. Some patients will drink a barium meal, or have an IV administration of contrast agent, to improve the image. Generally, CT is also preferred for finding brain bleeds, pneumonia, and most cancers.

Concentration []

A term to describe various types of density, electrolytes per unit of volume, or gas partial pressure. In pharmacology, concentration is defined as the ratio of solute to its solution. A high ratio means the solution is more concentrated; if the ratio is low, then the solution is diluted. With weight/volume drug values, concentration refers to the ratio of solute to solvent. When using molar measurements, concentration is the term used to describe molarity, which is moles of solute (drug) per litre of solvent.

Concentration Effect

The higher the concentration of an inhaled agent (FI), the quicker the alveolar concentration (FA) approaches FI. See *FA/FI ratio*.

Concentration Gradient

A higher concentration of particles in one space compared with another space. Particles passively (no energy needed) move from a higher to a lower concentration, to equalise the concentrations.

Congestive Heart Failure

Aka *Heart Failure*: Failure of the heart to pump sufficient blood volume for proper metabolism. Consequently, fluid builds up in the lungs, abdomen, liver, jugular vein (visible engorgement), and lower body. The main causes are hypertension, coronary heart disease, and diabetes mellitus.

Heart Failure Stages...

1: Risk of HF (Heart Failure), due to diabetes mellitus, hypertension, coronary artery disease, alcoholism, family history of cardiac problems, or some drugs. No symptoms.

2: Pre-HF, systolic left ventricle dysfunction, but symptoms only with physical activity.

3: Diagnosed with HF; symptoms from minor physical activity.

4: Suffering HF, cannot do any physical activity.

See Left/Right/Forward/Backward Heart Failure.

Conjugate

To join substances.

Conjugate Acid/Base

A conjugate base gains a proton (H+ ion) in a chemical reaction, whereas a conjugate acid donates the proton. When an acid dissociates in water, a chemical reaction causes the acid to donate an H+ ion (proton), leaving the conjugate base. These H+ ions are the cause of blood acidity. A relevant example is when CO_2 dissolves with water, to form carbonic acid ($H_2CO_3^-$), and then dissociates into an H+ ion and bicarbonate (HCO_3^-).

Consolidation

See Pulmonary Consolidation.

Continuous Positive Airway Pressure (CPAP)

In spontaneous ventilation, a CPAP mask system maintains constant positive airway pressure, typically 10 cmH_2O, until the end of expiration. Closing pressure holds open the alveoli, so that partial pressure of arterial oxygen is improved, reducing shunting, and making breathing easier. CPAP also increases FRC.

Conventional Mechanical Ventilation (CMV)

Invasive ventilation techniques, using ET or tracheotomy tubes.

Cook Airway Exchange Catheter

A long, flexible, hollow tube, designed to exchange an in-situ endotracheal or tracheostomy tube. Exchange can be used in the management of patients with significant tracheal deviation, such as with an enlarged thyroid gland. Additionally, the Cook Catheter may be used for jet ventilation, or for end-tidal carbon dioxide measurement. Some versions are hollow, and can be fitted with a *Rapi-Fit* adaptor, which allows connection to an oxygen supply.

Cooperative Binding

The affinity of O_2 (oxygen) binding to an Hb (haemoglobin) molecule increases as the Hb molecule fills with O_2. When none of the Hb molecule's 4 binding sites is occupied by O_2, binding is relatively difficult. When one O_2 molecule is bound to the Hb, it is easier for the second O_2 molecule to bind to the Hb. The ease of O_2 binding increases again for the third and fourth O_2 molecules.

Cor Pulmonale

Enlargement (hypertrophy) and eventual failure of the right ventricle, caused by hypertension of the pulmonary arteries (pulmonary hypertension). The patient must be protected from hypoxia, acidosis, hypercapnia, and avoid nitrous oxide.

Cormack and Lehane Grading

A laryngoscopic scoring system, of the laryngeal view, based on the visibility of the Glottis and Epiglottis.

Grade	*Laryngoscopic view*
I	Glottis
II	Part of glottis
III	Epiglottis – but not Glottis
IV	Epiglottis not visible

Corneal Abrasion

A scratch on the eye, which can occur during anaesthesia, because the patient has lost their protective reflexes. Prevented with eye tape, padding, goggles, or Lacri-Lube.

Coronary Artery Bypass Graft (CABG)

A procedure to treat narrowing (stenosis) of coronary arteries, by creating bypasses around the obstructions, with arteries or veins from elsewhere in the body, so improving blood flow to the heart.

Coronary Arteries

During the heart's relaxation phase, the coronary arteries supply all but the inner part of the heart with oxygenated blood.

Coronary Heart Disease

Aka *Ischaemic Heart Disease:* Atherosclerosis (narrowing or clogging) of the coronary arteries. Main risk factors:

- Diabetes
- Hypertension
- Sedentary lifestyle
- Smoking
- High cholesterol

Coronary Thrombosis

A thrombus (blood clot) inside a heart artery, which impedes blood flow, and might cause a myocardial infarction.

Coronavirus

A family of crown shaped viruses that cause respiratory tract infections, spread by touch and through the air (cough, sneeze). Effects can be mild to lethal, and typical symptoms are coughing and a high temperature. Examples are *Severe Acute Respiratory Syndrome*, *COVID-19*, and *Middle East Respiratory Syndrome*.

Corticosteroid

Aka *steroid*: Anti-inflammatory agents e.g., Dexamethasone. Asthmatic patients use inhalers which contain corticosteroids.

Cost-

Referring to the ribs.

Costal Breathing

A shallow mode of breathing, using the intercostal (rib) muscles. At expiration, air leaves the lungs passively (lung elastic recoil).

Cough Reflex

The protective and reflexive (automatic) action of expelling bronchial secretions or foreign bodies in the airway, triggered by the secretions/foreign bodies being detected by airway receptors.

COVID-19 (SARS-CoV2)

Coronavirus 19 is a strain of coronavirus, discovered in 2019 – hence the 19. See *Coronavirus*.

CPAP

See Continuous Positive Airway Pressure.

CPEX (CPET) Test

A Cardiopulmonary Exercise Test (non-invasive) determines respiratory and cardiac efficiency, by measuring gas volumes whilst the subject rides a stationary bicycle, and breathes through a circuit. Results help guide the choice of ventilation regime, and predict how the patient will recover from surgery.

Crackles

Bibasilar Crackle are abnormal "crackling" breathing (especially inhalation) sounds, from the base of the lungs, heard on auscultation, and indicating interference with normal air flow. Common causes include pulmonary oedema (fluid or mucous in the alveoli), or atelectasis (inability of the alveoli to inflate).

Creatinine

Compound waste product of muscle metabolism (cells and *creatine phosphate*); levels determined by age, gender, BMI, and race. Unhealthy kidneys excrete less creatinine (so blood levels rise). High levels associated with higher stroke or cardiac arrest risk. Serum range: 60-110 micromole/L (0.7-1.2 mg/dL).

Crenation

The shrinking of cells, due to water leaving the cell, by osmosis, when exposed to hypertonic interstitial fluid.

Cricoid Cartilage

Ring shaped cartilage, inferior to the cricothyroid membrane. The Cricoid is the first and only complete ring of cartilage in the respiratory system.

Cricoid Pressure (Sellick's Manoeuvre)

Application of pressure to the anterior arch of the Cricoid cartilage, to temporarily occlude the lumen of the oesophagus (upper end), preventing aspiration of stomach contents into the lungs. Typically used during *Rapid Sequence Induction*, or during normal intubation, when the lower oesophageal (cardiac) sphincter is expected to be incompetent. A light force is required when the patient is drowsy, and 30-40 newton (3-4 kg) when unconscious.

Contra-indications

- Cricotracheal injury
- Active vomiting
- Unstable Cervical Spine injury

Note 1: The airway and breathing are higher priorities than the application of cricoid pressure.

Note 2: Obstetric patients are especially susceptible to aspiration during anaesthetic induction.

Cricothyroidotomy/Cricothyrotomy

Emergency procedure, to provide a temporary airway. Used in *Can't Intubate, Can't Ventilate* situations, and in upper airway obstruction: An opening is made through the cricothyroid membrane, so that a size 6 ET (endotracheal) or tracheostomy tube can be inserted, thereby allowing a route to ventilate the patient. Cricothyrotomy is quicker than a tracheotomy, and incurs less bleeding. See Appendix A36 (pg 415).

Critical Care Levels

Classification of patients according to condition and needs, with ward allocation suitable for relevant support and monitoring.

Level	Patient type
0	Low risk and acute ward
1	Re-classed down from higher level, or condition may deteriorate; acute ward with advice from CCT (Critical Care Team)
2	Re-classed down from higher level, or needs postoperative care, or more detailed monitoring or intervention for failing single organ system
3	Intrensive care: Advanced respiratory support, or basic respiratory support and monitoring for two or more failing organ systems

Cross Matching

The testing of compatibility between a sample of blood from a donor, and the blood of a recipient. The mixed blood is analysed, by microscope, for clumping. An absence of clumping indicates a successful match. The process takes approximately 40 minutes.

Croup

Acute inflammation and obstruction of the trachea and larynx, particularly in children, producing a cough and rasping, caused by allergy, infection, or new growth.

CRT

1. Capillary Refill Time   2. Cardiac Resynchronisation Therapy

Cryoprecipitate

Product (yellow) when solids form after thawing Fresh Frozen Plasma, and collected by centrifuging, before re-freezing @ -30° C. Rich in Factor VIII, Factor XIII, Von Willebrand Factor, **Fibrinogen** (more concentrated than in FFP), and Fibronectin. Used to treat haemophilia and fibrinogen deficiency (< 200 mg/dL). Also given to a patient who is bleeding, and with a fibrinogen level below 1.5 g/litre. ABO type is preferred, but not essential. Cross matching is not required. Dose: ~40 ml/kg. Use blood giving set with 170-200 micron filter. Give immediately after thawing, or store for max 4 hours @ ambient temperature. Reactions: anaphylaxis, *Transfusion Related Acute Lung Injury*.

Crystalloids

Intravenous extracellular volume expanding fluids, which cross semi-permeable membranes. Crystalloids, which are isotonic with extracellular fluid, can be used to correct electrolyte imbalances.

Three of the most commonly used perioperative crystalloids are Plasma Lyte, Hartmann's Solution, and 0.9% Sodium Chloride.

CSF

See Cerebrospinal Fluid.

ctHb

Total concentration of haemoglobin (Hb) in blood, includes: O_2Hb and dyshaemoglobins. It is the measure of the potential oxygen carrying capacity of the blood. Men: 129-166 g/litre. Women: 114-152 g/litre. In anaemic patients, ctHb is lower, but the oxygen saturation value is unaffected.

ctO_2 (O_2ct)

Volume of oxygen dissolved in plasma and bound to haemoglobin: $O_2Ct = (1.34 * Hb * SaO_2) + (0.003 * paO_2)$ ml. 9-22 ml/100 ml.

Cubital Fossa

The triangular depression at the bend of the elbow, which contains the median cubital vein (connects basilic and cephalic veins) - commonly used for venepuncture.

Cyanosis

Blue discolouring of the skin, nail beds, and mucus membranes, due to deficient oxygen in the blood.

Central Cyanosis: Blue discolouring of the lips and tongue, typically caused by respiratory and cardiac problems, which allow poorly oxygenated blood to enter the arterial circulation.

Peripheral Cyanosis: Blue discolouring in peripheral sites, such as the finger tips and toes, caused by reduced peripheral circulation, or reduced blood oxygenation.

Cycling

Describes how a ventilator switches from inspiration to expiration, using one of several ventilation types:

Time: In pressure-control, where an absence of the patient's effort to breathe, within a specific time, causes a ventilator "breath".

Flow: In pressure-support, a reduction of the peak inspiratory flow cycles the ventilator into commencing expiration.

Volume: In volume-control, the ventilator switches to expiration after a specific gas volume has been delivered.

Cyclizine

An anti-emetic agent, with an intravenous dose of 50 mg (12 yrs +) or 0.5–1 mg/kg (children). Side-effects include: Apnoea, bronchospasm, arrhythmia, hypertension, or hypotension.

Cyst-

Referring to the bladder.

Cystic Fibrosis

A genetic condition where mucous accumulates in the lungs, digestive, and other organs, resulting in frequent lung infections and digestive problems.

Cystogram

Procedure to observe how the bladder fills and empties.

Cystoscopy

The insertion of a cystoscope into the bladder, via the urethra.

-cyte

Suffix denoting a cell or cellular.

Cyto-

Prefix denoting a cell or cellular.

Cytosis

Movement of molecules in and out of cells. **Endocytosis**: cells absorb molecules; **Exocytosis**: molecules move out of the cells; **Transcytosis**: molecules move within the cell.

Cytotoxic

A toxic effect on cells.

Dalteparin Sodium (Fragmin)

Low-molecular-weight heparin, providing an anticoagulant and antithrombotic (anti blood clotting) function. Dalteparin prevents blood clots from developing, and prevents existing clots from growing, but it does not break down existing blood clots. Typical treatments include deep vein thrombosis, pulmonary embolism, unstable angina, and coronary artery disease.

Dantrolene Sodium

Emergency muscle relaxing drug, used to prevent muscle spasm in cases of Malignant Hyperthermia, by halting muscle contractility. Initial dosage is 2-3 mg/kg, reconstituted with sterile water. Contraindications: liver dysfunction, COPD, severe heart disease.

Dead Space

The parts of the airway space that do not take part in gas exchange:

◇ **Equipment**: Gas delivery circuitry, from the anaesthetic machine or other ventilation equipment, external to the patient.

◇ **Alveolar**: Alveoli which are ventilated (contain oxygen) but not perfused (no blood flow).

◇ **Anatomic**: The conducting zone of the airway, superior to the respiratory bronchioles.

◇ **Physiologic**: Sum of the alveolar and anatomic dead spaces.

An increase in dead space causes increased pressure of arterial carbon dioxide partial pressure ($paCO_2$), respiratory acidosis, hypoxaemia, and cardiac arrhythmias.

Dead Space Ventilation

The volume of breathing gas (eg, air) that is inhaled, but does not take part in gas exchange, because it does not reach the alveoli (stays in dead space), or reaches alveoli that are not perfused.

Decompensated Shock

During shock, when blood volume drops below ~30%, the compensatory shock mechanisms are unable to maintain life sustaining organ perfusion.

Decompensation

When the body is experiencing an abnormal or harmful condition, other mechanisms compensate (eg, acid-base balance) to correct the system. If the body stops compensating (fatigue?), it is termed “decompensation”. In heart failure, the body tries to compensate for degraded circulation with more frequent (tachycardia) and more forceful contractions. Eventually, the compensation can no longer cope with the problem, hence decompensation.

Decompression Sickness

A physiological assault on a diver, caused by “ascending” from deeper water without allowing enough time for dissolved gases to come out of solution from the blood, and expired. An episode is referred to as a "bend" (singular). See Appendix A37 (pg 418).

Decubitus Ulcer

Aka *Pressure Sore*: An injury to the skin and underlying tissues, due to prolonged pressure on the relevant body part, especially on the bony projections of hips, elbows, spine, and ankles, which reduces proper blood circulation.

Deep Extubation

Removing the endotracheal tube when the patient is breathing spontaneously (paralysis reversed), but still anaesthetised, and before the return of upper airway reflexes. VERY IMPORTANT: Before removing the tube, the airway must be suctioned, and an airway inserted. If the patient reacts to the suctioning, anaesthesia is too light, so more propofol or opioid must be given, before re-attempting to suction the airway. Deep extubation reduces the chance of coughing (does not prevent laryngospasm), and is used when the coughing that accompanies the return of airway reflexes might be undesirable in, e.g., intracranial, eye, or ear surgery. Not advisable in RSI, high BMI, or difficult intubation cases.

Deep Vein Thrombosis (DVT)

A thrombus (clot) in a lower limb vein, indicated by local pain and swelling, that can be caused by immobility, such as after a long flight. If below the knee, in the veins of the calf, it is termed a **Distal DVT**. A thrombus in the upper leg, such as in the Iliac, Popliteal or Femoral vein, is termed **Proximal DVT**, and gives a higher risk of pulmonary embolus, which can be fatal. To prevent recurrence, and embolisation, Heparin is given for immediate effect, and Warfarin for longer term. Mechanical prophylaxis is by means of compression (TED) stockings, to increase flow velocity, and intermittent pneumatic compression cuffs (Flowtrons).

Defibrillation

Delivery of an electric shock to a fibrillating (twitching) heart, to try to stop the fibrillation. Usually, a 200 joule charge is given, using a biphasic technique (shock is given in both directions), so that a smaller charge can be given than with a monophasic charge, so potential for heart muscle damage is reduced.

Dehiscence

The rupture of a wound along the line of sutures.

Dehydration

When the body (mainly intracellular) is depleted of fluid. Can cause hypovolaemia, and metabolic acidosis due to reduced glomerular filtration and H+ excretion. **Causes**: diarrhoea, vomiting, excessive sweating, diuretics, diabetes mellitus. **Symptoms**: darker urine and oliguria, fatigue, dryness, high urea and/or creatinine. **Treatment**: Slow infusion of 5% glucose.

Delayed Sequence Intubation (procedural sedation)

A procedural sedation, to preoxygenate the patient before intubation, when he/she cannot tolerate a normal preoxygenation, due to agitation or phobia, etc., or because the patient cannot tolerate an extra pre-intubation procedure, such as placement of a nasogastric tube. **Steps**: 1. Position the patient 30° head up 2. Give ketamine (preserves airway reflexes and respiratory drive) over 30 seconds 3. Place nasal cannula (15 L/min) 4. Pre-oxygenate for 3 minutes 5. Give suxamethonium or rocuronium 6. Intubate.

Delta (Δ) Anion Gap

Calculation of what acid-base disturbance is present, in addition to metabolic acidosis, derived by [Anion Gap (AG) increase from normal] MINUS [bicarbonate (HCO_3^-) decrease from normal]:

(AG-12) – (24-HCO_3^-), shortens to **AG + HCO_3^- - 36**.

* **Gap** < **-6** means rise in AG is less than fall in bicarbonate, so a **NAGMA** is present.

* **Gap between -6 and 6** means this is only a **NAGMA**.

* **Gap** > **6** means increased AG is greater than the fall in bicarbonate, so a **metabolic alkalosis** might be present. See *HAGMA*, *NAGMA*.

Delta (Δ) Ratio

A calculated value that can reveal the cause of a metabolic acidosis, and if there is a mixed disturbance, by resolving the Increase in Anion Gap / Decrease in bicarbonate (HCO_3). See Appendix A38 (pg 420).

Deoxyhaemoglobin (HHb)

Haemoglobin not bound with oxygen. Former name: *Reduced Hb.*

Depolarising Neuromuscular Block

Persistent depolarization of skeletal muscles, making the muscle fibre resistant to further stimulation by acetylcholine. Suxamethonium is a depolarising neuromuscular blocking drug.

Deposition

A direct change of phase of a substance from gaseous to solid.

Dermatome

An area of skin supplied by a single spinal nerve. Each nerve relays sensation from its region of skin to the brain. Pain in a dermatome, without, heat of infection, can indicate spinal damage. Application of cold to a dermatome indicates level of nerve (afferent) block. See *Bromage Scale*.

Desflurane

Volatile anaesthetic agent that can increase heart rate and blood pressure, with the quickest onset and recovery of all agents. Its low *oil:gas partition coefficient* (28) means it is less potent than either Isoflurane or Sevoflurane, and does not easily become absorbed into fatty tissues, such as the brain. MAC, for a healthy young adult, is approximately 6%, and the *blood:gas partition coefficient* of 0.45 means it has low solubility - the main factor in producing quick onset and offset of anaesthesia. Desflurane vapourisers are **pressurised** (Iso/Sevo not) to two times ambient pressure, and warm up to the working temperature of 39° C.

Dexamethasone

A steroidal drug, to reduce inflammation and post operative nausea and vomiting. Also used to treat asthma, arthritis, coronovirus, and skin problems. Contraindications: diabetes mellitus, hypertension, osteoporosis, duodenal and peptic ulcers.

Dextrose

Synonymous with glucose, and is chemically identical, the only difference is that it is made from rice and corn. See *Blood Sugar*.

Diabetes Insipidus

Excessive urine production due to under production of Vasopressin.

Diabetes Mellitus (DM)

A disease where the body cannot properly respond to, or produce enough insulin to help glucose enter the cells. DM patients should have their blood sugar levels measured shortly before anaesthesia, and during surgery. Insulin and dextrose solutions must always be immediately available. See Appendix A39 (pg 421).

Diabetic Coma

An emergency condition where the diabetes mellitus sufferer has hyperglycaemia or hypoglycaemia.

Diabetic Ketoacidosis (DKA)

Metabolic acidotic condition where low levels of insulin means the DM sufferer cannot utilise glucose for energy, because the glucose stays (and builds up) in extracellular fluid, rather than entering cells, and causes the cells to metabolise fat instead, producing high levels of acidic ketones in the bloodstream as a result {DKA also causes dehydration, →hypotension}. DKA is defined by: pH < 7.3, HCO_3^- < 18 mmol/L, blood glucose > 13.9 mmol/L. The resultant ketone bodies are used as energy. DKA **symptoms** are: polyuria, polydipsia, polyphagia, hypotension, dry mucous membranes, lethargy, confusion, vomiting, abdominal pain, tachypnoea, hyperglycaemia, high ketone level in urine, tachycardia due to dehydration, Kussmaul breathing, fruity or nail varnish breath (acetone exhaled). If blood gas shows HAGMA and high glucose level, it is probably a diabetic ketoacidosis. **Triggers**: MI, stroke, trauma, pregnancy, pancreatitis, pneumonia, UTI, steroids, sympathomimetics. Note: alcoholism can also cause ketoacidosis, without involvement of glucose imbalance. **Treatments**: rehydration, potassium, insulin.

Diameter Index Safety System (DISS)

Gas specific pipeline connection system, up to 14 bar, to connect to anaesthetic machines and other gas delivery systems.

Diamorphine Hydrochloride (Heroin)

A powerful and quick acting opioid (opiate), often used in spinal anaesthesia, and sometimes in pulmonary oedema. Diluted to 1 mg/ml with normal saline.

Diaphoretic

Inducing perspiration.

Diastole

The phase in the heart cycle when cardiac muscle is relaxed, blood is drawn into the chambers, and blood pressure is at its lowest.

Diathermy

Device for tissue coagulation and cutting, with minimal blood loss, by very high frequency alternating current, through a hand-held probe. High frequency does not interfere with normal body systems – heart signals etc. Monopolar technique consists of an active (diathermy tip) electrode, and a return (indifferent) electrode (adhesive plate), which is placed on a well vascularised part of the patient, close to the operation site. The bipolar technique has a current return lead in parallel with the active lead, and the circuit is completed by tissue between the tips of the instrument. As a rule, monopolar diathermy must not be used any closer than six inches (15 cm) to a pacemaker – if at all.

Diclofenac Sodium (brand name Voltarol)

A non steroidal anti-inflammatory drug, to treat mild pain and inflammation. Diclofenac inhibits effects of COX (cyclo-oxygenase) 1 and 2 enzymes. *Side effects* include hypertension, peripheral oedema, headache, diarrhoea, nausea, constipation, and vertigo. *Contra-indications* include ischaemic heart disease, congestive heart failure, hypertension, asthma, stomach ulcer, allergies, pregnancy, liver or kidney disease, and blood clotting disorders.

Dicrotic Notch

The jagged turn, on the downward slope of an arterial line trace, indicating pressure is temporarily greater in the aorta than in the left ventricle, due to increased peripheral vascular resistance when the aortic valve closes. In a hypovolaemic patient, the notch is small. Image: see Appendix A13 (pg 366).

Difficult Intubation

If intubation proves difficult, a difficult airway algorithm must be followed. See Appendices A40 (pg 424) & A50 (pg 441).

Diffusion

The net passive migration of particles – atoms, molecules or ions - from regions of higher to lower concentrations. Also defined as the intermingling of particles resulting from random thermal agitation, as in the dispersion of a vapour in air. When two gases combine, the particles diffuse quickly eg, oxygen and nitrous oxide together, and will be a smoothe mixture. Diffusion is faster with: larger surface areas, larger concentration gradients, higher temperature, and smaller molecules. See *Fick's Law*.

Diffusion Deficit

Pathology where the interface (alveolar epithelial cells - interstitial space - capillary endothelium) between alveolar gas and capillary blood is dysfunctional, creating degraded gas exchange and low arterial oxygen partial pressure (paO_2).

Diffusion Hypoxia (Fink Effect/Third Gas Effect)

The effect of emerging from administration of an anaesthetic which included N_2O (nitrous oxide), where the anaesthetic gas mix is replaced by air. A large concentration of N_2O moves from blood to alveoli (because N_2O has low blood solubility), and so dilutes concentration of alveolar oxygen CO_2, and so might produce hypoxia and reduced respiratory drive. As mitigation, oxygen is administered. Diffusion hypoxia can be thought of as the reverse of the *Second Gas Effect*.

Diffusion Limitation

Conditions that give reduced diffusion (transfer) from alveoli to capillaries, and leading to hypoxia. Examples: asbestosis, pulmonary oedema, and pulmonary fibrosis.

Diffusion Limited Gas Transfer

The rate of gas flow from alveoli to the capillaries is determined by the rate of diffusion across the blood-gas barrier, as described by Fick's Law. Increasing blood flow (perfusion) has little effect on gas transfer. See also *Perfusion Limited Gas Transfer*.

Dilling's Formula

Paediatric drug dose formula: age (years) * adult dose/20.

Diluent

A substance which dilutes (lowers) the concentration of a solution.

Dilutional Anaemia

An increase in plasma can reduce concentrations of Hb, RBCs, and haematocrit, without reduction in those entities.

Dilutional Coagulopathy

Loss, consumption, or dilution of platelets when the haemorrhaging or trauma patient is given fluids (such as crystalloids), that do not contain coagulation factors. Treatment: raise the fibrinogen level.

Displacement Volume (DV)

Volume of a fluid displaced when an object (solute) is placed into a carrier fluid (solvent). A real world example is when a bath is run, the water level marked, you step into the bath, then mark the new water level. The volume of water that occupies the area between the two marked levels is the volume which has been displaced by YOUR body, i.e., your displacement volume. **Eureka**!

In pharmacology, displacement volume is that which is occupied by a powder when reconstituted with a solvent. For example, if 250 mg of a drug has a displacement volume of 0.2 ml, and 4.8 diluent is added to it, the solution formed will be 250 mg in 5 ml. In most instances, the displacement volume is so small, it can be discounted - for calculation purposes. For example, if a drug has a DV of 0.02 ml per mg, and 1 mg must be reconstituted to a volume of 10 ml, then 9.98 ml of solvent is required, if exactly 10 ml of solution is to be produced but, in practice, 10 ml solvent is added.

DISS

See Diameter Index Safety System.

Disseminated Intravascular Coagulation

A condition, often occurring alongside septic shock, where the proteins controlling blood clotting are too active, with the result that small clots develop and block smaller vessels. The excess clotting depletes the body of its clotting factors, and platelets, to the extent that excessive bleeding can run uncontrolled.

Dissociative Anaesthesia

A model of intravenous anaesthesia which causes sedation,

amnesia, and a sense of detachment (dissociation) from reality, but does not require loss of consciousness. See also *Ketamine*.

Dissolve

When a solute forms into a homogeneous (1 type) mixture with another substance (solvent), the solute is said to be dissolved in the solvent, such as when with salt is added to water. This occurs because the solute breaks down from a large crystalline formation, into sodium and chloride ions, which are then enveloped by the H2O molecules (compounds).

Distributive Shock

Aka vasodilatory shock; peripheral vasodilation causes relative hypovolaemia. Example types: Septic, Neurogenic, Anaphylactic.

Diuresis

A significantly increased level of urine production.

Diuretic

An agent, such as Furosemide, which increases urine excretion.

Dolorimetry

The measurement of pain, using a dolorimeter (instrument).

Doppler Guided Fluid Management

See CardioQ Doppler Monitor.

Dorsal

Orientation towards the spine, back or an upper surface.

Dose Response Relationship

Correlation between the dose of an agent and its therapeutic or toxic effect.

Double Lumen Endobronchial/Endotracheal Tube

Combined bronchial and tracheal tube set, for thoracic surgery, where either lung can be isolated (clamped proximal to the gas supply), whilst the other lung is ventilated. Left-sided tubes are commonly used, because the first bronchus of the right lung is too close to the carina to allow enough distance for the bronchial tube to safely ventilate the other lobes – the tube might sit inside the first lobe. In the left lung, the distance between the carina and first lobar bronchus is great enough for the tube sit above the first bronchus, thereby ensuring that all lobes are ventilated. The tracheal cuff is of high volume, the bronchial cuff is low volume, requiring only 2 ml air to inflate. Positioning the bronchial tube (blue coloured) is achieved with the use of a stylet, and confirmed with a bronchoscope. Adult sizes (French gauge): Males; 39-41. Females; 37-39. See Appendices A41 (pg 425), A113 (pg 537).

Doxapram Hydrochloride

A stimulant, that increases respiratory rate, and which may be given when the patient takes too long to commence spontaneous breathing, after recovering from an anaesthetic.

Drip Rate Calculation

Drip rates can be solved by the simple equation: **vg = rt**.

Where **v** represents the volume of fluid to infuse, **g** is drops per ml of the giving set, **r** is the infusion rate, and **t** is the infusion time.

Drop Factor (gtt)

Drops per ml of fluid administration sets. Abbreviated from "guttae" (Latin for "drop"). Often used, particularly on infusion set packaging. Note: "gtt" also refers to *glucose tolerance test.*

Common drop factors:

- ◇ 10 drops/ml (blood)
- ◇ 15 drops/ml (blood)
- ◇ 20 drops/ml (crystalloid)
- ◇ 60 drops/ml (microdrop, Burette)

Drug Absorption

Pharmacokinetic process describing the time needed for uptake of a drug across various barrier sites, and absorption into the bloodstream, whence it crosses cell membranes to reach its site of action. Absorption types are: ① **Passive diffusion** (drug molecules move from high to low concentration areas, without need of energy); ② **Facilitated passive** (passive movement assisted by the substrate molecule taxi service); ③ **Active transport** (energy moves the drug against concentration gradients); ④ **Pinocytosis** (energy assisted drug encapsulation by cells). Drug absorption can be affected by its: lipid solubility, physical form (gas, liquid, solid) administration route, and method (tablet, transdermal), molecular size, concentration, and excipients.

Drug Administration

See Appendix A42 (pg 426).

Drum Cartridge Catheter

A catheter used in central vein cannulation, where the vein is cannulated with an introducer. The needle is removed, and is replaced by the drum cartridge catheter, which is left in place.

Drug Clearance

The vascular volume that is cleared of a drug, per unit of time.

Drug Distribution

Pharmacokinetic process that describes how an absorbed and unmetabolised drug is dispersed throughout the systemic circulation, and distributed to tissues, determined by eg, pH, perfusion, permeability of cell membranes, and molecule size.

Drug Elimination (Clearance)

Pharmacokinetic process of metabolising and removing drugs from the kidneys (mostly), liver, skin, glands, or lungs.

Dura Mater

Latin: *Hard Matter*. The thickest, toughest, and outermost of the three meninges (up against the arachnoid mater, with *subdural space* between), through which a spinal needle is pierced, to infiltrate anaesthetics for spinal block. The dura should NOT be pierced when passing an epidural needle.

DVT

Deep Vein Thrombosis.

Dys-

Difficult.

Dyshaemoglobins

Haemoglobin types that cannot transport oxygen: carboxyhaemoglobin (COHb), methaemoglobin (MetHb), sulfhaemoglobin (SulfHb).

Dysphagia

Difficulty in swallowing that can produce intubation problems, and requiring difficult airway equipment on standby. Some patients develop post-extubation dysphagia.

Dysrhythmia

Alternative term for arrhythmia.

Dyspnoea

Breathlessness, caused by eg, cardiorespiratory disease, pain, metabolic acidosis, or anxiety. According to the British Thoracic Society, "Oxygen is treatment for hypoxaemia, not breathlessness".

Dysuria

Difficulty or pain in passing urine.

D5NS

Abbreviation for 5% concentration dextrose in 0.9% normal saline.

D5W

Abbreviation for 5% dextrose in water.

Early Warning Score

A *Track and Trigger* system. See *NEWS2*.

Ecchymosis

Skin discolouration caused by bruising/bleeding.

ECF

Extracellular Fluid.

Eclampsia

Hypertensive disorder and toxaemia of pregnancy: acute and life-threatening, characterized by convulsions, usually in a patient who has developed pre-eclampsia (hypertension and fluid retention). Other cerebral signs may precede the convulsion, for example: nausea, vomiting, headache, and cortical blindness. Organ symptoms may also be present, including abdominal pain, liver failure, pulmonary oedema, and oliguria.

Ectopic

Ectopic: away from the normal place, as with *ectopic heartbeat*, where a discernible heartbeat occurs earlier than usual, due to a premature atrial or ventricular contraction. An occasional ectopic beat may be harmless, but investigations may be necessary, if a significant condition is to be identified. Causes can be: alcohol, caffeine, exertion, stimulant drugs, stress, and tobacco. The sufferer may experience dizziness, or awareness of an unusual heart rhythm. Also, *ectopic pregnancy*, where the fertilised egg is outside of the womb, usually in a fallopian tube.

Effective Dose

The amount or concentration of a drug which produces the required therapeutic effect, in a particular proportion of patients taking the drug. See also *Median Effective Dose*.

Efferent

From the centre to the periphery.

Efferent limb

The part of a breathing circuit that carries expired gas away from the patient. Efferent reservoir systems (D, E with Jackson Rees modification of Ayre's T piece) have a reservoir bag in the efferent limb, and work well with controlled ventilation, but need high gas flows with spontaneous ventilation.

Effusion

Liquid discharge from a cavity.

Electrocardiogram (ECG)

Trace of the heart's electrical activity, starting at the SA (sinoatrial) node, then the AV (atrioventricular) node, Bundle of Hiss, and Purkinje Fibres, causing ventricular contraction. Electrical activity towards the heart causes positive deflection (up stroke) in the corresponding lead. Electrical activity away from the heart causes negative deflection in the lead. Overall direction of electrical activity is towards leads I, II, and III. Heart rate per minute is calculated by dividing 300 by the number of large squares between R waves (1 large square is 0.2 second). See *PQRST*.

Electroconvulsive Therapy (ECT)

Treatment for psychiatrist led cases, where the anaesthetised patient receives a small electric current, through the brain, which triggers a short seizure. The aim is to alter the brain chemistry for specific mental health issues. See Appendix A44 (pg 428).

Electroencephalogram (EEG)

A recording of brain activity, through sensors on the scalp, in order to detect abnormalities, such as epilepsy.

Electrolyte

Any atom, molecule, or compound, found in the body, that has an electrical charge (ionised). Many electrolytes are formed when a compound (solute) is dissolved in water, and dissociates into its component ions, cations and anions, so that the solution becomes electrically conductive. Electrolyte balance is governed by the kidneys, hypothalamus, and hormones, such as ADH, PTH, and aldosterone. See Appendix A45 (pg 430).

Electromyographic Endotracheal Tube

An ET tube for thyroid surgery, which allows monitoring of the Recurrent Laryngeal Nerve, to prevent nerve damage.

Elimination Half Life

The time for half of the remaining drug, in the plasma, to be eliminated from the body. For example, if a patient is given a 200 mg dose of a drug, which has an elimination half-life of 4 hours, then 100 mg will be eliminated after 4 hours, another 50 mg is eliminated in the next 4 hours, an 25 mg in the next 4 hours.

Embolisation

Process of halting blood supply to part of the body, by blocking a blood vessel.

Embolism

Obstruction of a blood vessel by an embolus, which has travelled from its place of formation. Note: a gas embolism is associated with a diver surfacing too quickly, and nitrogen or helium coming out of solution too fast for the blood to take it to the lungs.

Embolus

A mass (clot, gas, thrombus, fat), which circulates through the bloodstream, until it stops at a narrow point, then causes an obstruction (embolism) to circulation.

Emergency Anaesthesia

An emergency case, such as a ruptured aortic aneurysm, demands immediate anaesthetic induction (RSI), and surgical intervention. Fluid loss must be countered, with blood replacement for haemorrhage, plasma for burns victims, and electrolyte solutions for intestinal losses. See Appendix A46 (pg 432).

EFONA (Emergency Front Of Neck Access)

Tracheotomy or cricothyrotomy for the compromised airway.

Emesis

Vomiting.

Emphysema

A progressively worsening type of COPD, where the alveoli lose their elasticity, and their walls become inflamed. Consequently, air becomes trapped in the lungs, producing hyperinflation and degraded gas exchange, so the sufferer has to breathe harder, with a characteristic shortness of breath. Type II respiratory failure is a consequence of emphysema. Typical sufferers are asthmatics, smokers and those who are subject to polluted air. **Symptoms**: productive (mucous) cough, painful breathing, cyanosis, wheezing, chest tightness. **Treatment**: Clean air, antibiotics, inhaled corticosteroids, bronchodilators (relax airway).

Empyema

A mass of pus in the pleural or other cavity.

End Tidal Carbon Dioxide ($EtCO_2$)

Exhaled carbon dioxide pressure, typically 35-45 mmHg. $EtCO_2$ partial pressure closely matches the partial pressure of CO_2 in the arteries ($paCO_2$). $EtCO_2$ increases when alveolar ventilation decreases (and vice-versa), and reduces with a reduction in cardiac output. Opioids increase $EtCO_2$ levels, but not enough to interfere with validating proper ventilation, coincidental with intubation.

Endoscopy

Viewing the inner cavities of a patient, using camera equipment.

Endothelium

The single layer set of endothelial cells lining the inner wall of blood and lymphatic vessels, controlling exchange of substances between the vessel and surrounding tissue.

Endotracheal Tube (ETT)

Single-use hollow pvc tube that is usually passed through the larynx to the trachea, via mouth or nose, to provide ventilatory gases, and seal the airway from pollution from regurgitated stomach liquid. A seal is made by inflating a cuff, with the tip of the tube sitting ~ ½ inch (1.25 cm) above the carina. *{**Covid** caution: Inflate the cuff BEFORE attaching FGF}* The tube is formed to match the anatomical curvature of the airway, and is of a length which allows shortening (reduces resistance to gas flow), by cutting off a section at the airway attachment (proximal) end. For adult females, a typical size would be internal diameter 7 mm, with placement to a depth, at the lips, of 21 cm. For males, the internal diameter might be 8 mm, to a depth of 23 cm.

Other features include:

- Depth markings (cm)
- Bevelled end – to reduce the possibility of occlusion
- Murphy eye – mitigates against the end being occluded
- X-ray detectable line – to verify placement and depth
- Internal and external diameter indications
- A transverse black line indicates the level of the vocal cords
- An inflatable cuff, to seal the trachea. Plus inflation port.
- A pilot balloon, to correspond with the cuff pressure

Note: Some paediatric tubes do not have inflatable cuffs.

Enter-

Referring to the intestines.

Enteral

Enteral nutrition refers to a method of feeding which uses the gastrointestinal tract to deliver a patient's caloric requirements.

Entonox (gas and air)

A brand name for a mixture of 50% oxygen and 50% nitrous oxide, by volume. Used for pain relief in conscious patients.

Enzyme

A protein which catalyses a reaction, e.g., acetylcholinesterase, which decomposes the acetylcholine neurotransmitter.

Ephedrine

A sympathomimetic vasopressor, for hypotension (safe for use in pregnancy - does not reduce placental blood flow). Typical bolus is 100 microgram/kg, up to 5 mg.

Side-effects

- Tachycardia
- Hypertension
- Irritability
- Nausea
- Anxiety

Contra-indications

- Arrhythmia
- Diabetes mellitus
- Hypertension
- Hyperthyroidism
- Cardiovascular disease

Epicardium

Outer layer of the heart wall.

Epidermis

The outermost of the two skin layers.

Epidural Block

The blocking of nerve roots that exit the dura, by placement of a catheter into the epidural space, allowing the anaesthetist to administer an analgesic. The epidural should NOT pierce the dura mater (a test dose can prove NOT intrathecal or intravascular). Used in procedures involving the lower limbs, pelvis, perineum and lower abdomen. Commonly used to alleviate pain in childbirth, usually started during labour, and given before the neck of the womb has started to dilate. See Appendix A47 (pg 434).

Epidural Space

Epidural: "Outside the Dura Mater": The space between the dura mater and the tough (gritty feel) ligamentum flavum (Latin: yellow ligament) of the spinal wall. Contains CSF, spinal nerves and arteries, extradural venous plexus, fat and lymph tissue, spinal nerve roots, and dural sac.

Epigastric

Above the navel.

Epiglottis

Leaf shaped cartilage which sits on top of the larynx, behind the root of the tongue, and attached to the thyroid cartilage; prevents food from entering the larynx/trachea. If inflamed, the condition is called *epiglottitis*, and ventilation might be affected.

Epileptic Fit

A neurological disorder marked by recurrent sensory disturbance, loss of consciousness, or convulsions. See Appendix A49 (pg 439).

Epistaxis

Bleeding from the nose.

Equivalent (equiv, Eq)

Amount of a substance that reacts with a mole of another substance, in a particular chemical reaction, such as when releasing hydrogen ions (H+). Equivalents are still used in some countries for blood gas reports, but the use is outdated, and has been mostly replaced by molar concentration.

Erythrocyte (Red Blood Cell, RBC)

Created in red bone marrow, RBCs contain haemoglobin molecules (270 million/cell), which transport oxygen and carbon dioxide, constitute ~ 45% of whole blood. and must be stored at 4° C. RBC cells may be transfused into a patient if it is necessary to restore oxygen carrying capacity. See Appendix A20 (pg 375).

Erythromycin

A macrolide antibiotic which slows or stops the growth of bacteria, and is often used in patients with Penicillin allergy.

Esmolol Hydrochloride

Beta blocker used for hypertension, and an antiarrhythmic (narrow complex tachycardia). Quick onset and short duration.

ETT

See Endotracheal Tube.

Etomidate

Quick acting induction agent, at 0.3 mg/kg, which does not adversely effect haemodynamic stability (no hypotension), so may be suitable for cardiovascular and haemodynamically unstable patients. Does not cause respiratory depression; can cause PONV.

Eupnea

See Quiet Breathing.

Eutectic Mixture of Local Anaesthetic (EMLA) Cream

Mixture of lignocaine and prilocaine. Applied 1-5 hours prior to venepuncture. Once removed, the anaesthetic wear off is 20-30 minutes. The cream can cause vasoconstriction, so *Ametop cream* is often preferred. Only suitable for children over 1 year old.

Eversion

Turning something inside out.

Evisceration

The displacement of tissue or organs from a body cavity, such as during transplantation.

Evulsion

A forcible extraction.

Excipient

An inert (should be) substance, which helps to deliver a product in a more suitable form. For example: a binding agent in a pharmaceutical product, to stop it from falling apart.

Expiratory Reserve Volume

Maximum volume of air that can be forcefully expired, after a normal breath out.

Exsanguinate

Latin: *Bloodless*. Squeezing blood, distal to proximal, out of a limb, prior to applying a tourniquet, such as in "regional" blocks.

Extension

The straightening of a joint.

External Respiration

Gas exchange between alveoli and blood. Oxygen moves down a concentration gradient from the alveoli (104 mmHg, 13.8 kPa) to the pulmonary circulation (from 70-100 mmHg, 9-13.3kPa), whilst carbon dioxide moves down its concentration gradient from the bloodstream (45 mmHg, 6 kPa) to the alveoli (40 mmHg, 5.3 kPa).

Extracellular Fluid (ECF)

The fluid outside of cells, comprising ~ ⅓ of total body fluid, within three compartments: **intravascular**, **interstitial**, and **transcellular**.

Extracorporeal

Something that occurs or is located outside of the body.

Extracorporeal Membrane Oxygenation (ECMO)

ECMO is a life support technique, where the circulation system is extended, by peripheral or central cannulation, and blood is pumped to a "lung" reservoir (membrane), at a rate of 3 – 6 litre/minute, so that gas exchange may be realised, by adding oxygen, and filtering out carbon dioxide. ECMO may be used in cases of severe respiratory or cardiac failure, or when a patient is waiting for heart or lung transplantation.

Extra-pulmonary (Cardiac) Shunt

Venous blood bypasses the lungs, and goes straight back into the systemic circulation without being oxygenated.

Extravasation

The infiltration (leaking/tissuing) of an agent from a vein and into surrounding tissue. Extravasation may also describe the shift of cells out of a blood vessel, during an inflammatory episode.

Extubation

Removal of an endotracheal tube, following a general anaesthetic, and when the patient can start to breathe spontaneously.

Main extubation criteria for the patient include:

- √ Neuromuscular blockade is ended or has been reversed
- √ Breathing 100% oxygen
- √ The airway has been adequately suctioned
- √ Regained airway reflexes
- √ Weaned from (doesn't need) ventilator support
- √ Opens their eyes
- √ Follows voice commands (open eyes, hand squeeze)

Exudate

Serous (fibrin, leukocytes, serum) fluid and cells that have escaped from blood vessels, and leaked into surrounding tissues. Exudate may or may not be clear, and might be seen at sites of injury. Unlike transudate, exudate is not filtered of the above cells.

FA/FI Ratio

Ratio between alveolar (FA) and inspired (FI) gas concentrations, which rises faster as ventilation increases; increasing FI speeds up the fraction of alveolar concentration (FA), ie, the *concentration effect*. A higher Blood:Gas Partition Coefficient (higher solubility) of an inhalational agent causes a greater uptake by the capillaries, but a slower rise in FA/FI ratio. {Relevance: nitrous oxide use}

Face Masks

Different styles of face mask are used, according to the particular purpose, and to provide the required combination of breathing gases and fraction of inspired oxygen (FiO_2). Prior to anaesthesia and intubation, a soft seal mask, with adjustable mask-to-face cuff pressure, is used, so that no room air is entrained. For spontaneously breathing patients, post-anaesthesia (or on wards) patients will be given masks that allow room air entrainment, classed as either *Fixed* or *Variable Rate Performance Masks*.

Failed Intubation

If endotracheal intubation attempts fail, and surgery is not essential (emergency), wake the patient up, using the protocol in Appendix A50 (pg 441).

Fascia

The sheets of connective fibrous tissue which surrounds muscles, blood vessels, and nerves, to connect or separate structures.

Fasciculations

Isolated muscle contraction (twitching), such as what results from administration of Suxamethonium (succinylcholine).

Fasting

Preoperative fasting, for elective surgery, to mitigate against the possibility of aspiration of gastric contents. Minimum times are:

Adults: 2 hours for water; 6 hours for solids and milky drinks.

Children: Same as adults + Breast milk for 4 hours.

Febrile Convulsion

A seizure (rarely serious) occuring in a child with a fever over 39° C

(102.2° F). See Appendix A51 (pg 442).

Fentanyl

Class A opioid, 100 times the strength of morphine. Dose 1 microgram/kg from 50 microgram/ml supply. See *Opioids.*

Ferguson Mouth Gag

A device for keeping the mouth open, during surgery, or intubation, but is very rarely used, or encountered.

Fibreoptic Intubation

Camera assisted placement of a railroaded ET tube, using a flexible or rigid (Bonfils) bronchoscope, such as when the patient has limited movement of the jaw, or when the mouth/pharynx are within the operating site. See Appendix A52 (pg 443).

Fibrillation

Rapid and irregular quivering and vibration of muscle fibres, such as with *Ventricular Fibrillation*, is a cardiac arrest situation.

Fibrin (Factor Ia)

A sticky insoluble fibrous protein which forms a mesh over platelets, trapping them to form a blood clot over a wound. Together, the fibrin and platelets help to stop bleeding.

Fibrinogen (Factor I)

A soluble glycoprotein, produced by the liver, contained within plasma, essential for blood clotting, when thrombin converts fibrinogen into fibrin. Fibrinogen stimulates platelet clumping: platelets bind to collagen that becomes exposed, due to rupture of the endothelial lining of blood vessels. Range: 200-400 mg/dL. (IV form is Fibrinogen Concentrate)

Fibrinolysin

An enzyme which promotes the dissolution of blood clots, by breaking down fibrin.

Fibrinolysis

A normal body process whereby *fibrinolysin* is used to keep blood clots (thrombi) from growing. Primary fibrinolysis refers to the normal breakdown of fibrin (a protein) in blood clots. Secondary fibrinolysis is the breakdown of blood clots due to a medical disorder, medicine, or other cause, and which may cause severe bleeding. Blood clots form on fibrin. Fibrinolysis can increase under certain conditions, such as:

- Bacterial infections
- Intense exercise
- Cancer
- Intense exercise
- Low blood sugar
- Low O_2 to tissues

Fibrinolytic

Other name for Thrombolytic.

Fibrosis

Scar tissue: The accumulation of fibrous connective tissue to an organ, resulting from a repair process.

Fick's Law

Describes how rate of gas diffusion across a surface (eg membrane) is proportional to surface area and difference in concentrations, and is inversely proportional to surface thickness.

Filtering Facepiece (FFP) Respirator

A facepiece and filter equipment to protect the wearer against 3 levels of hazard: **FFP1** for low levels of dust, droplets and water mist; **FFP2** a higher level from FFP1; **FFP3** high level dust, asbestos, biological agents, and infectious droplets. Compare with a simple surgical facemask which only protects against droplets.

Fink Effect

See Diffusion Hypoxia.

FiO_2

See Fraction of Inspired Oxygen.

First Pass Metabolism

The metabolising of part of an oral medication, before it gets into the general circulation. Consequently, some of the administered drug may be wasted. The drug is mostly metabolised by the liver, and transported there, by the portal vein, from the intestinal tract.

Fixator

A metal rod placed through a bone, for support and stability.

Fixed Acid

A **non-volatile** (not breathed out) **metabolic** acid (eg, ketones, lactate, phosphate, and sulphate), produced in incomplete metabolism. All acids produced in the body, except carbonic acid (H_2CO_3) are fixed acids, and are removed by the kidneys.

Fixed Rate Performance Masks

Face mask devices, such as Venturi, that deliver a pre-set fraction of oxygen (FiO_2).

Flagyl

See Metronidazole.

Flexion

Bending at a joint so as to “un-straighten” the body part, as when bending the knees to sit down.

Flow Control Valve

Regulates gas flow to the patient: O_2 valve (grooved) left most.

Flow Rate

The flow rate of a fluid product, such as blood, can be determined by the *Hagen-Poisseuille* equation, defined as:

Flow rate (Q) = $(\Delta P * \pi * r^4) / (8 * l * \eta)$

ΔP	=	Relative Pressure difference.
r^4	=	Tubing internal radius, to power 4.
l	=	Length of the tubing.
η	=	Viscosity coefficient of the fluid.

The significance to fluid administration can be shown by the numerator ($\Delta P * \pi * r^4$) line of the equation, which illustrates how flow rate can be increased by increasing the pressure (gravity or pressure bag), or using tubing with a larger internal diameter.

The denominator ($8 * l * \eta$) line, shows how flow is increased by a reduction in tube length, or reducing the viscosity of the fluid product, which may be achieved by warming the product.

Fluid Balance

Maintenance and management of fluid input and output, to promote homoeostasis. Normal (adult) fluid intake is approximately 30 ml/kg, and urine output is 0.5 - 1 ml/kg/hour. Patients with kidney or liver problems need special consideration for fluid management, and should not be allowed to become “hypo” or “hyper” -volaemic.

Fluid Challenge

A technique to determine whether or not a hypotensive patient is hypovolaemic, and might be successfully administered with fluids, with the aim of increasing stroke volume. The patient is given 500 ml of fluid (crystalloid) over 20-30 minutes. If the patient responds positively to the challenge (cardiac index increases by 10% +), it indicates that the patient has a preload (cardiac muscle stretch) reserve and, consequently, will probably have further increases in cardiac output, when more fluid is administered.

Fluid Compartments

Body fluids exist within four spaces: 66% of the total volume is **intracellular** (in cytosols of cells), 25% is **interstitial** (bathes the cells), 7% is **intravascular** (in plasma and lymph), 2% is **transcellular** (eyes, joints, CSF).

Fluid Losses

Urine output of a normal adult is 50 ml/hour. Normal daily fluid exchange of a 70 kg man is 3 litres.

Fluid Shift

The movement of fluid between compartments, such as between intracellular fluid and interstitial spaces, governed by differences in osmotic pressures.

Fluid Warmer

For surgery of more than thirty minutes, hypothermic patients, and for administration of blood, a fluid warmer is fitted between the fluid source and patient ends of a giving set, so that the fluid is warmed to ~37° C. When blood is given, the extra heat makes the blood less viscous, which means the blood will flow more quickly.

Flumazenil (Romazicon)

A competitive antagonist of benzodiazepines, which might be used to counter the sedative effects of, for example, Midazolam, by initial 10 second bolus of 200 microgram (iv).

Flying Squad Blood

Emergency supply of "O" Rh negative blood, used before grouped and cross matched blood products are available.

FO2Hb

Fraction (95-98%) of O_2Hb to total Hb (inc dyshaemoglobins).

Forward Heart Failure

The left ventricle fails to pump out sufficient blood into the aorta for proper metabolic needs.

Fossa

A hollow in a structure, such as a bone.

Fowler's Position

Type of beach chair position, for shoulder and ENT surgery.

Fraction of Inspired Oxygen (FiO_2)

The fraction of the inspired breathing gas that is oxygen. In atmospheric air, the FiO_2 is ~ 0.21 (21%). When an anaesthetised patient is breathing a mixture of gases, which will be oxygen plus, for example, air and a volatile agent, the FiO_2 is that volume of oxygen (including the oxygen in the administered air) expressed as a fraction of the total gas flow. As a rough guide, paO_2 (arterial O_2 pressure) will be 8-10 kPa less than the % FiO_2 e.g., if FiO_2 is 50%, paO_2 will normally be 40-42 kPa; an alternative rough estimate is given by $paO_2 = 5 * FiO_2$, in mmHg, with 50% FiO_2 producing

paO_2 of 250 mmHg. Administered FiO_2 is not usually greater than 0.5, otherwise the patient may suffer oxygen toxicity.

Fragmin

A trade name for *Dalteparin Sodium*.

Fremitus

Vibrations on the chest, when the patient coughs or speaks, heard by auscultation or palpation.

French Gauge

Aka *Charrière's System*: Measuring system to indicate the OD (Outer Diameter) of a catheter, where the number refers to multiples of ⅓ mm. For example, 6 Fr means an OD of 2 mm.

Fresh Frozen Plasma (FFP)

An unconcentrated form of plasma (yellow) - the liquid portion of blood that has been frozen and preserved at -30° C. Formed from whole blood by centrifugation and separation within 6 hours of donation. One unit contains 150-300 ml of plasma, including antithrombin III, and clotting factors: II, VII, VIII, IX, X, XI, which can be used to supplement (but given before) red blood cells, or to correct a significant bleeding problem of unknown cause. FFP is also used to correct disseminated intravascular coagulation (system wide blood clots). FFP is usually given in a 1:1 ratio with Red Blood Cells. FFP must be ABO compatible but, if the blood group is unknown, give AB+ (AB doesn't have anti-A or anti-B antibodies, so is universal donor). Rh and cross matching are unnecessary. Thawed FFP is best used immediately (use giving set with 170-200 micron filter), or stored at 4° C and infused within 24 hours, otherwise, return to the blood bank, within 30 minutes of removal from the fridge. Dose: group compatible 10-15 ml/kg body weight (3-4 units for an adult). Infusion rate is 10-20 ml/kg/hour, over 30 minutes. Use blood giving set with 170-200 micron filter. May be used with a pump or rapid infuser IF manaufacturers allow it. FFP is not normally virally inactivated, so is not as safe as saline, gelatin, or human albumin solutions. Caution: FFP may trigger severe allergic reactions.

Fresh Gas Flow (FGF)

The volume/minute of mixed breathing gases, delivered to the breathing circuit, from the anaesthetic machine.

Fried's Formula

A paediatric (infant to 2 years) drug dose formula, when specific instructions are absent: age (months) * adult dose / 150.

Full Blood Count (FBC) Test

Count of red and white blood cells, platelets, haemoglobin, and haematocrit, mean cell volume, mean cell haemoglobin - to determine renal disease, infections, clotting disorder, anaemia, leukaemia, B12 deficiency. {**Lavender sample bottle cap**}

Functional Residual Capacity (FRC)

The volume of gas, present in the lungs, at the end of passive expiration – when the opposing elastic recoil forces of the lungs and chest wall are in equilibrium. The FRC is the combined total of the Expiratory Reserve and Residual Volumes, and is the lung O_2 store. When upright, the FRC (adult) is ~ 3 litres; When supine, the FRC drops to ~ 2.2 litres. PEEP and CPAP increase FRC, but anaesthesia reduces FRC by ~20%. Note: a higher FRC increases induction time.

Factors that reduce Functional Residual Capacity

- Obesity
- General anaesthetic

☙ Pregnancy ☙ Supine and Trendelenburg positions

Fundoplication

Surgery for gastroesophageal reflux disease (GORD). If done laparoscopically, the technique is *Nissen Fundoplication*. Ventilation is by ET tube. RSI may be required. See also *Stretta*.

Furosemide

Diuretic for hypertension, oedema, or heart failure.

Gamgee Tissue

Surgical dressing invented by Dr. Joseph Sampson Gamgee, Birmingham, in 1880. An absorbent gauze and cotton tissue, to cushion wounds. Gamgee is used for highly exuding wounds, such as cavity and surgical wounds, and can also be used for basic padding, but is not designed for pressure point protection.

Gas Cylinder Colours

Gas	*Cylinder colour*	*Shoulder colour*	*Pin index*
Air	Grey	Black & white	1,5
Carbon dioxide	Grey	Grey	1,6
Entonox	**Blue**	**Blue** & white	Central
Heliox	**Brown**	**Brown**	2,4
Nitrous oxide	**Blue**	**Blue**	3,5
Oxygen	**Black**	White	2,5

Gas Exchange

The net diffusion (passive) of gases, down concentration gradients. In the alveoli, oxygen diffuses to the bloodstream, where the partial pressure of oxygen is lower; CO_2 diffuses in the opposite direction, because the partial pressure of CO_2 is lower in the alveoli than in the blood. Effective gas exchange can be maintained by airway patency, higher inspired oxygen concentration, absence of shunting, proper alveolar ventilation and external respiration.

Gas Induction

Anaesthetising the patient by volatile agent (sevoflurane), rather than by intravenous injection of, for example, Propofol.

Gas Laws

See Boyle's Law, Charles's Law, Gay-Lussac Law.

Gas Scavenging

Anaesthetic gases that escape from a breathing circuit (after expiration), pollute environmental air, and can produce transient and chronic toxic effects to anyone breathing these gases and vapours. For that reason, in the UK, *Control of Substances Hazardous to Health Regulations* classify anaesthetic gases as being a danger to health, so their dangerous effects must be mitigated against by use of gas scavenging systems, which collect and dispose of these gases, either passively or actively (pumps), using equipment attached to anaesthetic machines.

Gas Supplies

Typical supplies to a theatre are: Air, Oxygen, and Nitrous Oxide, at 4-5 bar (400-500 kPa), relative pressure.

Gas Trapping

The abnormal retention of breathing gas (eg, air) in the lungs, when an exhalation is incomplete, as occurs in COPD and asthma.

Gastroesophageal Reflux Disease (GORD)

Condition where stomach contents tend to ascend the oesophagus.

Gay-Lussac Law

$P_1/T_1 = P_2/T_2$: At constant volume, gas **P**ressure is proportional to **T**emperature (kelvin).

General Anaesthesia (GA)

GA is where the unconscious patient loses protective airway reflexes (patency), particularly the cough reflex, so blood and secretions remain un-cleared from the pharynx and vocal cords, increasing the probability of laryngospasm, and cause a barrier to ventilation. Tracheal secretions may progress to the lungs, and produce bronchospasm and alveolar pollution. GA can also pose a risk, due to the cardiac depression and pulmonary atelectasis that the anaesthesia produces. Generally, GA produces a fall in blood pressure and, consequently, an increase in heart rate.

-genesis

A suffix for words which describe the creation or development of a biological condition or entity. Examples are: Osteogenesis (formation of new bone), Glucogenesis (formation of glucose from glycogen), and Angiogenesis (development of new blood vessels).

Gentamicin

Antibiotic for serious chest, urinary tract, and neonate infections.

Gestational Diabetes

High blood sugar (glucose) level, occurring during pregnancy.

Giving Set

A gravity powered intravenous fluid administration system, with a drip (or drop) rate controller. *Microdrip* sets produce small drips, and *macrodrip* sets produce larger drips. Giving sets are designed to administer colloids, such as blood, or crystalloid liquids, such as Normal Saline solution. For blood giving sets, the drip controller will, typically, administer 10 drips for each millilitre of blood, and will have an incorporated 200 micrometre filter. The normal drip rate for crystalloid giving sets is 20 drops/ml. In paediatric cases, a more fine administration is required, so a Burette is used. Note: Giving sets are packaged with labels which state their drip rate factors, or drops per ml, sometimes denoted gtt/ml.

Glasgow Coma Scale

System to rate a patient's consciousness level, based on: **Eye** opening, **Motor** response, **Verbal** response. Lower than eight indicates the need for intubation. See Appendix A53 (pg 444).

Glidescope

Video laryngoscope (Verathon) that provides a consistently clear, real-time view of the airway and for first pass endotracheal tube placement. SVGL (standard)=reusable; cVGL (cobalt)=disposable.

Global Alveolar Hypoventilation

Less than normal amount of oxygen is available to ALL of the alveoli, rather than just some, with inevitable respiratory acidosis, and a $paCO_2$ increase of 1 mmHg for every 1 mmHg increase in paO_2. Causes include: upper airway obstruction, obesity, CNS injury/disease, drug induced respiratory depression, neuromuscular problems, chest injury/deformity.

Glomerular Filtration Rate (GFR)

Gold standard for kidney health: Calculation of blood flow through the kidneys, and how well they filter blood. Poor kidney function can produce metabolic acidosis, which must be managed by the anaesthetist. A normal value is 60 ml/min or more.

Glottis

The part of the larynx that contains the true vocal folds (cords) and the space between them. Image: Appendix A65 (pg 466).

Glucagon

Pancreas produced polypeptide, which helps break down glycogen in the muscles and liver, thereby raising the blood sugar level.

Glucose

See Blood Sugar.

Glyceryl Trinitrate (GTN)

A quick acting agent, to relieve angina, cardiogenic shock, and left ventricular failure, by widening the coronary arteries. A sublingual tablet or spray takes effect within a few minutes. GTN cannot be given orally, because it is made completely inactive by first-pass metabolism.

Glycogen

The glucose that is not currently needed for energy production but, instead, is stored for later use, in skeletal muscle and liver.

Glycopyrrolate

An antimuscarinic (muscarinic receptor antagonist) which inhibits the parasympathetic action of the acetylcholine neurotransmitter, when it binds with muscarinic receptors. Intra-operatively, used to counter bradycardia (4 microgram/kg), and muscarinic effects of neostigmine – when reversing neuromuscular blockade.

Side-effects

- Arrhythmias
- Nausea
- Coughing

Contra-indications

- Peptic ulcer
- Prostate problems
- Glaucoma
- Ulcerative colitis
- Myasthenia Gravis
- Intestine obstruction

Glycolysis

The first phase of anaerobic breaking down glucose by enzymes, to release energy and pyruvic acid: one glucose molecule converts to two molecules of pyruvic, two H+ ions, and two water molecules.

Goitre

Neck swelling due to enlargement of the thyroid gland, making intubation difficult.

Graft

A process where tissue is transplanted from a donor site. Similar to a flap, but without also transferring blood vessels.

Groshong Line

Similar to a Hickman line, but with a 3-way tap for venous access.

Group and Save

The determination of a patient's ABO blood group, and screening serum for the presence of antibodies to common red cell antigens, which cause transfusion reactions. For a patient who is not expected to need a blood transfusion, the group testing will save time, in case a transfusion does become necessary, because only a cross match test will then be needed. See Appendix A21 (pg 378).

GTN

Glyceryl Trinitrate.

GTT

(1) *Glucose Tolerance Test*: A test to determine how well the body metabolises sugar, by measuring glucose levels before and after the patient consumes a glucose drink. A sufferer of diabetes mellitus, for example, may have a glucose level which is 50% higher (12 mmol/litre) than a non-diabetic (7.7 mmol/litre).

(2) A giving set drop factor, or drops per ml, where "gtt" is abbreviated from the latin: *guttae*, meaning "drop". A giving set will deliver so many drops per ml, and denoted as "gtt/ml".

Guedel Airway

An oropharyngeal airway adjunct (and bite block), for unconscious patients, to prevent the tongue from falling back and blocking the airway, which would otherwise impede ventilation. Without the guedel, extra gas pressure might be needed in order to provide ventilation, and the extra pressure may force gas into the stomach, with the result that reflux could occur.

Haem-

A compound that contains iron, and functions to bind oxygen to the haemoglobin molecule but, generally, refers to the blood.

Haematocrit (Packed Cell Volume, Hct)

The fraction of blood that is red blood cells (RBCs), eg., if there is

50 ml of RBCs in 100 ml blood, haematocrit is 50%. Reflects blood viscosity, and haemoglobin level. A low level, eg, anaemia, causes hypoxia. Ranges: 0.4 - 0.5 (men), and 0.37 - 0.45 (women).

Haematology

The study of blood composition. Normal (adult) ranges:

Substance	*Males*	*Females*	*Units*
Haemoglobin	130-180	115-165	gram/litre
Platelets	150-450	150-450	10^9/litre
Red blood cells	4.5-6.5	3.8-5.8	10^{12}/litre
White blood Cells	5,000-10,000	5,000-10,000	microlitre

Haematoma

A swelling that contains clotted blood.

Haemodynamics

The part of physiology concerning pumping and flowing of blood.

Haemodynamic Monitoring

Monitoring of cardiovascular state, either invasive (real-time) or non-invasive (non real-time). Invasive techniques include arterial and central lines; Non-invasive techniques include blood pressure cuffs and fluid balance measurement.

Haemoglobin (Hb)

Protein molecule within red blood cells (~270 million/cell), which give them their colour, and by which 10% CO_2 (*carbaminohaemoglobin*) and 98% of oxygen (*oxyhaemoglobin*) is transported. The fraction of total haemoglobin that carries oxygen is the measurement for oxygen saturation. Normal range of arterial haemoglobin is 140 to 180 g/litre (4.7-6.1 million cells/microlitre) for men, and 120 to 160 g/litre (4.2-5.4 million cells/microlitre) for women. A low Hb count may be due to internal bleeding, iron deficiency, thalassaemia, inflammation, cancer, infection, vitamin B6 or B12 deficiency, hypothyroidism, pregnancy, heart or kidney or liver disease. High Hb levels can be due to: smoking, hypoxia, dehydration, lung disease, excess red blood cell count. Red cells are given when the Hb concentration is < 70 g/litre. Note: If Hb level is normal, but some of the Hb is defective (can't bind wth O_2), oxygen saturation (SaO_2) will be low, but paO_2 may be normal, because paO_2 is measured in the plasma, not in Hb. See *ctHb, MetHb, HHb.*

Haemoglobin Electrophoresis

A system to determine what types of haemoglobin are contained within a blood sample, particularly useful when carbon monoxide (CO) poisoning is suspected, because CO binds to haemoglobin (Hb) in preference to oxygen, which means that even if the patient has a normal level of Hb, the CO will prevent some oxygen from binding to the Hb, and so the patient could become hypoxic.

Haemolysis

Decomposition or bursting of red blood cells.

Haemopneumothorax

The simultaneous occurrence of pneumothorax and haemothorax.

Haemoptysis

Coughing blood from the lower airway. Some causes: bronchitis, infection, a blocked airway, pneumonia, or pulmonary embolism.

Haemorrhage

Blood loss *on the body surface is external haemorrhage; if the bleeding is inside the body, it is internal haemorrhage.* Platelets aggregate at site of injury, causing a plug and local vasoconstriction, and prevent capillary bleeding. To arrest significant haemorrhage, RBCs, FFP (contains clotting factors), and Platelets are given.

Normally, the body has a balance of coagulation and clot breakdown (fibrinolysis) factors. **Signs**: Sweating, pale skin, cyanosis, hypotension, shallow breathing, confusion, headache, nausea. See Appendix A54 (pg 446).

Haemostasis

The process of blood clotting, and the subsequent dissolution of the clot, following repair of the injured tissue.

The process is comprised of four main steps:

Step 1: *Vascular constriction;* to limit the amount of blood flowing to the injured area.

Step 2: *Primary haemostasis;* platelets are activated by thrombin, and clump (aggregate) at the site of injury (endothelium), and adhere to form a temporary platelet plug, or thrombus.

Step 3: *Secondary haemostasis*; the coagulation cascade starts, and a fibrin mesh (the clot) fixes the platelet plug in place.

Step 4: The clot dissolves after the vessel has been repaired.

Haemostat

A clamp to stop bleeding.

Haemothorax

An accumulation of blood in the pleural cavity, typically caused by penetrating or blunt trauma. Some signs include:

- Breathing difficulty
- Chest pain
- Pallor
- Reduced breath sound
- Tachycardia
- Fever
- Cold sweat
- Fatigue

Treatment may be by chest drain or thoracotomy.

HAGMA

High Anion Gap Metabolic Acidosis, where Anion Gap > ~20 mmol/L, caused by kidney failure, ketoacidosis, lactic acidosis, toxins, paracetamol or aspirin overdose, accumulation of organic acids, and inability to excrete H+. See *Anion Gap* + Appendix A9.

Haldane Effect

The phenomenon where increased concentration of oxygen reduces the binding affinity of Hb (haemoglobin) with CO_2, and why, in the oxygen rich alveoli, Hb binds more readily with oxygen, in preference to CO_2. In contrast, at the tissues, where there is a much lower oxygen concentration, Hb has 3 times more affinity for binding with CO_2 than oxygen. See also *Bohr Effect*.

Half Life

Time taken for a particular property of a substance to reduce by half. After two half life periods, the substance will decay (or transform) to one quarter of its original value, and will decay by half again, every half-life period thereafter. In drug administration, half life factors are related to the drug in plasma. For example, if a patient is given a 40 mg dose of a drug, which has a metabolic half-life of 6 hours, 20 mg of the drug will be still "active" after 6 hours; 10 mg will be active after 12 hours, 5 mg will be active after 18 hours, and so on. It takes about five half life periods before a drug loses its effect.

Haloperidol

Anti-psychotic agent for eg, schizophrenia.

Harmonic Scalpel

Surgical tool which uses ultrasound energy to cut or cauterise bleeding vessels.

Hartmann's Solution

Crystalloid balanced salt solution, for general fluid replacement. Contains calcium, chloride, lactate, sodium, water. Not usually given to kidney transplant patients. Caution: Too much fluid can result in electrolyte imbalance, tachycardia, peripheral or pulmonary oedema, and raised jugular venous pressure.

Hb Testing

Testing Haemoglobin (Hb) levels in the blood, measured in grams per decilitre, or litre. A normal range for an adult male is 130-180 g/litre; for an adult female, the range is 115-165 g/litre. A low level can indicate anaemia.

HCO_3^-

See Bicarbonate.

Hct

See Haematocrit.

Head Tilt and Chin Lift

Manouevre to relieve upper airway obstruction, such as the tongue, and improve view of the vocal cords. Place the fingertips underneath the patient’s chin, and gently lifting upwards.

Heart Attack

See Myocardial Infarction.

Heart Block

A bradycardia, caused by interruption of electrical signals through the heart. For the three main types, see AV Block, Bundle Branch Block, and Tachycardia Syndrome.

Heart Failure (HF)

Alternative term for Congestive Heart Failure.

Heat and Moisture Exchanger (HME)

Attachement to a breathing circuit, at the patient end, to provide a degree of **passive** humidity control (when passive systems are used, such as in anaesthetic systems, the circuit is deemed to be of the *dry* type). Without an HME, the patient's mucosa and secretions could dry out, and cause plugging of the endotracheal tube. If **active** humidification systems are used, such as in ICU, they are termed *wet* circuits. In 2016, a patient died, at London Bridge Hospital, after an active humidifier was switched off, and the patient's endotracheal tube became occluded with dried out secretions, thus demonstrating the importance of humidification. If an HME device incorporates a microbial filter, it is termed an HME Filter.

HectoPascal (hPa)

100 pascals = 1 mBar = 0.75 mmHg = 1.02 cmH_2O.

HemoCue Hb Tester

A portable device, made by Radiometer, for measuring haemoglobin levels, in mmol/litre, or g/decilitre. Note: Radiometer also produce a HemoCue blood sugar (BM) tester.

Henry's Law

Describes the phenomenon where, at a constant temperature, the amount of a gas that can be dissolved in a liquid is proportional to the solubility of the gas, for that liquid, and the partial pressure of the gas. Henry's Law explains why, for example, isoflurane takes longer to start working than sevoflurane – isoflurane is more soluble in blood, it takes longer to be absorbed into the blood, than does sevoflurane, so it takes longer before isoflurane can start building its required concentration in the brain (anaesthesia).

HEPA Filter

High Efficiency Particulate Air Filter, which can block particles as small as 0.3 micron.

Heparin

Naturally occurring anticoagulant, which is added, for example, to the saline wash of a cell saver, and to arterial blood gas syringes. Heparin has an immediate effect, but only lasts 4-6 hours.

HHb

See Deoxyhaemoglobin.

Hiatus (Hiatal) Hernia

When part of the stomach squeezes up into the chest, through a hiatus (opening) in the diaphragm. Usually, the hernia moves up and down, in and out of the chest area – *sliding hiatus hernia*. If next to the oesophagus, it will be a *para-oesophageal hiatus hernia*. The operation to repair a hiatus hernia is a *fundoplication*.

Hickman Line

Inventor, Dr Robert Hickman: A soft central venous catheter, tunnelled along the chest and inserted into a large neck/groin/chest vein, with distal end fed to the superior vena cava and right atrium. A Dacron cuff (under skin) secures the line from dislodgement, and protects against infection. Used for administration of medications, and withdrawal of blood for analysis. The 1-3 lumens obviate the need to cause repeated needle assault to peripheral veins. Often used in chemotherapy and haematology patients, and some types used mainly for the purpose of apheresis or dialysis. Hickman lines may remain in place for extended periods. Insertion of a Hickman line is done under sedation or general anaesthetic. See Appendix A80 (pg 488).

High Dependency Unit (HDU)

A ward where patients need more focused care and monitoring than in a normal ward, but not as much as an Intensive Care Unit.

High Frequency Oscillatory Ventilation

Ventilation strategy using a cyclic "wave" of pressure variations, at a frequency up to 900 hertz (cycles/second), resulting in low tidal volumes. The aim is to reduce lung injury that might otherwise be caused by assisted ventilation, when high pressures and volumes would be needed in order to provide a proper level of gas exchange. Used in treatment for ARDS and air leak syndromes.

High Spinal Anaesthetic

Emergency state, with anaesthetic spreading high into the subarachnoid space, above T4, Symptoms are bradycardia and hypotension. To stop the spread, sit the patient up. For an obstetric patient, tilt the mother, left side down; give high flow O2; assess and support the breathing, and intubate if necessary. Treat **hypotension** with vasopressors (phenypelphrine, ephedrine), and **bradycardia** with a vagolytic (atropine). Increased intra-abdominal pressure and higher BMI both increase risk of high block. See *Total Spinal Block* and Appendix A56 (pg 452).

Histamine

A chemical that the immune system releases into the bloodstream when it detects substances that it considers threatening, especially those to which the individual is allergic. On release, histamine causes vasodilation, resulting in a lowering of blood pressure, and producing an increase in heart rate. Signs are skin redness and inflammation, typically on the face and chest. Histamine is an ingredient in wasp venom, and covers the surface of nettles.

Hives (Urticaria, Nettle Rash)

A recurrent eruption of irritating wheals, redness, an itchy rash.

HME

See Heat and Moisture Exchanger.

Homoeostatis

The body's process of maintaining an optimal state, by regulating bodily systems to counter effects, particularly from the external environment, which oppose steady and optimal conditions. In general, homoeostatic mechanisms can be likened to a room temperature thermostat, where sensors detect any out of normal range conditions, and counter them through a negative feedback system; when the room is too cold, the heating switches on; when the room is too warm, the heating switches off.

Hormones

Greek "impetus": A chemical released by a gland (endocrine system) in one part of the body, and travels to a target receptor on a cell in another part of the body, where it stimulates an affect. A hormone acts as a catalyst for cellular level chemical changes, necessary for homoeostasis, growth, development, and energy. Endocrine hormone molecules are released into the bloodstream. Exocrine hormones are secreted into ducts, and then flow into the bloodstream, or travel (by diffusion) from cell to cell, in a process known as paracrine signalling.

Horowitz Index

Alternative name for Carrico Index or P/F Ratio.

Hospital Acquired Infection

See Nosocomial.

Huber Tip

The long curved tip (to prevent piercing the dura mater) of a hollow needle, and bevelled to prevent the possibility of "coring" the tissue it penetrates. Found on Tuohy epidural needles.

Hudson mask

Variable rate simple face mask, of various types, for spontaneously breathing patients. Post-surgery, the "Hudson" type mask has holes in the sides, to allow entrainment of room air and evacuation of expired CO_2. To prevent rebreathing, flow rate should be 4-10 L/min, but a higher rate does not necessarily correspond with better tissue oxygenation. FiO_2 is dependent on PIFR, O_2 flow rate, respiratory rate, and mask reservoir space.

Human Albumin Solutions

HAS 4.5% is used as a plasma expander. HAS 20% is used for hypoproteinaemic (low protein) patients. HAS products are no more effective than cheaper colloid and crystalloid products.

Human Factors

The modern term for "ergonomics", with several definitions, such as: *The study of human behaviour with respect to their environments and situations.* In terms of safety analysis, Human Factor study is based on the *Dirty Dozen* behavioural and situational conditions. See Appendix A57 (pg 453).

Humidity

A value which describes the amount of water vapour in the air, measured in grams per cubic metre (g/m^3). Absolute humidity is the humidity value, without taking into account the ambient temperature. Relative humidity is the fraction of water vapour, compared with the maximum amount which the air could hold at its particular temperature. The ability of the air to hold moisture increases with temperature. In the operating theatre, a typical relative humidity is between 50% and 60%. (Note: low humidity increases the probability of static charge build-up)

Humphrey ADE Circuit

A relatively new type of circuit which can be switched between the Mapleson A, D and E systems.

Hydrocortisone

Corticosteroid for problems with the skin, joints, asthma, and adrenal glands. Also used in anaphylaxis and severe bronchospasm. Reduces inflammation and itching, but weakens the immune system, so used with caution.

Hydrogen Carbonate (HCO_3^-)

Commonly referred to as *Bicarbonate*.

Hydrogen Ion (H+)

A positive hydrogen atom (ion), consisting of a proton only. H+ ions are what make acidity in the body. H+ ions easily bond with other substances. Concentration of H+ ions is measured in mmol/litre (normally 35-45 nmol/L), is proportionate to acidity, with pH calculated as the negative log of the molarity of the H+ concentration. What this means is that the greater the hydrogen ion concentration, the greater the acidity, and the lower the pH.

Hydrothorax

A non-inflammatory condition – a type of pleural effusion (fluid within the pleural membranes) made of transudate (filtrateserous fluid leaked out of blood vessels). Causes: liver failure, kidney failure, or congestive heart failure.

Hyoid Bone

A landmark for intubation, the hyoid bone lies at the base of the mandible, between the mentum (chin) and thyroid. The hyoid consists of a central body, two Greater and two Lesser Horns. The Greater and Lesser horns serve as attachments for various muscles and ligaments, and act as a base for the tongue.

Hyaluronidase

An enzyme that breaks down hyaluronic acid, to help increase absorption of drugs (intramuscular, subcutaneous) into tissues, and to reduce tissue damage caused by drug extravasation.

Hyperaemia

Excess of blood in the vessels or organ of a specific body part, resulting from increased supply of blood, or decreased drainage (venal obstruction). Hyperaemia differs from haemorrhage, because the excess blood is internal to the vessels, as opposed to the broken vessels of haemorrhage. Prominent signs are:

- Lethargy
- Palpitations
- Weight gain
- Oedema
- Drowsiness
- Difficulty urinating
- Headaches
- Short of breath

Hyperaesthesia

An increased awareness of a particular sense organ, such as when a patient has an abnormally heightened sensation of pain.

Hyperalgesia

Excessive sensitivity to pain. If the sensitivity is due to repeated opioid use, the condition is called *Opioid Induced Hyperalgesia*.

Hypercalcaemia

A high level of calcium (3 - 3.5 mmol/litre) in blood serum, with attendant risk of cardiac arrhythmias. Symptoms include:

- Thirst
- Anorexia
- Hypertension
- Coma
- Nausea
- Pancreatitis
- Confusion
- Confusion
- Renal impairment

The most common cause is hyperparathyroidism.

In cardiac arrest, treat the underlying cause, give furosemide, and rehydrate with 5 litre of 0.9% saline IV, over 24 hours.

Hypercapnia (Hypercarbia)

Increased level of CO_2 > 45 mmHg (6 kPa) in arterial blood, causing over stimulation of the respiratory centre, and depression of the central nervous system, typically caused by hypoventilation, COPD, bronchospasm, or airway/circuit obstruction. **Signs**: vasodilation, tachycardia, hypertension, headache, confusion, drowsiness, lack of patient cooperation. **Treatments**: depending on severity, include supplemental oxygen, bronchodilators, antibiotics, and corticosteroids (reduces airway inflammation).

Hyperchloraemic Metabolic Acidosis (HMA)

Metabolic acidosis due to (1) low serum bicarbonate (with subsequent rise in chloride) caused by GI loss or kidney problems, or (2) loss of water in the kidneys is greater than loss of sodium. HMA differs from "normal" metabolic acidosis because it is not caused by excess acid production or retention.

Hyperglycaemia

Excess of blood sugar in diabetic mellitus (DM), greater than 7 mmol/litre during a fasting period, or greater than 11 mmol/litre within two hours of eating. The main cause of DM hyperglycaemia is inadequate insulin production, causing diabetic ketoacidosis.

Symptoms

Polyuria	**Drowsiness**	**Blurred vision**
Nausea	**Fruity breath**	**Recurring infections**
V thirsty	Weak pulse	Vomiting
Fatigue	Stomach pain	Dry mouth

Emergency treatment is to give fast acting insulin (eg, Actrapid).

Hyperkalaemia

An electrolyte emergency: an excess of potassium (K) > 5.2 mmol/L, which the kidneys are unable to excrete, resulting in arrhythmias and cardiac arrest (> 7 mmol/L). Insulin and glucose are given to shift potassium into cells. Calcium chloride (or gluconate) might also be given (iv or im) for hyperkalaemia, to reduce risk of VF. See Appendix A83 (pg 493).

Hyperlactaemia

Increase in lood lactate > 2 mmol/L. If concentration reaches 3-5 mmol/L, the condition is lactate acidosis (a metabolic acidosis). High lactate results from increased biological stresses, and increasing levels coincide with an increasingly worsening patient condition, such as: hypoxia in sepsis, diabetes, liver dysfunction, intoxication, and disease. Normal level is 0.6-1.4 mmol/L.

Hyperlipidaemia

An elevated level of cholesterol or triglycerides (fat) in the blood.

Hypernatraemia

Excess sodium in the blood (> 145 mmol/litre). **Caused** by dehydration, diarrhoea, diuretics, vomiting, kidney failure. **Symptoms**: *Lethargy ≈ Tremors ≈ Irritability ≈ Seizures.* **Treatment**: usually involves fluid based therapy.

Hyperosmolar Hyperglycaemia State

An emergency condition in Type 2 diabetics, with dehydration and high levels of blood glucose, of over 35 mmol/litre. Typically, the **cause** can be infection, myocardial infarction, trauma, alcoholism, missed insulin administration, or substance abuse. **Treatment** may include rehydration, and balancing electrolytes, especially potassium and sodium, followed by a course of insulin.

Hyperoxaemia

Oxygen toxicity caused by arterial oxygen partial pressure (paO_2) > 119 mmHg (16 kPa), causing the alveoli to collapse or fill with fluid. During myocardial infarction, too much oxygen can cause coronary vasoconstriction, resulting in reduced oxygen to cardiac muscle. Survivors of cardiac arrest have worse outcomes if hyperoxaemic, so aim for normoxaemia. **Signs**: chest pain, coughing, nausea, vertigo, face/hand twitches, dyspnoea, seizures.

Hyperoxia

Excess concentration or partial pressure of oxygen at the tissues, where prolonged exposure leads to oxygen toxicity.

Hyperpnoea

An abnormally increased rate and depth of breathing.

Hypertension

Blood pressure > 170+ mmHg for a particular category of person, according to age, weight, etc. Typical treatment is by a Beta-blocker, such as Esmolol, Atenolol, or Labetalol.

Hyperthermia

Excessive body temperature - above 38° C. Note: excess temperature results in an increase in MAC.

Hypertonic

Excessive tension of a blood vessel or muscle; a solution with higher osmotic pressure than normal body fluid. See also *Isotonic*.

Hypertrophic

An enlargement of an organ.

Hyperventilation

Deep and/or fast breathing, resulting in quicker than normal elimination of CO_2. Central chemoreceptors, which detect blood CO_2 levels, signal the medulla oblongata, which responds by reducing the respiratory drive, until the CO_2 level is back to normal. When hyperventilating to remove excess CO_2, exhaustion can result, then CO_2 rises rapidly, and can lead to respiratory failure. See Appendix A58 (pg 455).

Hypervolaemia (fluid overload)

Excess of fluid in the body, which might overload the heart, and can result in congestive heart failure. Typically caused by excess sodium, excess ADH, liver cirrhosis, or heart or kidney failure. **Signs**: Oedema, hypertension **Treatment**: Stop fluid admin, give furosemide (diuretic).

Hypoalgesia

A condition where the sufferer has a decreased sensitivity to pain. Causes can be due to use of opioids, the placebo effect, or underlying conditions, such as heart disease.

Hypocalcaemia

Deficiency of calcium, requiring rebalancing with intravenous calcium chloride, or calcium gluconate. Symptoms include: Twitching, seizures, bronchospasm, and muscle weakness. In cardiac arrest, give 10-40 ml of 10% calcium chloride.

Hypocapnia (Hypocarbia)

A low level of CO_2 (carbon dioxide) in the blood, partial pressure of arterial CO_2 < 34 mmHg (4.5 kPa), typically caused by hyperventilation. A normal partial pressure, at rest, is 40 mmHg (5 kPa). Hypocapnia can suppress breathing, and causes cerebral vasoconstriction, leading to cerebral hypoxia.

Hypoglycaemia

A low level of blood sugar (< 4 mmol/litre, 72 mg/deciLitre). Diabetics may become hypoglycaemic after taking too much insulin, or going too long without food.

Symptoms

Dizziness	**Shaking**	**V hungry**	**Tingling lips**
Fatigue	**Sweating**	**Dizziness**	**Pale, dry skin**
Irritable	**Tearful**	**Palpitations**	
Tachycardia	Anxiety	Headache	Shallow breathing

Immediate treatment is fruit juice or sugary sweets.

Hypokalaemia

Serum potassium < 3.5 mmol/litre, which can cause arrhythmias. Signified by prominent U waves. See Appendix A83 (pg 493).

Hyponatraemia

Low serum sodium concentration. Sodium regulates water levels in and around cells. A low sodium level causes cells to swell and rupture, is the most common electrolyte disorder, and may lead to heart failure. **Normal** level: 136-142 mmol/litre; **Mild** hyponatraemia: 130-135; **Moderate**: 125-129; **Severe**: less than 125. Endocrinologist advice may be needed for all but the mildest cases. *Causes* include heart failure, kidney or liver problems, diuretics, antidepressants, pain medication, severe vomiting or diarrhoea, oedema, hormonal weakness, and hypotonic fluids. *Symptoms*: Nausea, seizures, coma, fatigue, irritability, headaches. *Treatment*: Intravenous saline.

Hypoperfusion

Lower than normal blood flow to tissues, which can lead to ischaemia. Might be caused by cardiac problems, hypotension, or hypovolaemia. Signs can include cool skin, tachypnoea (rapid breathing), hypotension, and increased capillary refill time.

Hypopnoea

Shallow breathing, during sleep.

Hypotension

Blood pressure below the normal range for a particular category of patient. Low diastolic pressure suggests arterial vasodilation, as with sepsis or anaphylaxis. A small pulse pressure could be due to arterial vasoconstriction, such as with hypovolaemia, or cardiogenic shock. Unmanageable hypotension is deemed “refractory”, and might be seen in a surgical patient - probably due to sepsis, hypovolaemia, or metabolic acidosis. In trauma, target MAP is > 65 mmHg. Treated by fluids or vasoconstrictors.

Hypothermia

A treatable cause of cardiac arrest - low core body temperature, where heat loss is greater than production, resulting in impaired systemic function, particularly of respiratory and cardiovascular systems. Three classes: *Mild* = 32-35° C; ***Moderate* = 28-32°** C; ***Severe* < 28°** C. **Primary** hypothermia is caused by exposure to low temperatures; **Secondary** hypothermia is a side effect of organ dysfunction. See Appendix A59 (pg 457).

Hypotonic

The state where a substance has lower osmotic pressure, or tone, than a particular fluid. See also *Isotonic*.

Hypoventilation

Respiratory Depression: Inadequate alveolar ventilation, resulting in increased CO_2 concentration, and increased acidity. Central chemoreceptors detect the high level of CO_2 (in the form of carbonic acid and H^+ ions), that triggers an increased respiratory drive, which aims to flush out the excess CO_2. A-a Gradient is normal in hypoventilation. See Appendix A60 (pg 458).

Hypovolaemia

Absolute hypovolaemia is a reduction (mainly) in the intravascular blood volume, leading to hypoperfusion. Two root types are kidney dysfunction and not kidney dysfunction. Kidney problems may be due to failure to reabsorb salt and water in the tubules. Non kidney causes include: loss of fluids (sweating, burns, diarrhoea, vomiting, hyperventilation), or movement of fluid into 3rd spaces (cavities). Underlying causes should be addressed, e.g., re-hydrate with crystalloids. Up to 30% volume mqy be lost before symptoms appear. *Relative hypovolaemia* is an increase in vessel capacitance, making it difficult to pump the existing volume sufficiently. Treat with a blood product, colloid, 0.9% saline, or Hartmann's (balanced salt).

Early Signs

- Headache
- Thirst
- Fatigue
- Weakness

Severe Signs

See *Hypovolaemic Shock*.

Hypovolaemic Shock

Aka *Haemorrhagic Shock*: Inadequate tissue perfusion caused by a loss of 15-20% intravascular blood volume.

Progression: Increased heart rate, vasoconstriction, coagulation cascade starts, adrenal glands release aldosterone – kidneys reabsorb sodium, and retain water.

Symptoms: Pale, cold, clammy skin; Tachycardia; Hypotension; Tachypnoea; Low pulse pressure; Dry mucous membranes; Anxiety; Oliguria; Cyanosis; Chest pain; Abdominal pain; Slow capillary refill; Feinting.

Identification: Arterial blood gases; Lactate; Haemoglobin; Haematocrit.

Management: Ensure oxygenation. Establish 2 * large bore venous cannulae. Manage haemorrhage. Maintain systolic BP at > 80 mmHg, with 100 ml fluid boluses (unless brain trauma).

Hypoxaemia

When breathing room air, if partial pressure of arterial oxygen (paO_2) is less than 8 kPa (60 mmHg). *Note: If paO_2 and oxygen saturation (SaO_2) are normal, hypoxaemia can still occur, if haemoglobin (Hb) level is low.* Hypoxaemia can also occur if some Hb cannot carry O_2, eg, due to carbon monoxide poisoning (carboxyhaemoglobin).

Causes: V/Q mismatch, global alveolar hypoventilation, low inspired O_2 pressure (altitude), diffusion limitation, right-to-left shunt.

Symptoms: Tachycardia, tachypnoea, coughing, central cyanosis, sweating, wheezing, confusion, headache, irritability, lethargy.

Treatment: Oxygen, sit patient up.

Note: Hypoxaemia severity is given by the Carrico Index: a value less than 300 might indicate lung injury.

Hypoxia

Low concentration of O_2 (oxygen) at the tissue cellular level, resulting in cell death. Hypoxia is a late sign of airway obstruction, so O_2 saturation is not a real-time indicator of ventilation. See Appendix A61 (pg 460).

Hypoxic Drive

The stimulus to increase minute volume, in response to a low level of arterial oxygen saturation, detected by peripheral (aortic and carotid bodies), chemoreceptors. COPD patients, for example, no longer have the ability to detect carbon dioxide and, therefore, have a degraded *respiratory drive*, and rely (in theory) on the hypoxic drive in order to regulate their breathing.

Hypoxic Guard

A mechanical or electronic interlink device between an anaesthetic machine's oxygen and nitrous oxide flow controls, which aims to prevent administration of pure nitrous oxide, by maintaining an oxygen:nitrous ratio of 1:3. If the oxygen flow falls below 200 ml/minute, the nitrous flow shuts off.

Hypoxic Mixture

A concentration of breathing gases, from an anaesthetic machine, where the fraction of oxygen is too low to prevent hypoxia.

Hypoxic Pulmonary Vasoconstriction (HPV)

A reflexive, homoeostatic, contraction of pulmonary vascular smooth muscle, causing narrowing of pulmonary capillaries and arteries, in response to unventilated alveoli. HPV is the body's attempt to normalise the ventilation:perfusion ratio, by creating a pulmonary shunt - the diversion of perfusion (blood flow) to better ventilated parts of the lung. HPV is suppressed by volatile anaesthetic agents, but is not affected by TIVA.

Ibuprofen

An antipyretic, anti-inflammatory, and analgesic.

ICF

Intracellular Fluid.

ICD

See Implantable Cardioverter Defibrillator.

ICP

Intra Cranial Pressure, normally 5-15 mmHg.

ICU Bed

Before leaving theatre, patients destined for Intensive Care Units must be transported on special beds, checked for the following:

- Suction equipment
- Ventilator
- Ambu bag
- Oxygen cylinder
- Capnometer
- Monitoring
- Mapleson C circuit
- Pillow

Ideal Gas Law

PV = nRT

Equates properties of a gas according to the variables:

Pressure * **V**olume = **n** * unive**R**sal gas constant * **T**emperature

Note: "**n**" refers to the number of moles of gas.

I:E Ratio

See Inspiratory:Expiratory Ratio.

I-Gel

A second generation supra-glottic airway device, with built in suction tube and bite block. One of I-Gel's unique selling points is its thermoplastic properties, which enables it to mould itself to a patient's particular airway anatomy.

Iliac Arteries

Left and right branches from the Common Illiac artery, distal to the Abdominal Aorta. Internal Iliac artery supplies the Uterus/Prostate, bladder and buttocks. The External Iliac supplies the lower limbs.

Immunoglobulin (Ig)

Proteins, produced by WBCs, that serve as antibodies, by binding to antigens.

Implantable Cardioverter Defibrillator (ICD)

An ICD is implanted into patients who suffer arrhythmias. The ICD detects fibrillations, then responds with a defibrillating shock. Some ICDs also have a pacemaker function (CRT-D).

Implanted Venous Access Device (IVAD)

Implanted device, for long term use, with access via a port that is just under the skin, accessed by *Huber Needle*. The port holds a slowly released reservoir of injected agent. See also *Portacath*.

Increased Airway Pressure

During IPPV (intubated), a raised peak airway pressure (above 35 cmH_2O) can be a sign of an underlying problem, which must be addressed. Causes of increased peak airway pressure include:

- Obstructed airway
- Blocked ETT/circuit
- Poor lung compliance
- High tidal volume
- Pneumoperitoneum
- Trendelenburg position
- Bronchospasm
- Pathology
- Obesity
- PEEP high
- High inspiratory flow rate
- ETT internal diameter too small
- Tension pneumothorax
- Only one bronchus intubated

Induction

Inducing a patient into a state of anaesthesia. Verification is by ensuring an adequate level of E_TCO_2 (end-tidal carbon dioxide), ET tube condensation (synchronised with respiration), symmetrical chest movement, auscultation, and oxygen saturation.

Induction Agents

Drugs to induce patients into a state of anaesthesia. Examples...

Barbiturates:	Thiopentone, Methohexitone
Imidazole:	Etomidate
Phenol:	Propofol
Phencyclidine:	Ketamine

Infarct

The wedge shaped area of necrosis in an organ, caused by a failed blood supply, often caused by a blocked blood vessel.

Infection

An assault by bacteria, fungi, virus, or parasites, which interfere with normal body function, and result in inflammation or tissue damage. Infectious agents multiply and propagate until the body's defences, or medical intervention, destroy/remove the agents. Infection can degrade oxygenation, and can increase blood sugar.

Infection Signs

- Fever
- Chills
- Swollen lymph
- Aches
- Lethargy
- Inflammation
- Nausea
- Headache
- New cough
- Diarrhoea
- Sweats
- Poor breathing
- Temperature < 36° or > 37.5° C

Risks – see Appendix A62 (pg 462). Also, see Sepsis.

Infiltration (Tissuing)

Infusion or leaking of an agent – the *infiltrate* - from a vein into surrounding tissue. Infiltration can be caused when a cannula pierces the wall of a blood vessel, or slips out of the vein, probably due to the cannula not being secured properly. A sign of infiltration is swelling in the subcutaneous tissue, after injecting, but swelling does not always occur. It can take several days for the infiltrate to be removed by the bloodstream (or lymph) and, unless the drug has a relatively short half life, it may exert its effect at an unwanted time, such as when the patient is no longer under medical supervision. Infiltration also describes the application of a local anaesthetic around a wound.

Inflammation

The body's healing mechanism, following an injury. Typical signs:
- Pain
- Redness
- Loss of function
- Swelling
- Heat

Infusion

Administration of an agent/solution, by intravenous, epidural, arterial, or subcutaneous means, and at a predetermined rate – by volume. Controlled by gravity or pump system. If multiple infusions share the main infusion (common volume) tubing, 1-way valves should be placed in each upstream tube, to stop a downstream blockage from backing up the other tube.

Infusion Pump

A machine which infuses an agent at a pre-determined rate. The simplest classification is based on the delivery type: if infusion is governed by motorised continuous or pulsatile positive displacement of a syringe plunger, it is a syringe pump, otherwise it is a volumetric pump, where the contents of a bag or bottle are delivered by peristaltic (usually) compression of the tubing, which forces the fluid towards the patient's cannula.

Inhalational Anaesthetics

Anaesthetic agents (vapours and gases) that enter the bloodstream from alveoli, as opposed to the intravenous route. Common examples: sevoflurane, desflurane, isoflurane, and nitrous oxide. **Side effects** include respiratory depression, decreased systemic arterial resistance (BP), PONV, reduced blood flow in the brain, myocardial depression, reduced blood pressure, and depressed metabolism of glucose. Efficacy of an inhalational agent is realised by its partial pressure in the central nervous system, so it is absolute, and not relative pressure that determines the value of partial pressure. Setting a vapouriser at 1% at Standard Temperature and Pressure will produce a higher partial pressure of the agent (in the alveoli, arteries, CNS) than a 1% setting if the vapouriser is at a higher altitude. Consequently, vapourisers must be calibrated for their mean ambient pressures.

Innervation

Nerve supply, or stimulation.

Inotrope

Any drug that affects the force of muscular contractions, especially of the heart. Inotropes are irritants, so must usually be given centrally, and should be given as an infusion, not bolus, due to high potency. See Appendix A63 (pg 463).

INR

See International Normalised Ratio.

Insensible Fluid Loss

The loss of fluid, which cannot be measured, such as from respiration and perspiration.

Inspiration

The active process of drawing air into the lungs. The inward movement of air (or other breathing gas) is a result of the relative lower pressure, in the lungs, than ambient pressure. This lower pressure is caused by the increase in effective lung volume, which occurs after the diaphragm and intercostal muscles contract.

Inspiratory Capacity

The maximum volume of air that can be inspired; the sum of Tidal and Inspiratory Reserve Volumes.

Inspiratory:Expiratory (I:E) Ratio

The ratio between the time spent on inspiration and respiration, typically 1:2 i.e., an expiration lasts twice the time of an inspiration. In periods of high exertion, oxygen demands may alter the ratio to 1:1. For asthmatics, the ratio may be 1:3 or 1:4.

Inspiratory Pause

Time between the end and start of an inspiration.

Inspiratory Reserve Volume

Maximum volume of air that can be breathed in, above Tidal Volume.

Insufflation

The filling of a body cavity with low pressure gas, such as carbon dioxide, during endoscopic procedures, to give working space.

Insulin Shock

A diabetic emergency caused by having too much insulin in the blood, resulting in hypoglycaemia (low blood sugar). **Symptoms**: dizziness, tachycardia, anxiety, hunger, headache, tremors, coma. Emergency **action** is to give a sugary drink, sweets, or administration of glucagon.

Integumentary System

The skin, sweat glands, hair, nails, and other external (mostly) elements of the body, which serve to provide protection against environmental factors, such as extreme temperature, infection, and mechanical damage.

Intercostal Muscles

The muscles found between the ribs (inside of the ribcage), that extend from the front of the ribs, and go around the back, past the bend in the ribs. The nipple, located in the 4th intercostal space, can be used as a "landmark" for rib location.

Intercostal Retraction

The sinking in of the intercostal muscles, when taking a breath, due to a reduced pressure in the lungs, in respiratory distress, caused by airway blockage or infection.

Intermittent Positive Pressure Ventilation (IPPV)

Intermittent inflation of the intubated patient's lungs (increases FRC), by a ventilator, controlled by pressure or volume; and not synchronised with patient's breathing efforts.

Justifications

- ◇ Anaesthetised patients - with muscle paralysis
- ◇ Acute respiratory or ventilatory failure
- ◇ To prevent hypoxia
- ◇ Chest injury and lung contusion (bruising)
- ◇ Coma with breathing difficulties (drug overdose?)

Internal Respiration

Exchange of gases (oxygen, CO_2) between blood and tissue cells.

International Normalised Ratio (INR)

The ratio of how long it takes a patient's blood to clot (prothrombin time), compared with a standard value - the *Mean Normal Prothrombin Time*. A normal reading would be 0.8–1.1 (taking 12-14 seconds). INR is of special significance to surgical patients, who may be undertaking anti-coagulation therapy; value for a Warfarin patient would be 2-3.5. Note: the higher the INR value, the longer it takes for a clot (thrombus) to form.

International Unit (IU)

A quantity of a substance which produces a particular biological effect, agreed upon as an international standard. The mass or volume of a substance, which constitutes one IU, varies, based on the substance being measured, and the variance is based on the biological activity or effect, for the purpose of easier comparison across substances. International Units are used to quantify the potency of vitamins, hormones, some medications, vaccines, blood products, and similar biologically active substances.

Interosseous

Between bones, such as interosseous injection, where peripheral or central venous access is not available. Typical access is via the antero-medial aspect of the upper proximal tibia.

Interstitial Fluid (Tissue/Third Space)

24% of total body fluid, bathing the cells, and allowing exchange of nutrients (water, glucose, minerals, hormones, neurotransmitters, electrolytes) and metabolites between cells and capillaries.

Intracellular Fluid (ICF)

The fluid within cells, comprising ⅔ total body fluid volume.

IntraLipid 20%

Fresenius Kabi owned trademark for an intravenous lipid emulsion, used to treat toxic reactions to local anaesthetics (1 ml/kg, over 1 min, increased to 2 ml/min), and to provide parenteral (IV) nutrition. IntraLipid contains soy bean oil, glycerin, and egg phospholipids. It is thought that the emulsion neutralises the anaesthetic effect by "capturing" its molecules.

Intramuscular (IM)

Inside (intra) a muscle: Injecting (1-1.5", 25-38 mm, 20/22 G) a drug into a muscle gives a more sustained absorption and steady infusion than if given IV, are also quicker to give, and do not need as much skill. Technique: Z-Track, and check for blood aspiration.

Intraoperative Awareness

Becoming aware during general anaesthesia due to, for example, inadequate levels of anaesthetic agents, whilst still being under the influence of a neuromuscular blocking agent. Paralysis means that the patient can hear what is happening around them, but is unable to communicate their awareness.

Signs of Awareness

Eyelash reflex	Hypertension	Muscle contraction	Reduced lung compliance
Responsive pupils	Sweating	Tachycardia	Tears

Risk Factors

25-50 years	Female	Muscle relaxants
Obesity	Obstetric case	Trauma

Intraosseous Cannulation

A method of establishing vascular access via a bone (marrow), especially when normal intravenous access is not possible. Typical sites for intraosseous cannulation, are: Proximal Tibia, Proximal Humerus, Distal Tibia, and Distal Femur.

Intrapleural Pressure (P_{ip})

Pressure within the pleural cavity, which is always lower than atmospheric and alveolar pressures - prevents atelectasis.

Intrapulmonary (Intra-alveolar) Pressure (P_{alv})

The pressure exerted by gases in the alveoli; higher than intrapleural pressure.

Intrapulmonary (Alveolar) Shunt

A Ventilation/Perfusion mismatch (v/q=0) condition where alveoli are perfused (have blood flow), but not ventilated (lack oxygen), resulting in de-oxygenated blood continuing to the systemic circulation. Causes include oedema, atelectasis, alveolar consolidation (alveoli with blood, pus, tumour), and pneumonia.

Intrathecal

Theca - Sheath: Inside the *subarachnoid space*. Drugs can be introduced intrathecally, to reach the CSF, and then act on the nervous system; for chemotherapy, anaesthesia, or pain management. The intrathecal route bypasses the blood-brain barrier, so may be useful with drugs with low lipid solubility. See also *Spinal Block*.

Intravascular Fluid

Fluid component of plasma and lymph. 6% total body fluid.

Intravenous (IV)

Route for drugs that exert their effect quickly, and avoid First Pass Metabolism. Some drugs are given IV, because they are too irritant for intramuscular or subcutaneous administration. IV administration set types: filtered, vented, non-vented, gravity.

Intrinsic PEEP (Auto PEEP)

In IPPV, a "breath" delivered before complete exhalation of the previous breath, causing over-inflation and not allowing the lungs to completely deflate after the breath, possibly resulting in barotrauma. Causes: large tidal volume, prolonged inspiration, or a restrictive airway. Compare with *breath stacking*.

Intubating LMA

A laryngeal mask airway, allowing single-handed blind insertion of an endotracheal tube, without the need to move the patient's head, or place fingers inside the patient's mouth. Used in difficult airway situations, or when the patient may have cervical spinal injury. The LMA section serves as a guide for a reinforced ET tube to be placed, without having to displace the anatomy. If the patient suffers from an oesophageal or pharyngeal abnormality, then intubation via the ILMA is contraindicated, unless used in an airway rescue situation.

Intubation

Insertion of an endotracheal tube into the trachea. An intubation attempt should not last longer than 30 seconds, and should normally be stopped if oxygen saturation drops below 95%. After intubation, patency may be confirmed by:

√ Equal bilateral chest rise and fall

√ Water vapour within lumen of tube during exhalation

√ Normal end tidal carbon dioxide waveform and value

√ Visualisation of the tube passing through vocal cords

√ Auscultation for equal bilateral breath sounds

√ No breathing sounds over the stomach

√ Depth of tube at incisors (21:women, 23:men)

√ Normal airway pressure

√ Normal tidal volume

√ No gastric contents in tube

√ Tube cuff pressure: 20-25 cmH_2O

√ Reservoir bag moves in sympathy with lungs (+ feel)

Inverse Ratio Ventilation

Ratio of inspiratory to expiratory times, with inspiration longer than expiration, such as 3:1, as for poorly compliant lungs.

Ion

An atom or molecule which has either lost or gained an electron(s), giving it a positive (cation) or negative (anion) charge.

Ionic Compound

A compound, such as NaCl (saline), containing ions that are held together by electrostatic forces (ionic bonds). In water, the compound dissociates into its ions, making the solution electrically conductive, so the ions are termed *electrolytes*.

IPPV

See Intermittent Positive Pressure Ventilation.

Irritant Agent

When a drug/agent leaks from a vein into surrounding tissue (extravasation), but causes shorter lasting and less severe damage than a vesicant agent, it is termed an *irritant*. See also *Infiltration*.

Ischaemia

Deficient blood supply (perfusion) to an organ, caused by, for example, a blocked artery. Without proper blood perfusion, tissues can die due to lack of oxygenation.

Ischaemic Heart Disease

See Coronary Heart Disease.

Iso-

Equal (pressure, temperature, concentration,...).

Isoflurane

Potent volatile anaesthetic agent, that is irritating to the airway. The MAC value of 1.2% (30 year olds) illustrates why it is more potent than either sevoflurane or desflurane, and is due to it having the highest *oil:gas partition* coefficient of 98, which means more of it is absorbed by the brain, where it exerts its effect. With a *blood:gas partition* coefficient of 1.4, isoflurane also has the highest blood solubility of all volatile agents, making it the slowest to achieve onset and recovery of anaesthesia – it has to "fill" the blood space before it can build concentration in the brain. See also *Volatile Anaesthetic Agents*.

Isotonic

Substances having equal osmotic pressure. Isotonic solutions e.g., 0.9% saline solution and blood, do not result in net movement of water (no osmosis) between them. Therefore, if extracellular fluid is isotonic with a cell that it is in contact with, no fluid will flow between the cell and extracellular fluid. Alternatively, if a fluid, such as pure water, which has lower tonicity (hypotonic) than the cell, comes in contact with the cell, water will flow into the cell, in an attempt to balance the two concentrations. Conversely, a fluid with higher tonicity (hypertonic) than the cell, such as sea water, will cause a net movement of water out of the cell, thereby producing a state of cellular dehydration.

Isotope

Any instance of a particular atom with different number of neutrons to other instances of the same type of atom.

-itis

Inflammation.

Jaw Thrust

Technique of opening the airway, which might be occluded by the tongue. Unlike the Head Tilt - Chin Lift method, a jaw thrust may be used when the patient is suspected of having a spinal injury.

Jet Ventilation (Lung Protective Ventilation)

Jet or *high frequency ventilation*, is a type of mechanical ventilation that produces high respiratory rates (150+ breaths/min) and very small tidal volumes. The low airway pressure generated makes Jet systems suitable for upper respiratory tract and ENT procedures. High frequency ventilation (HFV) is thought to reduce ventilator-associated lung injury. There are different flavours of HFV, and each type has its own advantages and disadvantages. The types of HFV are characterized by the delivery system and the type of exhalation phase. See Appendix A64 (pg 465).

Joule

Newton Metre: S.I. derived unit of energy, defined as the work done when a force of one newton acts on an object for a distance of one metre. **Note**: Anyone taking part in defibrillating a patient should understand the concept of energy measurement (joules).

Jugular Venous Distension (JVD)

The prominent distension (swelling) of the right internal jugular vein, caused by pressure in the superior vena cava, such as when the patient has cardiac tamponade or tension pneumothorax. Image: See Appendix A55.

Junctional Circuit

The expiratory valve is next to the next to FGF inlet.

K-Band

Urgo Medical elasticated, breathable, comfortable bandage, to wrap dressings, and to prevent children pulling out cannulae.

Ketamine

A non-competitive antagonist (NMDA-glutamate receptor) that causes dissociative ("zombie") anaesthesia: eyes may remain open, with an increase in saliva, BP, cardiac output, and tachycardia, but does not cause respiratory depression or unconsciousness. Contraindicated in hypertensives. Causes bronchodilation, so may be suitable for asthmatics. Is cardiovascular stable, so may also be suitable for patients with history of heart failure. Ketamine crosses the blood-brain barrier quickly, so has a quick onset, and short ½-life. It is the only sedative to produce analgesia. Secretions may mean patient needs pre-medication with glycopyrrolate or atropine, and suction. Adult dose: 1–2 mg/kg.

Ketoacidosis

See Diabetic Ketoacidosis.

Ketone

Water soluble molecular byproduct of the liver breaking down fat and protein, used for energy when glucose is lacking (eg, during fasting), or when lack of insulin prevents metabolism of carbohydrates, and uses fat instead. Ketones (measured in urine) lead to ketoacidosis. **Signs**: frequent urination, stomach pain, fruit smelling breath, nausea, confusion, thirst, hyperglycaemia.

Ketosis

A non-harmful high level of ketones in the blood, caused by fasting, alcohol, and low carbohydrate diets.

Kussmaul Breathing

Laboured and deep breathing pattern, a sign of acidosis, and caused by inadequate hydrogen ion (H+) buffering, often resulting from metabolic acidosis. Commonly seen in patients who are suffering from diabetic ketoacidosis, with kidney dysfunction.

Kussmaul's Sign

Increased pressure and distension in the jugular veins, during inspiration, caused by right ventricle or other cardiac myopathy.

Labile Hypertension

Labile is something that is not constant, but changes easily. Labile hypertension means the patient's blood pressure changes back and forth between between normotension and hypertension. Similarly for labile HYPOtension.

Lack circuit

Functionally coaxial Mapleson A afferent reservoir circuit, similar to the Magill system, but with the expiratory valve at the machine end. Fresh gas flows up the outer sleeve, expired gas flows down the inner tube, to the exhaust valve.

Lacri-Lube

Brand/generic name for eye ointment, to protect against corneal abrasion, when an anaesthetised patient is put in the prone position, and to stop a dry cornea sticking to the inner eyelid.

Lactate

{Lactic acid minus a proton} Previously thought to be a toxic end-product of metabolism, caused by hypoperfusion and hypoxia, but now known to be an ionic end product of glycolysis: cells produce energy by converting glucose into pyruvate, which is then converted into Acetyl Coenzyme A – the body's main energy source. In the absence of oxygen, pyruvate is converted into lactate, to enable breakdown and oxidisation of glucose, to produce energy, with excess lactate converted into glucose (liver). Increased physiological stress increases lactate levels. Normal blood levels are:

Arterial:	0.5 - 1.6 mmol/litre
Venous:	0.5 - 2.2 mmol/litre

Above 2 mmol/litre suggests septic shock (or hypoperfusion). At 4 mmol/litre or higher, the patient requires immediate ICU care.

Above 5 mmol/litre, signs are tachycardia, tachypnoea, confusion, and Kussmaul breathing.

Lactic Acidosis

A serum lactate level > 4 mmol/litre, that is a common cause of high anion gap metabolic acidosis (HAGMA). Lactic acidosis occurs because of lactate over-production, or there is a problem in liver metabolism. There are two types: **Type A** *lactic acidosis* occurs in poor tissue perfusion issues, such as in anaemia, CO poisoning, dehydration, airway inflammation or obstruction, hypoperfusion, hypovolaemia, or when the patient is hypoxic, such as during shock (septic, haemorrhagic, or cardiogenic). **Type B** can occur when tissue perfusion, oxygenation, BP, volume, and Hb are normal, and is due to toxin ingestion, alcoholism, drug use, genetic problems, infection, sepsis, short bowel syndrome, pancreatitis, kidney or liver disease, or other metabolic issues. **Signs:** lactate > 2 mmol/L, ph < 7.35, $paCO_2$ < 42 mmHg, abnormal breathing, tachycardia, disorientation, jaundice, muscle or abdominal pain, fatigue, headache, nausea, diarrhoea.

Laminar Flow Ventilation (Unidirectional airflow)

A type of ventilation where filtered **High Efficiency Particulate Air** is uniformly forced down and outward, away from the operating table, with the object of reducing the number of airborne pathogens in the immediate vicinity of the surgical field and, thereby, reducing the possibility of surgical site infection. A significant goal of a laminar flow system is to reduce pathogens from one of the main sources, which is of human (staff) origin. Laminar flow aims to continuously flush clean air over the surgical field, with up to 300 air changes per hour.

Laparo-

Referring to the abdomen.

Larson's Manouevre

A method of treating or preventing laryngospasm, especially at extubation, by applying pressure to the *laryngospasm notch.*

Laryngeal Handshake

Technique of locating the cricothyroid membrane, particularly for emergency front of neck access (FONA).

Laryngeal Mask Airway (LMA)

An LMA is a supraglottic (above the larynx) device that sits in the hypopharynx, in spontaneous ventilation. The tip of the LMA sits against the valve at the top of the oesophagus, thereby providing a partial seal against regurgitation and pulmonary aspiration. One advantage over bag/valve/mask ventilation is the reduced possibility of insufflating the oesophagus, which might otherwise cause gastric distension. Additionally, an LMA does not irritate the throat as much as an endotracheal tube. An LMA is unsuitable for patients who are obese or at risk of aspiration.

Laryngo-Tracheal Mucosal Atomization Device (LMA)

The *LMA MADgic* is a narrow and malleable stylet, 6" (15 cm) long, to administer a fine atomized spray of anaesthetic (phenylephrine/cocaine) to the upper airway and vocal cords. The device can be fitted to a luer-lock syringe. See also *Mucosal Atomisation Device.*

Laryngoscope

Endoscopic instrument to aid visualisation of the airway during intubation. Several types of laryngoscope blade are available, with the curved Macintosh blade being used for standard intubation. Sizes range from 0 (neonate) to 4 (large adult).

Blade types:

- Macintosh (curved) - standard use
- McCoy - hinged curved tip, to lift epiglottis
- Polio (120°) - obese and large breasted patients
- Magill (straight) - for infants (U shaped cross section)
- Miller (straight with curved tip) - for infants (large epiglottis)

A Macintosh blade is positioned in the vallecula, anterior to the epiglottis, lifting it out of the visual path, while the Miller blade is positioned posterior to the epiglottis, trapping it to expose the glottis and vocal folds. Other common types of laryngoscope are fibreoptic and video aided systems (C-MAC, Airtraq, Glidescope).

Laryngoscopy

Process of obtaining a view of the larynx, with a dedicated laryngoscope or other optical device. During intubation, laryngoscopy can induce a blood pressure increase, which may be nullified by giving extra induction agent, or quick acting opioid.

Laryngospasm

The partial or full reflexive, protective, spasmodic closing of the vocal cords. Most dangerous when the patient is semi-conscious, because the protective reflexes are heightened, and the reflexes to re-open the vocal cords are minimal. See Appendix A65 (pg 466).

Larynx

Tube shaped structure between the pharynx and trachea, marked by the two vocal cords (V shaped), with glottis between them. Composition is muscle and cartilage (thyroid, epiglottis, cricoid, two each of arytenoid, corniculate, cuneiform), ligaments, and membranes. Typical larynx lengths: males: 44 mm (1.75 inch), females: 36 mm (1.5 inch). The larynx is responsible for making sound, the cough reflex, and protecting the lower respiratory tract. See *Image*, Appendix A65 (pg 466).

Laser Endotracheal Tube

An armoured ET tube, used specifically when there is risk of tube damage, by laser, during microlaryngeal procedures of the airway. If an ordinary ET tube is used, the laser light can puncture the tube, and initiate a fire (fed by the oxygen supply) which is being fed through the tube to the patient. Some regulatory bodies recommend that, for extra fire safety, the cuff of a laser ET tube should be filled with water (plus methylene blue), rather than air.

Left Heart Failure

A congestive condition, where the **left ventricle** (LV) fails to pump sufficient blood into the systemic circulation (aorta). Consequently, blood builds up in the lungs, causing pulmonary oedema. **Systolic** failure (reduced ejection fraction) is when the LV cannot contract properly. **Diastolic** failure means the LV is stiff, and cannot fully relax between beats, which prevents complete filling. **Symptoms**: vertigo, central cyanosis, bronchospasm, "crackles", couch, bubbly sputum. *Forward* and *Left* Heart Failure are synonymous.

Left to Right Shunt

Condition where some of the blood, which should have passed from the left side of the heart into the systemic circulation, flows back to the right side of the heart, typically because of a faulty valve, a hole in the septum between the two atria or ventricles, or perforated aorta. A consequence may be higher blood volume and pressure in the pulmonary than the systemic circulations.

L.E.M.O.N.

An acronym for one type of pre-anaesthesia assessment system, to help predict difficulty of intubation, based on:

- **L**ook for external signs, eg, obesity, anatomical problems.
- **E**valuate: 3-3-2 finger rule (3 mouth opening, 3 thyromental distance, 2 between the hyoid bone and thyroid notch).
- **M**allampati grade
- **O**bstruction of airway

- **N**eck mobility

Leucocyte (Leukocyte)

White blood cells (WBCs) that patrol the bloodstream to find pathogens, and ingest or produce antibodies against them. See Appendix A20 (pg 375).

Leucocytosis (Leukocytosis)

An increase in white blood cells (leukocyte), often during infection.

Leucodepletion (Leukodepletion) Filter

A fine filter (40 micron) which removes leukocytes from blood, particularly a patient's salvaged blood, with the intention of preventing re-infusion of malignant cells, fat, and small aggregates. Typical cases that warrant leukocyte filtration include:

Sickle cell anaemia	Leukaemia
Organ transplantation	Infection

Leucopenia (Leukopenia)

A decrease in white blood cell count.

Levobupivacaine

A version of bupivacaine, but less cardio and neuro toxic, and produces less depression of myocardial contractility. For spinal anaesthesia.

Lidco-Plus (Lithium Dilution Cardiac Output) Monitor

A monitor that provides continuous haemodynamic status of high risk patients, so helping guide fluid and drug management, achieved by analysing the arterial pressure waveform, to produce an estimation of cardiac output, from which, stroke volume and systemic vascular resistance are derived.

Lidocaine/Lignocaine Hydrochloride 1%/2%

A short duration (0.5-3 hour) local anaesthetic with 2 minute onset. Dose is 1 mg/kg. Also used to treat ventricular tachycardia.

Ligand

A molecule (drug, neurotransmitter, hormone) that binds with a receptor, to cause or inhibit an action. A particular type of ligand may bind with several types of receptor, which is one of the reasons why side-effects occur.

Lingual

Relating to the tongue.

Lipid Emulsion

Lipid: Fatty acids - oils or fats - not soluble in water. At room temperature, *oil* is liquid, and *fat* is solid. ***Emulsion***: A colloid formed by combining several immiscible liquids – one does not dissolve the other (not a homogenous mixture). See *IntraLipid*.

Liver Function Test

Measurement of enzymes and proteins, to determine how well the liver is working. A damaged liver releases enzymes into the blood, and the level of proteins produced by the liver begins to drop.

LMA

See Laryngeal Mask Airway.

Loading Dose

Initial administration of a large dose of a drug that reaches a therapeutic level quickly, and which is larger than subsequent doses. E.g., induction with 200 mg (loading dose) propofol, followed by a 50 mg maintenance dose, a few minutes later.

Local Anaesthetic

A type of (vasodilating) anaesthetic that is injected into a specific part of the body, to stop localised pain impulses being sent to the brain. To minimise risk of toxicity, the maximum volume of injection is given as (dose per kg * patient weight) divided by (10 * % concentration). See *Lidocaine, Bupivacaine, Marcaine.*

Local Anaesthetic Toxicity

An adverse reaction to a local anaesthetic, such as Lidocaine. See Appendix A66 (pg 469).

Lower Airway Obstruction

Obstruction below the larynx, caused by foreign objects, blood, secretions, pneumonia, asthma, bronchiole constriction. **Signs** include agitation, distress, expiratory stridor/wheezing, and chest expansion. **Treatment** may include intubation, Positive End Expiratory Pressure, oxygen, salbutamol (for bronchospasm).

Lower Oesophageal (Cardiac) Sphincter

Ring of muscular tissue, at the distal end of the oesophagus (entrance to stomach), acting as a 1-way valve, allowing food to enter the stomach, but preventing contents from backing up into the oesophagus, where it could move up and into the trachea, to pollute the lungs. Paralysing agents, such as atracurium, relax the muscle and, thereby, suppress the 1-way valve effect.

Luer Lock Syringe

A syringe with a screw fitting, making it a secure fit to a fluid line.

Luer Slip Syringe

The standard "push-fit" syringe.

Lumen

Latin for "an opening". The space inside a tubular structure, such as the inner tube of a Bain circuit, or the distal end of an ET tube.

Lung Compliance

The elasticity of the lungs is described as the change in lung volume per change in pressure, normally 100-200 ml/cmH_2O. A decreased compliance can result in a higher peak airway pressure.

Lyse

To undergo "lysis" - to break down cells.

-lysis

A suffix to indicate a decomposition or breaking apart of something, such as blood cells (haemolysis).

MAC

See Minimum Alveolar Concentration.

MAC Awake Concentration

The anaesthetic concentration level at which a patient does not respond to verbal commands, such as "open your eyes" in 50% of patients. Approximately 1/3 – 1/2 MAC level.

Magill Circuit

This is the original Mapleson A system, comprising a three way T shaped tube, which is connected to the fresh gas outlet (FGF), a reservoir bag (90° to FGF), a corrugated reservoir tube and, at the other end, an expiratory valve, then the patient connection.

Magill Forceps

Blunt forceps, an aid to nasal intubation, placement of throat packs, and removal of visible foreign bodies in the pharynx.

Magnesium (Mg) Sulphate

Important for heart health, bone production, nerves, glucose levels, polarity of cell membranes, and decreasing pulmonary vascular tone. Mg can alleviate eclampsia, enhance analgesia, relieve asthma (bronchodilates), cause vasodilation, and normalise arrhythmias. Mg can produce hypotension or hypokalaemia. In cardiac arrest, 2 g IV is given to counter VT. Calcium gluconate (10 ml 10% w/v) might be given in cases of magnesium toxicity.

Magnetic Resonance Imaging

Device that uses magnets and radio waves to produce internal body images. MRI is superior to CT for examination of the spinal cord, blood vessels, internal organs, and brain tumors.

Malignant Hypertension

A sudden onset of a very high blood pressure, which might be higher than 180/120, and could cause organ damage. **Symptoms** include: blurred vision, nausea, confusion, nose bleed, headache, vertigo, chest pain, arrhythmia, numbness, tingling, seizure, and ruptured capillaries in the retinas. **Treatment** includes intensive care, nitroglycerin, beta-blockers, and ACE inhibitors.

Malignant Hyperthermia

An abnormality of skeletal muscle fibre metabolism. The most common triggers are Suxamethonium (succinylcholine) and volatile agents; also lignocaine, atropine, diazepam, pancuronium, phenothiazines, and stress. See Appendix A67 (pg 470).

Maintenance Dose

The administration of a drug dosage that is equal to the steady state rate that the drug is being metabolised.

Mallampati Classifications

Airway grading scheme for anticipation of endotracheal intubation difficulty. **Class I**: Hard palate, soft palate, uvula, faucial pillars. **Class II**: Hard palate, soft palate, most of uvula, faucial pillars. **Class III**: Hard palate, soft palate, base of uvula. **Class IV**: Only hard palate visible. Image: see Appendix A6 (pg 348).

Mandible

The lower jaw bone.

Mannitol

An osmotic diuretic, which is used to reduce intracranial pressure, intraocular pressure, cerebral oedema, and oliguria in patients with inadequate kidney function.

Manometer

A device for measuring pressure; sometimes used to determine the cuff pressure of a laryngeal mask airway or endotracheal tube.

Manual In-Line Stabilisation (MILS)

Technique to prevent patient head movement, by pressure to the occiput (back of head) and mastoid processes (behind ear), whilst the anaesthetist intubates. Image: see Appendix A46 (pg 433).

MAP

See *Mean Arterial Pressure* and *Mean Airway Pressure*.

Mapleson Circuits

Semi-closed (reservoir, partial rebreathing) class of breathing circuits, with types A-E. With F added later.

Mapleson A (Magill) Circuit

An afferent reservoir circuit, which eliminates CO_2 efficiently, but needs high Fresh Gas Flow (FGF) in controlled ventilation. Ideal for spontaneous ventilation. Requires a FGF matching minute volume, to avoid functional re-breathing. Dead space is minimised by having the expiratory valve close to the patient. Does not have an efferent limb. A *Lack* circuit is a co-axial Mapleson A.

Mapleson B Circuit

Junctional afferent reservoir circuit, suitable for resuscitation and patient transfers, because the bag and valve are close to the patient. Requires FGF of 1.5 - 2 times minute volume to avoid functional re-breathing. (Does not have an efferent limb)

Mapleson C Circuit

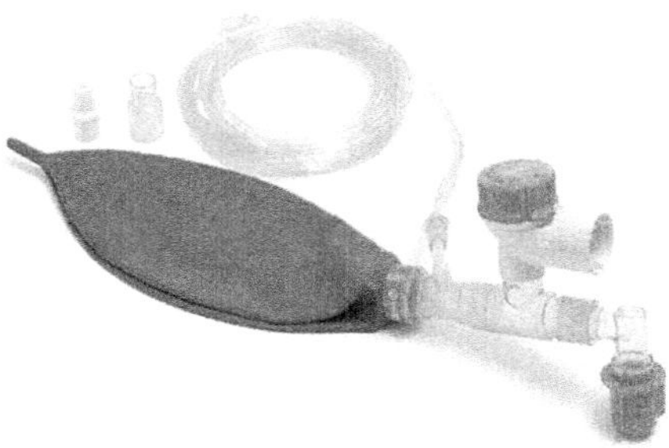

Junctional afferent reservoir circuit, incorrectly known as a Waters circuit. Essentially, Mapleson B, without the extra tubing in the expiratory limb. For short term use, such as resuscitation and patient transfers, because it is compact, and gives good feedback. Needs FGF 1.5-2 * minute volume (V_E) to avoid re-breathing. (Has no efferent limb.) Warning: In critical care setting emergency intubation, a high FGF can nullify E_TCO_2.

Mapleson D Circuit

An efferent reservoir (bag in the efferent limb) circuit, which needs high gas flows in spontaneous ventilation, so performs best with controlled ventilation. Requires FGF of 2-4 times minute volume to avoid functional re-breathing.

Mapleson E Circuit

A valveless and bag-less circuit, with low breathing resistance; for spontaneous or assisted ventilation. Derived from the Ayre's modification of the original T-piece, having reservoir tubing added to the expiratory limb. Requires high gas flow.

Mapleson F Circuit

Not strictly a Mapleson class, but refers to the Jackson-Rees modification of the Ayres's T-piece system, which connects an open ended bag to the efferent (expiratory) limb of a circuit. Gas escapes via the open end of the bag. A minimal resistance circuit that allows intermittent positive pressure ventilation, by occluding the tail of the bag (finger and thumb), and squeezing the bag. There is also a version with a closed end bag and an APL valve.

Marcaine

A brand name for *Bupivacaine* Hydrochloride.

Marcain Heavy

Hyperbaric version of 0.5% w/v marcaine, used in spinal blocks, with 80 mg/ml glucose added to give it a density higher than CSF, so that it will more readily succumb to gravity when spreading in the intrathecal space, reducing the risk of a high spinal block.

Mastoid Process

The cone shaped prominence behind the earlobe, to which neck muscles attach.

Mater

Any of three meninges. See *Pia, Arachnoid,* and *Dura Maters*.

Maxilla

Upper jaw bone.

Maximum Safe Concentration

The mean (from a trial population) maximum plasma concentration of a drug, above which it will start to become toxic.

McCoy Laryngoscope

For difficult airway situations, where the epiglottis obscures the view of the vocal cords. The tip of the blade is hinged, and manipulated by a long lever, so that the epiglottis can be lifted to reveal the view of the vocal cords that the anaesthetist needs.

Mean Airway Pressure (MPAW)

Mean airway pressure, during one cycle of mechanically assisted ventilation. Typically, 10-15 cmH_2O. *Note:* Some anaesthetic machines measure airway pressure in hPa (hectoPascals); multiply hPa by 1.02 to give cmH_2O. For such a small difference, it is reasonable to convert 1 to 1.

Mean Arterial Pressure (MAP)

During a single cardiac cycle, MAP is approximately the sum of diastolic and 1/3 pulse pressure (75-100 mmHg). More formally, MAP is the product of cardiac output and systemic vascular resistance, plus central venous pressure. For accuracy, the mean pressure can be calculated by taking the mean value from the integrated (summed) values of the pressures during one cardiac cycle. MAP is an indicator of perfusion.

Measured Flow Vapouriser

A vapouriser that has separate carrier gas and anaesthetic agent supplies, as opposed to *variable bypass* vapourisers where part of the carrier gas is channelled through a volatile agent chamber. An example vapouriser is the Ohmeda 885A.

Median Effective Dose (ED_{50})

Describes the drug dose that produces a desired effect in 50% of the population. The ED_{50} is the principle on which minimum alveolar concentration is formed.

Median Lethal Dose (LD_{50})

The drug dose that produces death in 50% of the population.

Mediastinum

The central section of the thorax, between the lungs, containing the heart, oesophagus, aorta, trachea, and thymus.

Medulla

Soft inner part of an organ e.g., kidney (outer part is the cortex).

Membrane

The very thin protective layer which surrounds a biological element, such as a cell, or blood vessel, through which some entities may pass. If a membrane is selective about what it lets through, it can be described as semi or selectively permeable.

Membrane Selectivity

Refers to how a membrane is permeable to only some cells.

Mendelson's Syndrome

Aspiration pneumonitis (alveoli inflammation); caused by pulmonary aspiration, during anaesthesia.

Meninges

Singular: *meninx*. Three membranes that surround and protect the brain and spinal cord. See *Pia*, *Arachnoid*, and *Dura maters*.

Mento-

Referring to the Mentum (chin).

Mesentery

Double layer of tissue that extends the peritoneum, and supports the intestines by attaching them to the abdominal wall.

Metabolic Acidosis

Accumulation of acid due to: increased acid production or ingestion, decreased acid secretion, GI or renal loss of bicarbonate. Metabolic acidosis can lead to an acidaemia (arterial pH < 7.35), where bicarbonate (HCO_3^-) ion level would fall below 22 mmol/L (22 mEq/L). A severe metabolic acidosis can cause HCO_3^- to fall below 12 mmol/L. **Causes**: increased acid production or ingestion, serum bicarbonate loss from the GI tract (NAGMA) by e.g., severe diarrhoea, sodium chloride, and inability of the kidneys to excrete excess H+ ions. Reasons for the acidosis include lactic acidosis, fasting, alcohol, toxins, anaerobic metabolism (e.g. in sepsis), severe dehydration, and ketoacidosis. **Symptoms**: tachycardia, tachypnoea, palpitations, fatigue, headache, Kussmaul breathing (diabetics), nausea, loss of appetite, confusion, breathing difficulty, vomiting. Common **treatment** is to give sodium bicarbonate to buffer (mop up) H+ ions, and address the underlying cause.

Metabolic Acidosis: Respiratory Compensation

The body's respiratory response to metabolic acidosis, with the aim of bringing pH back to the normal range, with reduced respiratory CO_2 level calculated by *Winter's Formula*:

$paCO_2 \sim (1.5 * HCO_3^-) + 8 +/- 2$ mmHg

If the blood gas $paCO_2$ is lower than expected, the patient may also have a primary respiratory alkalosis; alternatively, a higher than expected $paCO_2$ value means there may be a mixed respiratory/metabolic acidosis. Note: compensation does not swing to a respiratory alkalosis, so an alkalotic swing will probably be due to mixed acid/alkali cases.

Metabolic Alkalosis

The process that leads to alkalaemia (pH > 7.45), where serum bicarbonate can climb above 26 mmol/L (26 mEq/L). Two types:

① H+ ions lost due to vomiting, dehydration, or NG suctioning.

② Increased bicarbonate in the blood, or it shifts from blood into the cells.

Caused by: burns, severe vomiting (causes hypokalaemia and hyponatraemia, and loses H+ ions), kidney excretion (perhaps from diuretics) of H+, dehydration, diuretics, bicarbonate infusion, NG tube (removes H+ from stomach), hypovolaemia. **Signs**: vomiting, seizures, confusion, twitching, numbness, and tingling. Low potassium and low chloride are often associated with metabolic alkalosis. If a patient has metabolic acidosis, and vomits (lose H+) excessively, they can have both metabolic alkalosis and acidosis. Often associated with low potassium and chloride levels.

Metabolic Alkalosis: Respiratory Compensation

An expected respiratory acidotic compensation (to normalise pH) in metabolic alkalosis, calculated as:

$$paCO_2 \sim (0.7 * \{HCO_3^- - 24\}) + 40 \text{ mmHg} +/- 3$$

If blood gas $paCO_2$ is lower than expected, there may be a mixed respiratory/metabolic alkalosis. Conversely, a higher than expected blood gas level of $paCO_2$ suggests a mixed metabolic alkalosis/respiratory acidosis.

Metabolise

Verb: to change a substance by biological and chemical reactions.

Metabolism

The complete set of biological processes and chemical reactions that cause build up (anabolism) and break down (catabolism) of molecules. Metabolism also concerns the provision of energy (from food), and the synthesis of new bodily tissues.

Metabolites

Substances produced by metabolic processes.

Metaraminol

Sympathomimetic vasoconstrictor, for hypotension. Intravenous bolus dose is 0.5 mg from a 1 in 2,000 (10 mg in 20 ml NS) solution. For infusion, 15-100 mg. Can cause headache and ↑ BP and, rarely, extravasation and skin exfoliation at cannula site.

Metastasis

The spread of a disease condition, from its point of origin, to another part of the body. Usually refers to spread of cancer cells.

Methaemoglobin (MetHb)

Haemoglobin that cannot bind with oxygen: 0-1.5% of total.

Metformin

Prevents and treats Gestational and Type II diabetes.

Metoclopramide

Antiemetic. Contraindicated in GI bleeding, pregnancy, renal failure, liver failure, and bradycardia.

Metronidazole (Flagyl)

An antibiotic, commonly used for prophylaxis and treatment of anaerobic bacterial infections of the: respiratory tract, pelvis, vagina, pressure sores, and brain. (Brand name is *Flagyl*)

Microlaryngeal ET Tube (MLT)

A long but small diameter (4, 5, 6 mm) flexible endotracheal tube, designed for laryngeal surgical procedures.

Microlaryngoscopy

Endoscopic examination of the larynx (voice box).

Midazolam

A benzodiazepine sedative and anxiolytic, often used in local/regional anaesthesia. Can cause respiratory arrest (used in USA to perform executions), so Flumazenil should be immediately available. Dose: 1-3 microgram/kg, 1 in 1,000 w/v concentration. Onset: 90 secs. Duration: 25 mins. Contraindicated for conscious sedation of patients with respiratory failure.

Middle East Respiratory Syndrome (MERS-CoV)

A coronavirus, first identified in Saudi Arabia (2012), that affects the respiratory system. The original major reservoir of infection is probably dromedary camels. Transmission is by close contact.

Midline Catheter

Similar to a PICC line, but shorter, and terminating at the axillary vein, not the superior vena cava.

Miller Blade

Straight laryngoscope blade, used when a Macintosh blade fails to provide a good laryngeal view, such as with paediatric patients.

Minimum Alveolar Concentration (MAC)

The partial pressure of an anaesthetic agent, in the alveoli, which would prevent response to a standard surgical stimulus in 50% of a particular population of patients. MAC values are determined at Standard Temperature and Pressure. A lower MAC means higher potency. See Appendix A68 (pg 472).

Minimum Effective Concentration

The minimum plasma concentration of a drug that produces its intended effect.

Minute Ventilation

See Minute Volume.

Minute Volume (VE)

The volume of gas inhaled or exhaled from the alveoli in one minute: the product of respiratory rate and tidal volume: if, for example, the patient's tidal volume is 400 ml, and respiratory rate is 12, then Minute Volume is 4.8 litre. Anaesthetic drugs, with the exception of Ketamine, cause a reduction in Minute Volume.

Minute Volume Divider

Apparatus that ensures that Tidal Volume multiplied by respiratory rate equals the Minute Volume. If Minute Volume is eg, 4 litre, and the anaesthetic machine is set to deliver a Tidal Volume of 400 ml, then respiratory rate will be 10 breaths/minute.

Miosis

Constriction of the pupils.

Miscible

When two substances mix so they form a single (homogenous) substance. Oil and water are **im**miscible (don't mix).

Misoprostol

Prevention and treatment of stomach ulcers, initiates childbirth, treats post-childbirth bleeding.

Mitochondria

The “power station” of cells that use oxygen and glucose to make ATP (adenosine triphosphate), the source of energy supply.

Mitral Valve (bicuspid)

The one-way heart valve which allows blood to flow from the left atrium to the left ventricle.

Mivacurium Chloride

Short duration (10-25 min, twice suxamethonium) non-depolarising neuromuscular blocking drug. IV dose is 70-250 microgram/kg. Onset slower than for atracurium or vecuronium, but quicker spontaneous recovery.

Mixed Acid-Base Conditions

See Appendix A69 (pg 474).

Mixture

A substance produced from two or more other substances, where no chemical reactions occur, no chemical bonding takes place, and the component substances can be easily separated.

Modified Early Obstetric Warning Score (MEOWS)

Monitoring system to guide identification of deterioration in the expectant mother's condition.

Moffett's Solution

A topical solution, used in rhinological (nasal) procedures, consisting of adrenaline for vasoconstriction (reduces bleeding), cocaine for local anaesthesia, and sodium bicarbonate for decongestion. When applied nasally, the solution will be administered via a mucosal atomisation device (MAD) nasal cone.

Adrenaline	1 ml	1:1,000 w/v.
Cocaine	2 ml	10% w/v.
Sodium Bicarbonate	4 ml	8.4% w/v.
Normal Saline	13 ml	0.9%.

Moiety

In pharmacology, a *moiety* is a particular part of a drug molecule. An active moiety is the part of the molecule which is responsible for delivering the drug's intended function.

Molality

The number of moles of a substance contained in 1 kg of solution.

Molar Solution

One mole of solute per litre of solution.

Molar Volume (Vm)

Volume of one mole of a substance at Standard Temperature and Pressure, in m^3/mol (or litre/mol), determined by dividing molar mass by density. Molar volume of an ideal gas is 22.4 litre/mol.

Molarity

The number of moles of a substance, when contained in 1 litre of solution. Often referred to as *molar concentration.*

Mole

The S.I. unit of measurement for amount of a substance that contains as many elementary particles (atoms, ions, or molecules) as there are in Avogadro's Constant ($6.02214076 * 10^{23}$), which is also the number of atoms in 12 g of carbon-12 (^{12}C). In some countries, molar values are used, for example, when measuring blood glucose i.e., mmol/litre. Elsewhere, such as the U.S.A., blood glucose is measured in mg/dL (mg/100 ml). An understanding of molar measurement, allows the molar concentration of a solution to be converted to a mass/volume (commonly known as weight/volume) value. For example, 40 mmol of Potassium Chloride (74.55 g/mol), in 20 ml of solvent, has a weight/volume concentration of 14.9%.

Monocyte

The largest white blood cell (leukocyte) type; ingests bacterial cells.

Morbidity

The state of disease or poor health; the higher the morbidity the poorer the state of health. Not to be confused with "mortality".

Morphine

Gold standard for controlling pain; long lasting (3 hours) but slow onset opiate. **Side-effects**: respiratory depression, nausea, vomiting, constipation. **Dose** 0.1 mg/kg from 1 mg/ml w/v.

Motor score

Scheme to describe a patient's ability to mobilise the lower limbs.

0 : Can bend knees and lift legs

1 : Can bend knees and slide legs apart

2 : Can wiggle toes, but unable to bend knees

3 : Unable to move legs

Moulage

Simulated injuries for training purposes.

Mucosal Atomisation Device (MAD)

A soft cone shaped bean sized "sponge", fitted to a syringe, to provide a seal, when applied to a nostril, where an atomised agent, such as Moffett's, is sprayed to the nasal mucosa, which absorbs the agent. Commonly used in ENT cases. See also *Laryngo-Tracheal Mucosal Atomization Device*.

Multiple Organ Dysfunction Syndrome (MODS)

Deterioration of two or more organs, secondary to primary injury (such as burns, trauma, or sepsis), and which initiates systemic inflammatory response syndrome and tissue damage. See *SOFA*.

Muscarinic

A (cholinergic) receptor for acetylcholine. Parasympathetic muscarinic effects include: bradycardia, smooth muscle contraction, miosis, bronchiole constriction, increased tear duct and glandular secretions. Neostigmine has muscarinic effects, so is usually given with glycopyrrolate, a muscarine antagonist.

Muscle

Tissue that contracts to produce movement or constriction. ***Smooth*** muscle applies pressure to organs, when signalled by the autonomic nervous system, by nerve impulses or hormone "messages". For example, by controlling the level of contraction of the smooth muscle of blood vessels, blood pressure can be modified. ***Cardiac*** (heart) muscle (myocardium), automatically contracts and relaxes to create the process of cardiac rhythm, or heart beat. ***Skeletal*** muscle is attached to the skeletal system by tendons, and facilitates voluntary movement and posture.

Myalgia

Muscular pain.

Myasthenia Gravis

An auto-immune disease, which attacks Acetylcholine receptors at the neuromuscular junctions of skeletal muscles. Resultant failure of neuro transmission causes muscle weakness, often affecting muscles that control chewing, speaking, swallowing, and vision.

Myo-

Referring to muscle.

Myocardial Infarction (MI)

Heart attack: Necrosis of part of the heart muscle, due to interrupted blood supply, commonly following a coronary thrombosis (artery occlusion). An MI is an Acute Coronary Syndrome, and has three sub-types: **STEMI** (ST segment elevated

MI) - the most serious type; **NSTEMI** (Non ST segment elevated); **coronary spasm** (unstable angina), which is the least serious.

Myocarditis

Inflammation of the heart muscle, often caused by a virus.

Myocardium

Muscle tissue of the heart.

Myopathy

A disease state where muscular tissue is dysfunctional.

NaCl

The chemical compound of sodium chloride.

NAGMA

See Normal Anion Gap Metabolic Acidosis.

Naloxone (Narcan)

A competitive antagonist of opioid receptors, to counter opioid depression of the central nervous system: 400 microgram IV.

Nasal Cannula

A device that fits in the nostrils (via prongs), to provide low flow oxygen (20-40%) to a spontaneously breathing patient. For long term use, or when flow > 4 L/min, the oxygen should be humidified. Flow rates for oxygen concentration, L/min: 1 L=14%, 2 L=28%, 3 L=32%, 4 L=36%. See also Appendix A70.

Nasal Intubation

Intubation through the nose if oral intubation not possible, due to pathology, trauma, or poor mouth opening, or oral tube interferes with the surgical field. The tube may be polar (north/south facing), or armoured. Sprayed anaesthetic may be required, so have MAD nasal cone and MADgic LMA devices available.

Nasogastric (NG) Tube

Radio opaque tube that is passed through the nose and oesophagus to the stomach, allowing stomach contents to be drained into a bag, or aspirated by syringe. The tube weakens the gastroesophageal sphincter, and makes regurgitation of stomach contents more likely, shown by increased intragastric pressure (the basis of vomiting). Some NG tube types are used to provide nutrition, but not usually in theatres. Estimate insertion length by passing the tube from nose to ear, then to the xiphisternum, plus 2" (5 cm). To check proper placement requires X-ray, or using pH indicator paper to ensure pH is < 4. If the NG tube is in the trachea, pH will probably be ~6.6, or 7.38, if in a lung.

Nasopharyngeal (nasal) Airway

A nasal airway that is less likely to induce gagging than an oropharyngeal airway, and can be used (lubricated) in a conscious patient. It can be life-saving in a patient with a clenched jaw, trismus (lockjaw), or maxillofacial injuries.

National Early Warning Score

See NEWS2.

NCEPOD

National Confidential Enquiry into Patient Outcome and Death: A classification system for surgical patients:

Grade	*Type*	*Description*
1	Emergency	Operation within 1 hour. Resuscitation simultaneous with

		surgical treatment.
2	Urgent	Operation: 1 to 3 hours. Early surgery, but not life saving.
3	Scheduled	Operation within 24 hours. Delayed operation after resuscitation.
4	Elective	Operation at time to suit team and patient.

Nebuliser

A device to convert a liquid carrier of a drug, such as salbutamol or magnesium sulphate, to a fine mist, which is inhaled through a mask or ET tube, for the treatment of respiratory disorders.

Necrosis

Death of cells and tissues, typically due to poor perfusion.

Negative Pressure Leak Test

On an anaesthetic machine, this test identifies a gas leak upstream of the gas outlet. The patient circuit leak test will not detect the upstream leak, because there is a one-way valve between the patient circuit and the gas outlet.

Negative Pressure Pulmonary Oedema

A form of non-cardiogenic pulmonary oedema, caused by generation of negative intrathoracic pressure that is needed to overcome upper airway obstruction. May occur in otherwise healthy individuals, who can generate the high negative intrathoracic pressure.

Negative Pressure Wound Therapy

A dressing that involves use of a vacuum pump to draw out infected fluids from the wound.

Neoplasia

The formation of new abnormal cells, or an abnormal number of new cells, caused by a process which may be malignant.

Neoplasm

Cells produced by neoplasia.

Neostigmine Methylsulfate

An anticholinesterase solution (2.5 mg neostigmine + 0.5 mg glycopyrrolate) to reverse the effect of non-depolarizing muscle blockade agents, such as atracurium, by neutralising acetylcholinesterase. Results in a quicker reversal of blockade. Some muscarinic side-effects (antagonised by glycopyrrolate) include bradycardia, increased bronchial secretions and salivation. Onset is ~ 1 minute; duration is ~ 20 minutes. Neostigmine does not enter the autonomic nervous system ganglia, so cannot cross the blood-brain barrier. See *Anticholinesterase*.

Nephro-

Concerning the kidneys.

Nerve

Nerves (100s), found in the peripheral nervous system, are bundles of *neurons* (plus connective tissue and blood vessels). ***Afferent*** nerves send **sensory** information to the brain and spinal cord, and ***efferent*** nerves send **motor** information from the brain to effector muscles and glands. A nerve serves a specific region of the body. There are 12 pairs of cranial nerves, and 31 pairs of spinal nerves.

Nerve Blockade (Neural Block)

To allow painless limb surgery, without general anaesthesia, a regional technique can be used, where the patient is awake, but pain relief is enabled by blocking nerve transmission of a particular nerve, by the anaesthetist, who injects local anaesthetic around the relevant nerve plexus. See Appendix A90 (pg 503).

Nerve Plexus

A point where a number of nerves meet – like trains meeting at a station. The nerves supply the same area of the body so, collectively, they function as a single nerve supply. An example is the Brachial Plexus, which includes thoracic (T1) and cervical (C5-8) nerves – a common target in regional blocks for arm surgery.

Nerve Stimulator

Electrical stimulator for locating a nerve or nerve plexus when performing blockade for regional anaesthesia. Another type is for monitoring of **neuromuscular blockade** (See *Train of Four*).

Neuraxial Nerve Block

A regional anaesthetic (blockade) technique, where local anaesthetic is infiltrated around the nerves of the spinal canal, to provide caudal, epidural, or spinal anaesthesia.

Neuraxis

Referrring to the nervous system – brain and spinal cord.

Neuroleptic Drugs

Drugs which act on the nervous system.

Neuromuscular Blocking Agent/Drug (NMBA/D)

Muscle relaxants provide blockade to the neuromuscular junction, by competing with the acetylcholine neurotransmitter, thereby preventing normal receptor binding and resultant muscle depolarisation. Their purpose is to (1) enable muscle paralysis so that endotracheal tube placement can be made, by preventing muscle contractions, and (2) facilitate some types of surgery, where non-relaxed muscles might impede the procedure.

Neuromuscular Junction

The synapse between the pre-synaptic motor neuron and the post-synaptic muscle membrane, where neurotransmitters cross.

Neuron

Electrically excitable nerve cell, with cell body (soma), nucleus, dendrites, and an axon. The cell body receives impulses, via the dendrites, and the axon carries impulses away from the cell body, towards other neurons, glands, or effector cells. A neuron responds to a stimulus, by creating an action potential (impulse), which is propagated to its neighbouring neuron. Two types of neuron: *Sensory* neurons send signals to the spinal cord and brain; *Motor* neurons send signals from spinal cord and brain to muscles and glands. A group of neurons form a nerve.

Neurotransmitter

A chemical messenger, between nerve cells, which is released to carry signals between neurons. When a nerve impulse (action potential) arrives at a nerve's axon terminal, neurotransmitters are released, and they diffuse across the synapse between the neuron and the adjacent neuron. When the neurotransmitters bind with the receiving neuron's receptors, they exert their effect by exciting or inhibiting the receiving neuron. If the neurotransmitter is excitatory, such as adrenaline or noradrenaline, its purpose is to propagate an action potential. Inhibitory neurotransmitters, such as serotonin, prevent propagation of action potentials.

Neurotransmitter examples

☺ Substance P	☺ Dopamine	☺ Noradrenaline	
☺ Acethlcholine	☺ Adrenaline	☺ Histamine	
☺ Noradrenaline	☺ Serotonin	☺ GABA	☺ Serotonin

NEWS2

The latest version of the National Early Warning Score *Track and Trigger* system, produced by the Royal College of Physicians; uses physiological parameters to anticipate trends in the patient's condition (high score = high warning, and more vigilance needed).

Scoring parameters

- Respiratory Rate (RR)
- **SpO2 % 2***
- Systolic Blood Pressure
- ACVPU (CNS)**
- SpO2 % 1
- Air or O2
- Pulse (HR)
- Temperature

* **SpO2 % 2** Measurement if patient has hypercapnic respiratory failure (from blood gas), otherwise use **SpO2 % 1**.

** **ACVPU** If the patient has a newly confused state, or has become agitated, the ACVPU score should be set to 3.

Risk *Low:* Aggregate score of 0-4. *Low:* Score of 3 in any one parameter. *Medium*: Score 5-6. *High*: 7+. Risk of infection and score > 4 gives risk of sepsis. See Appendix A43 (pg 427).

Newton

The S.I. derived unit of force, giving a mass of 1 kg an acceleration of 1 metre per second per second (1 N = 1 kg * m/s^2). During rapid sequence induction, the amount of force to be applied to the cricoid cartilage, is deemed to be 30 newtons.

NICE Surgical Severity Grades

National Institute for Health and Care Excellence classification system for surgical severity. Grades and surgery examples:

1: MINOR: Excision of skin lesion, abscess drainage.

2: INTERMEDATE: Knee arthroscopy, Varicose veins, Tonsillectomy, Inguinal Hernia.

3: MAJOR: Lumbar resection, Hysterectomy, Thyroidectomy.

4: MAJOR+: Bowel or lung resection, Total joint replacement, Cardiac or Neuro surgery.

Nicotinic

Acetylcholine receptors on skeletal muscle end-plate neurons. Activation by acetylcholine causes depolarisation of cells, with resultant contraction of skeletal muscle.

Nissen Fundoplication

See Fundoplication.

Nitrogen (N_2, Nitrogen)

An inert gas, the most abundant in the atmosphere.

Nitrogen Narcosis

The narcotic effects felt when breathing nitrogen at a partial pressure in excess of approximately 4 bar, absolute. Divers, breathing air, will start to experience nitrogen narcosis at depths greater than 100 feet (30 metres). No medical intervention is necessary, because the narcosis reduces in line with the reduction in partial pressure of nitrogen, during ascent to surface pressure.

Nitrous Oxide (N_2O, Dinitrogen Monoxide), *Laughing Gas*

An inhalational gas, used to supplement other anaesthetic gases, such as Sevoflurane. N_2O depresses cardiac function, and has a low blood:gas partition coefficient (0.47, very absorbed by the blood) so has a rapid onset of action (rapid wash in/out). N_2O increases blood flow in the brain, so should be avoided in patients with high intracranial pressure. See Appendix A71 (pg 476).

NIV

Non Invasive.

NMBA

See Neuromuscular Blocking Agent.

Nociceptor

A pain receptor – sends "threat" information to the CNS.

N.O.D.E.S.A.T.

Nasal Oxygen During Efforts Securing A Tube: The attempt to extend the safe apnoea time by fitting the patient with a nasal cannula, at an oxygen flow rate of 15 L/min, during intubation attempts. Similar to the THRIVE concept, but without the "jet" type equipment required for higher flow rates.

Nomogram

A graphical system that enables the user to find a pre-calculated value, without having to perform a calculation, using intersecting values on a chart. Often used to determine drug dosages, from Body Surface Area, for paediatric patients.

Non-competitive Antagonist

A substance that binds to an allosteric (non-agonist) site on the receptor, and so prevents receptor activation (think of preventing a car moving by clamping a wheel).

Non-depolarising Neuromuscular Block

Non-depolarising muscle relaxant drugs (NMBDs), such as Atracurium, compete with acetylcholine (ACh) molecules, released at the neuromuscular junction, to bind with nicotinic receptors on the post synaptic membrane of the motor end-plate. These drugs **block** the action of ACh, which prevents depolarisation and contraction of the muscle. The blocking agents cause relaxation of the diaphragm, abdomen, and vocal cords, so the patient requires assisted ventilation, during anaesthesia. Muscle groups differ in their sensitivity to muscle relaxants; the ocular muscles, which are responsible for moving the eyes, are the most sensitive, followed by the muscles of the jaw, neck, limbs, intercostals, and abdomen. The diaphragm is the least sensitive muscle, which is why surgical patients sometimes hiccup, as an early sign that the relaxants are wearing off. The usual reversal agent for the block is Neostigmine.

Non Interchangeable Screw Thread (NIST)

Fitting between flexible pipeline and anaesthetic machine, with gas specific profile, to prevent connecting to the wrong flexible pipeline to the outlet. A one-way valve prevents back flow.

Non Invasive Positive Pressure Ventilation (NIPPV)

Delivery of positive pressure ventilation, to keep alveoli open, via a tight fitting face or nasal mask, or helmet, by two methods: **Type 1** - CPAP, and **Type 2** - Bi-level Positive Airway Pressure (BiPAP).

Non-rebreathing Circuit

Circuit where expired gases are expelled to the atmosphere, normally via a one-way valve. Non-rebreathing systems provide good control of inspired gas concentrations, since fresh gas is inspired in each breath, but they are less economical than re-breathing systems, because the minute volume of ventilation (or more) must be supplied to the patient to prevent re-breathing, and they contribute more to atmospheric pollution. They are also less forgiving of operator error, since an inadequate fresh gas supply will result in re-breathing. A design failure is that they do not provide a seal, with the result that ambient air will be entrained.

Non-rebreathing Mask

Provides a spontaneously breathing patient with an oxygen concentration (FiO_2) of 80-90% (if good seal), at a flow rate > 10 L/min, whilst exhausting expired carbon dioxide through 1-way valves in the side of the mask. The patient should not be left untended, in case the gas supply becomes disconnected, because the valves would prevent breathing of the room air. Some mask device types have an incorporated reservoir bag, which is also protected by a 1-way valve, so allowing the patient to breathe in, with minimum extra effort, due to minimal dead space. Non-rebreather masks should only be used for short periods, then replaced by eg, CPAP or intubation. Note: the bag should be inflated BEFORE being put on the patient, and should have a gas flow that is enough to prevent complete bag deflation. If the bag does not partially deflate when the patient breathes in, the gas flow must be too high, so must be reduced.

Non Steroidal Anti-inflammatory Drugs (NSAIDs)

NSAIDs are a widely used class of drugs, with three main uses:

√ Pain relief - particularly postoperatively

√ Reduce inflammation

√ Reduce temperature (fever)

See Appendix A72 (pg 477).

Noradrenaline (USA: Norepinephrine)

A hormone and sympathetic nerve neurotransmitter, whose action is opposite to acetylcholine. When blood pressure is low, due to vasodilation, the adrenal gland releases noradrenaline, which constricts blood vessels (α1 receptors). A pharmalogical noradrenaline infusion is often used for sympathomimetic purposes, such as with vasodilatory shock (acute hypotension), after the patient has been properly hydrated. Extravasation can cause tissue necrosis, so infusion through a central line is recommended. Administration by infusion is because noradrenaline has a short half life, and BP should be constantly monitored, so an arterial line is usually necessary for real-time BP values. To raise BP, noradrenaline is preferred over adrenaline because it binds mostly with α receptors, found in arteries, and has much less binding with β receptors, whereas adrenaline binds readily with α and β receptors. Noradrenaline can also be used to raise blood sugar levels, increase heart rate (β1 receptors), and increase heart contractility (β1 receptors).

Normal Anion Gap Metabolic Acidosis (NAGMA)

Metabolic acidosis with normal Anion Gap (4-12 mmol/L). In NAGMA, causes of the metabolic acidosis include: low bicarbonate (GI and renal loss) and replacement with Cl-, Addisons Disease, high chloride level, drugs, and Renal Tubular Acidosis. See *Anion Gap*, *Albumin*, and Appendix A9.

Normal Saline (NS)

An isotonic crystalloid: When sodium chloride (NaCl) is added to water, it dissociates into sodium (+) and chloride (-) ions, and forms a 0.9% weight/volume solution - isotonic with blood and body fluids. Molarity is 0.154. Being isotonic with blood, NS does not cause fluid shift in or out of cells, which is why it is called "normal", and making it useful as a drug diluent and line "flush". Too much NS can cause hyperchloraemic (metabolic) acidosis.

Normotension

A normal blood pressure reading: 120/80.

Normothermia

Normal body temperature; approximately 37 degrees Celsius.

Normoxaemia

A normal blood concentration of oxygen (paO_2), according to the patient and condition. Typically, 85-95 mmHg (11-12.5 kPa).

Nosocomial

A disease state, such as infection, which originates in hospital.

NRFit Connector

Braun small bore connector type devices (coloured yellow), specifically for neuraxial and regional anaesthesia - including slip, loss of resistance, and locking **syringes**; filter, epidural, and spinal **needles**; catheter **connectors** and **filters**. Purpose: dedicated connector type prevents inadvertent connection with Luer lock intravenous connectors. Specified by ISO-80369-6.

NSTEMI (Non ST Elevation Myocardial Infarction)

A heart attack, less serious than a STEMI, with less of the heart muscle affected, and only a partial blockage of the blood supply.

O_2Hb

See Oxyhaemoglobin.

Obesity

{BMI > 30} Obese patients experience reduced functional lung volume, and are more likely to pose anaesthetic problems, due to greater probability of: hypertension, gastroesophageal reflux, airway obstruction, quicker desaturation, sleep apnoea, hypercapnia, reduced FRC, vasoconstriction, difficult mask ventilation and intubation. **Prepare**: ramping aids, airways, bougies, suction catheters, video laryngoscope, hover mattress, etc., and possibility of intubation in sitting up position.

Obesity Hypoventilation Syndrome

A ventilation disorder, often caused by upper airway obstruction, as a consequence of obesity, where the patient also suffers type 2 respiratory failure (hypoxaemia plus hypercapnia). Sufferers are prone to chronic respiratory acidosis.

Obstructive Airway Disease

Conditions such as asthma, cystic fibrosis, emphysema, and bronchitis, where the volume of gas flow through the airway is limited by constrictions, inflammation, or pathological barriers.

Obstructive Shock

An obstruction in the heart's larger vessels that reduces cardiac output. **Causes**: aortic stenosis, pericardial effusion, pulmonary embolism, cardiac tamponade, or tension pneumothorax. **Symptoms**: breathing difficulty, increased respiratory rate, cyanosis, tachycardia, cold extremities, chest pain, and signs of congestion on the face and jugular vein.

Obtund

The numbing of tissue, in order to facilitate surgical or other manipulation. Obtunding the airway, for example, aids intubation.

Obturator

Something which closes an opening.

Occiput

The bone at the back and base of the skull.

Occult

Something "occult" is hidden from normal view. A blood test, for example, may reveal a condition not otherwise discernible.

Octopus Connector

A proprietary name (Vygon) for a multi lumen extension tube for intravenous catheters, with one-way valves and colour coded lumen constriction clamps.

Oedema

Excess interstitial fluid in tissues, causing swelling. **Peripheral** oedema is from accumulation of fluid in the hands or lower legs.

Lymphoedema: Lymph fluid in the interstitial space.

Lipoedema: A chronic condition where fat builds up in the legs and buttocks – rarely in the arms.

Gravitational: Build up of fluid in the lower body, due to immobility.

Lymphovenous: Oedema caused by problems with the lymphatic and/or venous systems. Compression, elevation, and exercise are typical treatments.

Caused by...

- Obesity
- Allergy
- Varicose veins
- DVT
- Immobility
- Pregnancy
- Right heart failure

Oesophageal Doppler

See CardioQ Doppler Monitor.

Oesophageal Intubation

Inadvertent placement of an endotracheal tube - into the oesophagus.

Indications include...

- Abnormal lung sounds
- Absent chest expansion
- Distended stomach
- Oesophageal sounds
- Abnormal and shrinking end tidal CO_2 values

If left uncorrected, the patient will become hypoxic, and deteriorate towards an emergency cardiac episode.

Oesophago Gastro Duodenoscopy (OGD)

An examination of the oesophagus, stomach, and duodenum by gastroscope, under sedation or general anaesthetic. If the patient is to be anaesthetised, intubation will be with a reinforced endotracheal tube, the patient's eyes will be protected by padding, and their head will be placed on an inco-pad protected pillow.

Oesophagoscopy

Endoscopic examination of the oesophagus.

Oesophagus (Gullet)

A muscular tube (8 inch, 20 cm), lined with mucosa, that allows the passage of food between the pharynx and stomach. Unlike the trachea, the oesophagus does not include cartilage.

Oil:Gas Partition Coefficient (OGPC)

The concentration of an inhalational agent in the brain (lipid/oil), compared with concentration in the alveolar space (gas phase), when pressures are equal. An inhalational agent must cross the blood-brain barrier, to reach the CNS, where it exerts its effect. An agent with high OGPC, such as Isoflurane, has high potency, because it reaches the CNS more easily, than agents with lower OPGC. MAC and OGPC values are inversely related.

Oliguria

Deficient elimination of urine, and one sign of poor perfusion or hypovolaemia: less than 500 ml/day for adults; 0.5 ml/kg/hour for children; less than 1 ml/kg/hour for infants.

-oma

Referring to a mass, such as a tumour.

Omentum

Layers of visceral peritoneum that store fat, and hold macrophages. **Lesser Omentum**: a double fold of peritoneum extending from the lesser curvature of the stomach and duodenum to the liver. The 4 layers of the **Greater Omentum** extend from the greater curvature of the stomach and duodenum, then fold back to attach to the anterior transverse colon.

Onco-

Refers to a tumour.

Oncology

The study of tumours.

Oncotic Pressure

Colloid osmotic pressure, exerted by plasma proteins (mostly albumin) in capillaries, that draws fluid inwards, as opposed to hydrostatic pressure, which exerts pressure outwards against the walls of the capillaries.

Ondansetron

An anti-emetic, given at induction of anaesthesia.

One-way Valve (USA: Check Valve)

A mechanical device that allows a fluid to move in one direction only. Also known as a *uni-directional* valve.

Opiate

A naturally occurring alkaloid from resin of the poppy fibre and sap. Used in the production of Morphine, Diamorphine (heroin), and Codeine, Methadone, Oxycodone. Opiates work by agonising the body's opioid receptors (mu, kappa, delta, and ORL-1) to produce narcotic sedation, and analgesia.

Opioid

A molecule that acts (ligand) on opioid receptors in the brain, digestive tract, and spinal cord, producing analgesia, caused by the release of dopamine (pleasure molecule), and suppression of gamma-aminobutyric acid. Opioid" refers to Class A drugs - any synthetic derivative of the poppy plant, that mimics the effects of natural opiates. The term "opioid" refers to both opioids and opiates. (Note: all opiates are opioids, because they act on opioid receptors, but synthetic opioids are not opiates). Opioid drugs act on opioid receptors, but start to work at different "speeds", because they have different levels of lipid solubility (lipophilicity), so cross the blood-CSF fluid barrier at different speeds; eg, alfentanil crosses the barrier quickly, but morphine is much slower, so takes longer before it starts to work. **Side effects** of opioids: respiratory depression, nausea, vomiting, arrhythmias, constipation, dry mouth, muscle stiffness, headache, palpitations, urinary retention, drowsiness, hypotension, itching. Synthetic opioids: fentanyl, hydrocodone, methadone, oxycodone, tramadol.

Opioid Overdose

Causes respiratory depression, signified by a low minute volume, with resultant hypercapnia.

Symptoms

- Pin-point pupils
- Slow respiratory rate
- Sighing
- Hypercapnia
- Hypoxia

Reverse with Naloxone. Stimulate respiration with Doxapram.

Optiflow

Nasal high flow therapy device, which delivers a 40 litre/minute flow of gas to the patient, and which has been optimally heated and humidified, for comfort. See Appendix A74 (pg 479).

Oropharyngeal Airway

When unconscious, the muscles in the jaw relax, allowing the tongue to obstruct the airway. An oropharyngeal (eg, Guedel) airway device maintains a patent airway, by preventing the tongue from covering the epiglottis, which could otherwise prevent breathing. Size is chosen by measuring from the corner of the mouth to tip of the earlobe. The airway is then inserted into the patient's mouth, facing backwards. Once contact is made with the back of the throat, the airway is rotated 180 degrees.

Ortho-

Greek for "straight".

Orthogonal

Involving right angles, such as when two things are perpendicular to each other.

Osmolality

The concentration of osmotically active particles, in a solution, measured as osmoles of solute per kg of solvent. It is osmolality in the blood which governs production of Anti Diuretic Hormone which, itself, stimulates reabsorption of water, with the consequent reduced concentration of plasma. A test of urine osmolality indicates the concentration of compounds, such as sodium urea, potassium, and glucose. The results can help to show effective kidney function, and any imbalance of electrolytes. Blood osmolality tests can indicate various conditions, such as *Diabetes Mellitus*, and excessive levels of, for example, sodium or calcium.

Osmolarity (Osmotic Concentration)

The concentration of osmotically active particles, in a solution. Measurement is given as osmoles of solute per litre of solution.

Osmole

Mole of a substance that contributes to osmotic pressure. If a molecule dissociates into separate particles, the osmotic pressure exerted by the separate particle types contribute to the osmole count. If the molecule dissociates into two moles of distinct particle types, and both substances contribute to osmosis, then there are two moles of osmotically active substances (2 osmoles).

Osmosis

The passive and net diffusion of solvent, such as water, through a partially permeable (for the solvent) membrane, from a low (more dilute) concentration of solutes, to a higher concentration. This movement, driven by the internal energy of the solute molecules, tends to equalize the concentration of solute on each side. Osmosis is a key factor in water balance, specifically in the nephrons, where osmosis controls reabsorption of water.

Osmotic Pressure

Pressure that would have to be applied to a solution to prevent the net flow of solvent across a semi-permeable membrane.

-ostomy

A surgically created opening.

-otomy

Referring to an incision to make an opening.

Oxford Help Pillow

Ramping and head support, to aid intubation of bariatric patients.

Oxide

A compound of oxygen bound to 1 other element. Examples: water (H_2O), carbon dioxide (CO_2), nitrogen dioxide (NO_2), carbon monoxide (CO), and N_2O (nitrous oxide).

Oximetry

Measurement of the fraction of Hb (haemoglobin) that is saturated with O_2 (oxygen), with four O_2 molecules per Hb, measured by pulse oximeter (estimation), or blood gas machine. The value (SpO_2) provided is referred to as “Sats”. A pulse oximeter gives a value of **SpO2** by passing two wavelengths (660, 940 nm) of light through the finger (or toe, earlobe, babies=foot), using an infrared electromagnetic wave sensor to detect the amount of light absorbed by oxygenated capillary blood, giving a value as a fraction of how much of the Hb is oxygenated. A blood gas machine measures oxygen saturation (**SaO2**) from a blood sample. A normal level of O2 saturation is 95-100%, but lower in patients with respiratory and cardiac disorders, or low pH. Hb concentration (ctHb) has no affect on O2 saturation, so a good sats value eg, 99%, does NOT always mean proper tissue oxygenation, such as in anaemia, where the number of Hb molecules (ctHb) is low. Oximetry is not accurate during cardiac arrest, and surgical dyes, such as methylene blue, can give false low readings. A basic oximeter does not detect Hb loaded with carbon monoxide (COHb), or methaemoglobin (defective Hb), which means if 10% Hb is COHb, 10% is methaemoglobin, and the remaining 80% is normal Hb, fully bound with oxygen, then the oximeter will read as 100% oxygen saturation, but the real value is only 80%, and the patient will be hypoxic. Anaemia can also give a false high reading, because a low level of Hb, which is 100% oxygen saturated, does not provide the full oxygen level the patient needs – so will be hypoxic. See also *CO-Oximetry, Oxygen Saturation*. Special CO-oximeters are needed for accuracy in patients with suspected CO (carbon monoxide) poisoning, or have methaemoglobin.

Oxygen (O2)

Element number eight on the Periodic Table which, when existing as a two atom molecule, provides life to many organisms, including humans. O2 constitutes ~ 21% of atmospheric air and, at *Standard Atmospheric Pressure*, has ~19.6 kPa partial pressure, and can support life within a range of 15–30 kPa (150–300 mBar) [the value of 19.6 kPa is derived from standard atmospheric pressure, minus water vapour pressure, times 21%: **101 – 7.4 = 93.6, * 0.21 = 19.6**]. At higher partial pressures, O_2 becomes toxic, with toxic effects increasing in severity as the pressure and/or duration increases. O_2 diffuses across the very thin alveolar/capillary membrane (blood gas barrier), but diffusion can be degraded (diffusion limitation) by damage or thickening to the membrane. O_2 is not very soluble in blood, and only 1-2% is dissolved in the plasma, so 98-99% O_2 molecules are transported by Hb molecules. It is the O_2 dissolved in plasma - not in Hb - that provides the reading for paO_2 (partial pressure of O_2 in arterial blood). A red blood cell carries 270 million Hb molecules, 100 ml of blood carries 12-18 g of Hb, and each Hb can hold 4 O_2 molecules. There is 15-22 ml O_2 per 100 ml blood.

Oxygen (O_2) Capacity

The maximum amount of O_2, in a particular volume of blood, if all of the haemoglobin (Hb) molecules were completely loaded by O_2 molecules (4 O_2 per Hb). The practical limit is ~ 1.34 ml O_2 per gram of Hb, or 20 ml per 100 ml of blood.

Oxygen Cascade

Step down cascade of oxygen pressure (pO_2) starts at inhaled atmospheric pressure, with a standard value being 160 mmHg (21 kPa). As the oxygen makes its way through the trachea, pO_2 pressure becomes diluted to 150 mmHg by the pressure of water vapour and carbon dioxide. When it reaches the alveoli, pO_2 drops to ~104 mg/Hg (14 kPa). By the time the oxygen reaches the arterial blood, its pressure has reduced again to 90-100 mmHg (12-13 kPa). In the mitochondria, the pressure is ~ 40 mmHg (5.3 kPa), and drops to 30-38 mmHg (4-5 kPa), in venous blood.

Oxygen Concentration (CaO_2)

Volume of oxygen per 100 ml of arterial blood, maximum 20 ml.

Oxygen Dissociation Curve

See Oxyhaemoglobin Dissociation Curve.

Oxygen Elevator

See Apnoeic Oxygenation.

Oxygen Flush

Low pressure facility, which flushes 100% oxygen to an anaesthetic machine's breathing circuit, bypassing flow meters and vaporisers.

Oxygen Saturation (Sats)

The % of haemoglobin (Hb) molecules that are bound with oxygen molecules. If all Hb molecules are bound with oxygen, saturation is 100%. For acutely ill patients, not at risk of Type 2 respiratory Failure, target sats is 94-98%. **SpO_2** refers to oxygen saturation in peripheral capillaries, measured by non-invasive pulse oximeter, whereas **SaO_2** refers to oxygen saturation of arterial blood, measured by blood gas machine. If all Hb molecules are "filled" with oxygen molecules (4 per Hb), an increase in inspired oxygen flow will not increase the oxygen carried by Hb – it is already 100% saturated. See also *Oximetry, SaO_2, and SpO_2*.

Oxygen Toxicity

Condition resulting from the harmful effects of breathing molecular oxygen at elevated partial pressures. Severe cases can result in cell damage and death, with effects most often seen in the central nervous system, lungs and eyes, through damage to lipids, proteins, and nucleic acids. Oxygen toxicity is a concern for those on high concentrations of oxygen - particularly premature babies - and those having hyperbaric oxygen therapy. If a greater oxygen concentration than 60% is given for over 24 hours, permanent alveolar membrane damage may occur.

Symptoms...

- Anxiety
- Vision changes
- Tonic-Clonic Seizure
- Vomiting
- Disorientation
- Breathing problems

Oxygenation

The process of providing tissues with oxygen. Increased fraction of inspired oxygen should cause increased arterial partial pressure of oxygen, whilst a decrease has the opposite effect. Oxygenating the patient's tissues is the anaesthetist's primary goal.

Oxygenation Index

A value, which illustrates how well the arteries have been oxygenated, for particular values of MAP (mean airway pressure) (cmH_2O), arterial oxygen partial pressure (paO_2, mmHg), and fraction of inspired oxygen: **MAP * 100 * FiO_2 / paO_2**. A high index, such as **10**, suggests poor respiratory function. A low value, such as **4**, means better function. If > 40, ECMO may be required.

Oxyhaemoglobin (O_2Hb)

A haemoglobin (Hb) molecule bound with oxygen molecules – to a maximum of four oxygen molecules per Hb.

Oxyhaemoglobin Dissociation Curve

The sigmoid curve (X axis=paO_2, Y axis=% Hb saturation) that illustrates how the binding of O_2 to Hb (haemoglobin) is a function of the partial pressure of the O_2 to which the Hb is exposed. The higher the O_2 partial pressure, the greater the O_2 affinity for Hb (cooperative binding) and, hence, increased O_2 saturation.

Increasing acidity shifts the curve to the right (Bohr Effect), which means that acidity reduces Hb's affinity for O_2, compensated by increasing higher O_2 partial pressure (pO_2).

Oxylog Ventilator 3000

A portable ventilator, produced by Drager, to allow transfer of ventilated patients between eg, ICU and Operating Theatre.

Oxytocin

A hormone, produced by the hypothalamus, released by the pituitary gland, is a chemical messenger in childbirth and lactation. Normally released towards the end of pregnancy, to stimulate smooth muscle of the uterus, causing contractions, so that the baby can be pushed out. See also *Syntocinon*.

P- (p-)

Prefix to indicate pressure, or partial pressure, of the succeeding term (choice of case is personal preference), for example: pAO_2 and PAO_2 refer to pressure of alveoli oxygen.

Pacemaker 1

Matchbox sized implanted device to detect when the heart is not beating at a proper rate or rhythm (eg, uncoordinated ventricular contraction), then sends a signal, through pacing leads, to 1 or 2 chambers, to stimulate a normal rhythm. Pacemakers can suffer electromagnetic interference, such as when diathermy (especially monopolar) is used, so the pacemaker may have to be put into a triggered or asynchronous mode, unless bipolar diathermy is deemed to be safe. See also *CRT-P*.

Pacemaker 2

The Sinoatrial Node.

Pachymetry

Measurement of a cornea's thickness, prior to ophthalmic surgery.

Packed Cells

See Red Blood Cells.

Packing

A technique to stop uncontrollable bleeding, by tightly placing gauze swabs into the wound, and up against the source of bleeding, whilst applying pressure to the bleeding vessel. Once in place, firm pressure is applied for 4-6 minutes.

PaCO2

See Partial Pressure of Arterial Carbon Dioxide.

Paediatric Anaesthesia

The different anatomy, physiology, psychology, and social needs of a paediatric patient require an anaesthetic regime different from that for adults, e.g., gas induction, local anaesthetic (and cream) for I.V. access, and specific equipment (Appendix A75, pg 481).

Paediatric Endotracheal Tube (ETT) Size

The size of an uncuffed paediatric ETT (children under 10 yrs) is determined by: (age/4) + 4. For cuffed tubes, subtract ½.

Palatine

Relating to, or attached to, the palate (roof of the mouth).

Pallor

An unhealthy and pale appearance.

Palpation

Using the hands/fingers in a physical examination.

Palpitation

Abnormal rate, force, or rhythm of the heart, felt by the patient. **Symptoms**: chest pain, breathing difficulty, dizziness. **Causes** include: hormonal changes, smoking, caffeine, low blood sugar, dehydration, anaemia, arrhythmia, stress, shock, and drugs.

Panendoscopy

Endoscopic examination of the upper airway: larynx, oesophagus, mouth, nose, or tongue. Biopsies are taken for examination.

PAO2 (pAO2)

See Partial Pressure of **Alveolar** Oxygen.

PaO2 (paO2)

See Partial Pressure of **Arterial** Oxygen.

Paracentesis

Perforation of a cavity, in order to drain off fluid.

Paracetamol

Antipyretic and analgesic, but no anti-inflammatory effects. At "step one" in the WHO analgesic ladder: An intravenous dose is given, perioperatively, for mild to moderate pain. Typical dosage is 15 mg/kg, to a maximum of 1 g. An overdose (delayed action) or staggered overdose causes a build up of *n-acetyl-p-benzoquinone amine*, which can damage the liver, and can be fatal.

Paraesthesia

Feeling of tingling, burning, or pins and needles, in a limb. Usually caused by pressure preventing normal flow of sensory information between a peripheral nerve, supplying a limb, and the sensory cortex. Removal of the pressure restores normal feeling.

Paraglossal Intubation

A technique for difficult intubations, obese patients, large tongues, or short and thick necks. A Miller (straight) blade is passed from the right corner of the mouth, between the tongue and tonsil, using leftward and anterior pressure to displace the tongue to the left of the laryngoscope (to improve the view, the assistant pulls the right corner of the mouth). In comparison with using a Macintosh blade, the paraglossal approach gives a better view of the larynx, at the expense of less space to manipulate the tracheal tube.

Parasympathetic System

That part of the *Autonomic Nervous System* which manages homoeostasis, conserves energy, slows the heart rate, increases the glandular and intestinal activity, and relaxes muscles in the gastrointestinal tract. It is the *Rest and Digest* mechanism.

Parenchyma

The parts of an organ that are functional, as opposed to structural or connective. In the lung, the parenchyma are those parts involved in the process of gas exchange.

Parenteral

Apart from the alimentary canal: Introduction of drugs, nutrients or fluids into the body by a route other than the mouth or rectum, e.g., intravenous or subcutaneous.

Paresis

Muscular weakness; partial paralysis.

Parietal

The wall of an organ, organ cavity, or outer surface of an organ.

Parotid

1. Near the ear.
2. Salivary gland in front of each ear.

Paroxysmal

Sudden violent attack or worsened condition; a seizure or spasm.

Partial Pressure (p, P)

The pressure of a gas, amongst a mixture of gases, which it would exert on its containing vessel if it, alone, were present in that volume. The sum of the partial pressures of all of the gases in their enclosing vessel gives the total pressure of that vessel. This is *Dalton's Law of Partial Pressures*. Partial pressure is denoted "p" or "P", followed by the symbol for the gas, e.g., **pAO_2** or **PAO_2** denotes partial pressure of alveoli (A) oxygen. {Note: choice of using "p" or "P" is personal preference} Air, for example, is a mixture of gases, of which, oxygen represents ~ 21%. If, at a given moment, the air pressure is 1 bar, then the pressure exerted by oxygen (only) will be 21% of 1 bar, which is 210 mBar.

> Note: It is not possible to understand respiration and circulation, or the mechanics of anaesthesia, without understanding pressure - and the gas laws.

Partial Pressure of Alveolar Oxygen (pAO_2)

Pressure exerted by O_2 in the alveoli, calculated (young healthy adult) with the *alveolar gas equation* to be ~104 mmHg (13.8 kPa), and which reduces with age. PAO_2 forms the upper end of the concentration gradient with arterial oxygen, and there is a pressure drop of about 4 mmHg as O_2 crosses into the pulmonary capillaries. Note: at mean atmospheric pressure, breathing 100% oxygen gives a pAO_2 of ~660 mmHg (88 kPa) but, at peak of Mt Everest, pAO_2 is 166 mmHg (22 kPa).

Partial Pressure of Arterial Oxygen (paO_2)

Pressure exerted by dissolved systemic arterial oxygen (the 2% of oxygen that is dissolved is plasma) that indicates the state of oxygenation, and how well the lungs are performing; measured by arterial blood gas analysis. PaO_2 is unaffected by Hb level. At rest, normal paO_2 is 80-100 mmHg (10.6-13.3 kPa) and, as a rule, paO_2 should be ~10 kPa less than FiO_2 % so, if breathing 40% FiO_2, paO_2 should be ~30 kPa (225 mmHg). Deoxygenated blood in pulmonary arteries is at 40-50 mmHg (5.3-6.7 kPa). Note: paO_2 might be normal, and SaO_2 100%, but if the Hb level is low, oxygenation will be abnormally low, which is why anaesthetists always check Hb values on arterial blood gas reports.

Partial Pressure of Arterial Carbon Dioxide ($paCO_2$)

Partial pressure of CO_2 dissolved in systemic arteries, with normal values of 40-45 mmHg (5.3-6 kPa), or 23-29 mmol/litre. A high value suggests minute volume might be too low. Alveoli $paCO_2$ is usually ~5 mmHg less than arterial. In pulmonary arteries, CO_2 pressure is ~50 mmHg (6.7 kPa).

Partition Coefficient (Distribution Coefficient)

Describes how the ratio of concentrations of a compound is split between two immiscible solvents (phases: liquid, gas, or solid), when the two phases have equal pressure and temperature.

Pascal

An S.I. derived unit of pressure, equivalent to the application of one newton of force per one square metre.

Patient Controlled Anaesthesia (PCA)

A safe intravenous infusion of an analgesic agent, such as Morphine or Fentanyl, controlled by the patient, using a dedicated pump. The PCA delivers a pre-programmed bolus, when the patient requires it. After the bolus is delivered, no more boluses are available (for safety) until a lockout period, also pre-programmed, has passed. In some cases, all analgesia is controlled by the patient; in other cases, the patient requested boluses are supplemented by a continuous infusion, which is known as the *background dose*. Antiemetics are usually given with PCA use. Naloxone (200-400 microgram, IV) should be available if respiratory rate drops below 8/minute.

PAW

See Airway Pressure.

PCA

See Patient Controlled Anaesthesia.

PDPH

See Post Dural Puncture Headache.

Peak Inspiratory Pressure (PIP)

The maximum lung pressure achieved, at the end of an inspiration. It is the resistive pressure, against which, the ventilation system must overcome, if ventilation is to be patent. A level of 35 cmH_2O might be considered a reasonable maximum value (adults), during assisted ventilation. PIP may be increased by bronchospasm, secretions, low lung compliance, and the patient biting down on, or occlusion of, the endotracheal tube.

PEEP

See Positive End Expiratory Pressure.

-penia

A reduced amount of cells, eg, leukopenia (low WBC count).

Percutaneous Endoscopic Gastrostomy (PEG)

A tube through the abdominal wall, to the stomach, to allow feeding and medications, so bypassing the mouth and oesophagus.

Per Rectum

Instruction to give a drug via the rectum.

Percutaneous

Through (per) the skin (cutis).

Percutaneous Coronary Intervention (PCI)

A non-surgical procedure, under local anaesthetic, to treat stenotic (narrowed) coronary arteries, which result from the build up of cholesterol laden plaques, due to atherosclerosis. A coronary artery is widened by angioplasty (balloon), and the widening is structurally maintained by insertion of a stent. Navigation to the target site is made by catheter, via an artery in the groin or arm. PCI is a common treatment for STEMI.

Percutaneous Endoscopic Gastrostomy (PEG) Tube

A PEG tube is a feeding tube, that passes between the abdominal wall and stomach, for children and adults, when they cannot receive adequate nutrition by oral means.

Perfusion

The passage of fluid over an organ, or through vessels/tissue, to allow gas exchange. Poor perfusion (from hypotension, vasoconstriction, septic shock, hypovolaemia) causes peripheral skin to become cool, pale, and sweaty. Poor perfusion to the brain is shown by confusion and anxiety, and can lead to shock.

Perfusion Index

The ratio of peripheral pulsatile to non-pulsatile blood flow, calculated with some pulse oximeters (with plethysmograph), with normal range 0.02-20%, showing weak to strong pulse strength.

Perfusion Limited Gas Transfer

The rate of gas movement from alveoli to the capillaries is mostly determined by the rate of blood flow (perfusion) through the capillary bed. With an unchanging blood flow, increasing the alveolar-capillary oxygen pressure gradient makes little difference to uptake of the oxygen. See also *Diffusion Limited Gas Transfer*.

Peri-arrest

Conditions which may precede or follow a cardiac arrest. Access Resuscitation Council guidelines.

Pericardial Effusion

Build up of fluid in the pericardium. Drainage is by pericardiocentesis. See also *Cardiac Tamponade*.

Pericardiocentesis (Pericardial Tap)

Aspiration, using needle and catheter, through the fifth intercostal space, to relieve a pericardial effusion.

Pericarditis

Inflammation of the pericardium, often caused by infection, and causing chest pain and high temperature, particularly when breathing in or lying down. Pericarditis can lead to pericardial effusion. Possible treatments: anti-inflammatories (eg, ibuprofen), steroids, or antibiotics (if bacterial infection).

Pericardium (Pericardial Sac)

The double layered fluid filled sac surrounding the heart and the proximal ends of the aorta, vena cava, and pulmonary artery. Functionally, the sac fixes the heart in place, prevents overfilling, acts as an infection barrier between the heart and other organs, and reduces friction as the heart moves within the thoracic cavity.

Perioperative Warming

One of the side-effects of anaesthesia is heat loss, due to reduction in the body's normal heat regulatory processes, and to the effects of peripheral vasodilation. To counter such heat loss, passive and active warming techniques are used for surgery lasting more than thirty minutes, or for shorter durations with patients who are more vulnerable to hypothermia. *Active* warming is when under body heating or forced air warming is used; *passive* warming is the use of insulating blankets. In all situations, it is the **core** body temperature which is of significance, because a properly warmed core will, itself, provide heat to the peripheries. If a patient's core temperature is below 36° C, prior to anaesthesia, then their core must be warmed sufficiently, before anaesthesia is performed.

Peripheral Nerve Block

Injection of local anaesthetic close to a peripheral nerve/nerve plexus, either for non-surgical, intra-operative, or postoperative analgesia. Intra-operatively, the block allows avoidance or reduced levels of opioids, and their attendant side-effects, especially nausea and vomiting. See Appendix A78 (pg 486).

Peripheral Nerve Stimulator

A device to assess nerve function in neuromuscular blockade, using a measurement technique called the *Train of Four*. An anaesthetist will monitor for three or four "twitches" before giving the NMB reversal agent (neostigmine). See *Train of Four*.

Peripheral Nervous System (PNS)

All of the neurons which are either partly or entirely outside of the central nervous system, and comprising the Sensory-Somatic and Autonomic systems.

Sensory-Somatic System: Controls glands and skeletal muscles, by use of motor neurons. Comprises 12 pairs of cranial nerves, and 31 pairs of spinal nerves.

Autonomic System: Controls the visceral organs.

Peripheral Resistance

The resistance posed by the arteries to the flow of blood. The three factors that affect resistance are:

- Vasoconstrictor (increase) and vasodilator (decrease) drugs.
- Blood viscosity – decreases with heat (hence less resistance).
- Sympathetic nervous system stimulation – constricts arteries.

Peripherally Inserted Central Catheter (PICC)

For long term (weeks/months) IV therapy and TPN feeding: A flexible, non-tunnelled (straight into vein), 1 or 2 lumen central venous catheter. Unlike other central lines, its point of entry is from the periphery of the body. Ultrasound can be used to make insertion easier, and X-ray used to confirm placement. PICC lines must be kept dry, and need daily flushing and cleaning. Duration up to 1 month. See Appendix A80 (pg 488).

Peritoneum

Serous membrane lining the abdominal cavity, and forming a covering for the abdominal viscera (organs). The **Parietal** Peritoneum lines the pelvic and abdominal cavities. The **Visceral** Peritoneum is the inner layer which covers the abdominal organs.

Perle

A capsule of medicine.

Permacath

A tunnelled catheter, containing two large bore lumens, where the red capped line is for taking blood for dialysis, and the blue line for returning the blood from the dialysis machine.

Permissive Hypoxia

An experimental lung protective strategy to treat severe ARDS patients with just enough oxygen to avoid hypoxic injury, whilst avoiding the potentially toxic effects of ventilatory support.

Pertussis (Whooping Cough)

Highly contagious infection of the lungs and airway.

PET Scan

See Positron Emission Tomography.

P/F Ratio

See Carrico Index.

pH (Potential or Power of Hydrogen)

A value, between 0 and 14, describing how acidic an aqueous solution is, derived from the negative $\log_{10}$ of the H+ ion concentration, in moles/litre of solution. At pH of 7, a solution has equal concentrations of free hydrogen (H^+) and hydroxyl (OH^-) ions, ~100 nanomoles/litre, making it "neutral". If pH is lower than 7, the solution is acidic; above 7 is basic (alkali). Normal biological pH range is 7.35-7.45; pH outside this range prevents normal enzyme function, and denatures proteins. pH 7.4 (physiologic pH) means [H^+] is ~40 nanomoles/litre. With pH < 7.4, (acidic), O_2 has reduced binding with Hb, the kidneys reabsorb bicarbonate (H^+ buffer), and excrete H^+. When pH is > 7.4, (alkali), the kidneys remove more bicarbonate, but fewer H^+ ions. There are three buffer systems for pH: HCO_3^- (main system), Haemoglobin, and proteins. See Appendix A79 (pg 487).

Pharmacodynamics

The physiological effects and biological mechanisms a drug has on the body. Observations of drug interactions, side-effects, and dose response relationships are used to decide *Therapeutic Index* and *Maximum Safe Concentrations*.

Pharmacokinetics

Describes the stages of what the body does to a drug, in terms of absorption, distribution, metabolism, and elimination. Use of pharmacokinetic knowledge allows safe administration of drug dosages for individual patients. Note that the "PK" name given to infusion pumps (TCI) refers to pharmacokinetic processes.

Pharyngoscopy

Endoscopic examination of the pharynx (throat).

Phases of Anaesthesia

Main stages of an anaesthetic event, where the anaesthetist aims to maximise the proportion of time that the patient is in stage 3.

Stage 1: From giving the *induction* agent to loss of

consciousness/amnesia; the patient is sedated.

Stage 2: *Excitement* - Assymetric breathing pattern, or apnoea; Hypertension; tendency to vomit; Fluctuating heart rate; Dilated pupils; Animation.

Stage 3: *Surgical anaesthesia* - From automatic breathing to loss of ability to breathe; Hypotension; Lower heart rate; No eye movement; Relaxation.

Stage 4: *Coma* or overly medicated. Cardiovascular and Respiratory failure, requiring immediate ventilatory support.

Phenylephrine

Intravenous sympathomimetic vasoconstrictor (alpha-1 agonist) – increases vascular resistance (should be available for hypotension in caesarian sections). Typically prepared (fridge) as a 100 ml of 1 in 10,000 NS solution: given as a 50 – 100 microgram bolus.

Phenytoin

Intravenous agent for tonic-clonic and focal seizures.

Phlebitis

Inflammation of a vein (phleb-), caused by blood clot, due to trauma, cancer, varicose veins, keeping stationary on long journeys, or infection. **Signs** are pain, reddening, and inflammation, close to the affected site. If near the skin surface, it is termed *superficial phlebitis*. Phlebitis in the deeper veins of the legs and arms is *deep vein thrombophlebitis/thrombosis* (DVT), and is more serious, because it can lead to pulmonary embolism.

Phlebostatic Axis

The junction of the 4th intercostal space and mid-axillary line, approximates to the right atrium.

Physiologic Dead Space

The total of alveolar and anatomic dead space volumes.

Physiological Shunt

Blood perfuses the lungs as normal, but does not get oxygenated, because the alveoli are not ventilated, so gives V/Q ratio of 0.

Pia Mater

Latin: "tender mother". The innermost of the three layers of meninges (membranes) that surround the spinal cord and brain. The spinal subarachnoid space, between pia mater and arachnoid mater, is the injection target for spinal block.

PICC Line

Peripherally Inserted Central Catheter.

Pierre Robin Syndrome

An anatomical deformity, where the patient has a small and recessed lower jaw, and an obstructive tongue. With respect to airway management and anaesthesia, the syndrome demands extraordinary planning and equipment.

PIFR

Peak Inspiratory Flow Rate.

Pin Index Safety System

Mechanical system to ensure correct fitting of gas cylinders (size E on anaesthetic machines) to their respective housings, according to ISO standard 407 for Small Medical Gas Cylinders. The positions of the holes on the cylinder valve correspond with pins fitted to the yoke, such as on an anaesthetic machine.

PIP

Peak Inspiratory Pressure, with a safe maximum of ~35 cmH_2O.

Plaque

See Atheroma.

Plasma

Clear, straw coloured liquid part of blood and lymph, comprises 25% of extracellular fluid, described as "blood after cells are removed. Contains serum, electrolytes, glucose, fats, proteins (fibrinogen, albumin,...), hormones, CO_2, oxygen, and clotting factors". See Appendix A20 (pg 375).

Plasma Cholinesterase

Another name for *Butrylcholinesterase*.

Plasmapheresis

Removal of the liquid (plasma) component of blood from the cells.

Plateau Pressure (P_{PLAT})

IPPV (intubated) airway pressure, during the inspiratory pause, which immediately follows *Peak Inspiratory Pressure* (P_{IP}), and matches alveolar pressure, determined by lung compliance. A safe maximum value (adults), against barotrauma, is ~30 cmH_2O. Reducing PEEP or tidal volume will reduce plateau pressure.

Platelets (Thrombocytes)

Colourless cell fragments that help blood clotting, by adhering to (plugging) the breached endothelium, to form a base from which a fibrin mesh forms. Stored at 22° C in bags (cloudy yellow) to permit gas exchange, and kept moving in an agitator. Shelf life: 3-5 days. For haemorrhage, acute leukaemia, and bone marrow transplantation. Ideally, use same ABO as patient, but not essential. Give over 30 mins, and before RBCs. Use platelet or blood giving set with 170-200 micron filter. Do not give through a giving set previously used for blood. Do NOT put through a pump or rapid infuser unless manufacturer allows it. Has risk of bacterial contamination. See Appendix A20 (pg 375).

Plenum Vapouriser

The vapouriser in standard hospital use, with high internal resistance for a volatile agent, such as sevoflurane, requires a driving gas, so that it is above ambient pressure, before it can go on to mix with oxygen. Plenum vapourisers provide more accuracy than the more portable *draw-over* vapourisers, which are driven by a patient's respiratory efforts (used by the military - Triservice).

Plenum Ventilation

A building ventilation system that produces turbulent air flows. The air is suppled via a ducting pipe system, **output** to a room, and then **returned** to the duct for filtering and recycling. In an operating theatre, a plenum system performs 20 air changes/hour, the airborne pathogens collide and mix, and are more likely to settle in a wound than when laminar flow systems are used.

Plethysmography

The non-invasive measurement of changes of volume in an organ, such as lungs and blood vessels. **Body Plethysmography** tests lung function, by measuring how much air the lungs can breathe in, and how much is left after a forced expiration. Results help illustrate affects of lung diseases and how they are changing. **Photoplethysmography** (PPG) is the technique that modern sats probes use to display waveforms of arterial blood flow (a graphical illustration of heart beat and Perfusion Index).

Pleura

One of a double layer of serous membrane that enclose a lung (visceral pleura) and line the inner chest wall (parietal pleura).

Pleural Effusion

Accumulation of fluid in the pleural sac (membranes that line the lung and wall of chest cavity). If the effusion is sufficiently large enough, it can act like a cardiac tamponade. Usually, pleural effusion refers to hydrothorax.

Causes: Heart surgery, heart failure, haemorrhage, pneumonia, kidney disease, pulmonary embolism.
Symptoms: Chest pain, dyspnoea, dry cough.

Treatment: Sitting up; thoracentesis (needle drainage).

Pleural Sac/Cavity/Space

The cavity, containing a small amount of lubricating fluid, between visceral and parietal pleura (double layered serous membrane), separating the lungs from other structures. During normal quiet breathing, the pressure in the pleural space is negative, with respect to ambient pressure.

Pleurisy

Inflammation of the pleura. DRY pleurisy is when pleural surfaces rub against each other, and which may be heard by auscultation. WET pleurisy is when fluids in the pleural cavity (pleural effusion) compress the lungs, causing pain and breathing difficulty.

Causes: Pneumonia, pulmonary embolism, lung cancer, arthritis.
Symptoms: Chest pain on inspiration, sometimes shoulder pain. Also, shortness of breath, dry cough.

Treatment: Treat underlying cause; NSAIDs; Antibiotics - if bacterial infection; Fluid extraction - if wet pleurisy.

Plexus

A network of nerves, veins, or lymphatics.

-pnea, -pnoea

Referring to the breath.

Pneumatosis

Gas abnormally trapped in body cavities or tissues. Gas in the wall of the bowel (intestine) is known as *pneumatosis intestinalis*.

Pneumocyte

Alveolar cells of two types: Type I allow gas exchange between alveoli and surrounding capillary bed. Type II cells secrete surfactant, to reduce the possibility of alveoli from collapsing.

Pneumonectomy

Surgical removal of a lung, or part of a lung.

Pneumonia

Acute respiratory infection, and inflammation of the lungs, that causes alveoli to fill with pus or fluid. If in both lungs, the condition is double pneumonia. The patient ventilates normally, but the pus prevents alveoli to capillary O_2 diffusion, so less O_2 in the blood, giving a higher A-a Gradient.

Symptoms: Cough, lethargy, green or brown expectoration, high temperature, breathing problems, chest pain, hypotension, tachycardia, nausea, tachypnoea.

Treatment: If the cause is viral - fluids and rest. If the cause is bacterial, give antibiotics.

Pneumonitis

Inflammation of lung tissues, caused when pathogens irritate the alveoli, causing an allergic reaction.

Pneumoperitoneum

Gas in the peritoneal cavity, which can result in adverse affects to the cardiovascular system. Commonly caused by organ perforations, such as with an ulcer or tumor. X-ray to confirm.

Pneumothorax

Gas trapped in the pleural space (twixt visceral & parietal pleura), which might cause lung collapse. If there is also mediastinal shift, it may be a Tension Pneumothorax. See Appendix A81 (pg 490).

POGO Score

Score representing the Percentage Of Glottic Opening (visualised).

Polar Endotracheal Tube

Pre-formed north or south facing ET tube, for oral or nasal intubation, designed to keep the ET tube free from the surgical field in maxillofacial procedures. Unlike "RAE" ET tubes, which are otherwise identical to standard ET tubes, the "Polar" tube (usually blue) is of the "soft seal" type - it has a relatively larger volume inflatable cuff, made from a softer material than ordinary cuffs, giving less chance of trauma or irritation to the airway.

Polycythaemia

A high Red Blood Cell count.

Polymorphic Ventricular Tachycardia (PVT)

A type of VT where the QRS complexes vary in amplitude, axis and duration; typically caused by myocardial infarction. A common treatment is magnesium.

Polyuria

Excess urination.

PONV

See Post Operative Nausea and Vomiting.

Poor Peripheral Perfusion

Poor perfusion (reduced blood flow) to the extremities can occur for several reasons: cardiac failure, shock, or exposure to cold temperatures, where the body attempts to retain core heat at the expense of the peripheries. The reduction in perfusion slows down capillary refill time to more than two seconds, and can produce a significant difference between core and peripheral (toe) temperatures, of at least six degrees celsius.

Signs of poor peripheral perfusion...

- Confusion
- Bradycardia
- Cramps
- Varicose veins
- Cyanosis
- Weak pulse
- Low sats
- Cold peripheries
- Leg ulcers
- Fatigue
- Numb/cold fingers/toes
- Restlessness
- Mottled/clammy skin

Portal

Referring to a vein which does not lead to the heart but, instead, has capillaries at each end, allowing blood to pass between organs.

Portacath

An implanted (tunnelled) central venous access device for patients who need long-term or continuous administration of chemotherapy; placed under the skin, on the chest, whereupon the catheter is fed to the entrance of the right atrium, via the superior vena cava. There is no exit site, because the whole system is under the skin, including a small chamber (port), which is used for blood withdrawals and injections. Saline and heparin flushes keep the line patent, and a local anaesthetic cream can be applied to the skin above the port, to make needle use less painful. Has less infection risk than other CVC lines eg, Hickman and PICC lines.

Positive End Expiratory Pressure (PEEP)

The minimum positive (above ambient) alveolar pressure that the ventilation machine allows, with the aim of preventing the alveoli from collapsing (atelectasis), which might occur at the end of an expiration. The result is that more alveoli can be available for ventilation and gas exchange; otherwise, if some alveoli suffer collapse, a "shunt" might occur. Optimal PEEP can be found by setting a PEEP of 25 cmH_2O, then incrementally reducing until the best SpO_2 and compliance are found. A side-effect of PEEP can be reduced systolic blood pressure. See also *Shunt*.

Positive Inotrope

See Appendix A63 (pg 463).

Positron Emission Tomography (PET Scan)

A scanner that produces 3-D images of the organs, and shows diseased cells, to reveal cancer, heart and brain disorders. Prior to imaging, the patient is injected with a radioactive tracer dye.

Posology

Drug dosage details and instructions.

Post Dural Puncture Headache (PDPH)

A consequence of accidentally puncturing the dura and arachnoid maters, when attempting epidural anaesthesia or lumbar puncture, and causing reduced CSF pressure due to leakage from the subarachnoid space and into the epidural space.

Post Obstructive Pulmonary Oedema

Sudden occurrence of pulmonary oedema, immediately following an upper airway obstruction. Type I means **inhalation** against an obstruction, and type II means **exhalation** against an obstruction.

Post Operative Nausea and Vomiting (PONV)

A side effect of general anaesthesia, suffered by 1 in 4 patients. If unmanaged, can lead to pulmonary aspiration. Younger patients are more susceptible than older ones, as are gynaecological, urological, strabismus correction, and middle ear surgery patients. Treatment is by antiemetics, dispensing a combination of agents, until efficacy is achieved. See Appendix A82 (pg 492).

Post Thrombotic Syndrome

Synonymous with *Deep Vein Thrombosis*.

Postictal State

The abnormal condition occurring between the end of an epileptic seizure, and return to baseline condition.

Postpartum

The period shortly after giving birth.

Postpartum Haemorrhage (PPH)

The loss of 500 ml or more of blood from the genital tract, within 24 hours of giving birth, commonly caused by *uterine atony*. This is one of the conditions where emergency anaesthesia may become necessary, and might include: RSI, arterial line placement, rapid fluid infusion, or cell salvage.

Postural Hypotension

Dizziness caused by low blood pressure, when standing up.

Postural Tachycardia Syndrome (PoTS)

Abnormal increase in heart rate after standing up.

Potassium (K)

The major intracellular electrolyte. Maintains resting membrane potential for normal contraction of the myocardium and other muscle cells, helps nutrients cross into cells, and waste move the other way. Serum range is 3.5–5.2 mmol/litre. Potassium is given in diabetic ketoacidosis, to help shift glucose into cells. Potassium Chloride, available as 20/27/40 mmol/L, is used to stop the heart, to necessitate heart surgery. See *Hyperkalaemia, Hypokalaemia.*

Potency

Describes the relative effectiveness of a particular agent, in comparison with similar agents. For example, isoflurane is more potent than sevoflurane, it has a lower MAC and higher oil:gas partition coefficient, so requires a lower partial pressure in the brain, and lower % flow, to achieve its anaesthetic effect. Note: potency is directly proportional to lipid solubility.

Potentiation

The interaction of two or more pharmacological agents, which result in a response which is greater than the sum of the individual responses of those agents.

PQRST Wave

ECG waveform which reflects the phases of heart activation, from the sinus node, across the atria, atrioventricular node, and ventricular septum.

- P wave: Atrial depolarisation (contraction)
- QRS complex: Ventricular contraction
- T wave: Ventricles repolarising (relaxing)

The Q wave is negative (downstroke), the R wave is the 1st positive (upstroke) wave after the Q wave, and the S wave is the 1st positive wave after the R wave. The J point is the start of the ST segment, and is raised in ST elevated myocardial infarction.

PR

See Per Rectum.

Prandial

During the process of eating a meal.

Pre-eclampsia

Hypertension and proteinuria (excess protein in the blood), often with oedema, during pregnancy. In severe pre-eclampsia, symptoms may include heartburn, vision problems, headache, abdominal pain, and swelling in the face, feet, and hands. Pre-eclampsia requires immediate response, otherwise the foetus may suffer hypoxia induced neurological injury.

Precipitate

Deposition of solid matter, previously in solution. More formally: a *precipitate* is formed by transforming a dissolved substance into an insoluble solid or suspension, from a solution. In general, one phase ejects another phase, e.g., a liquid phase ejects a solid substance, or a gas ejects a solid or liquid. See *Cryoprecipitate*.

Precordial Thump

An attempt to interrupt an arrhythmia, such as Ventricular Fibrillation, by a single fist strike, to the centre of the patient's sternum. The thump might be effective if made at the onset of a witnessed and monitored adverse rhythm (VF/pVT), and a defibrillator is not immediately available. The latest resuscitation guidelines de-emphasise use of the precordial thump.

Precordium

The part of the thorax over the heart.

Pre-oxygenation

Administering oxygen to a patient, prior to anaesthesia, with the intention of replacing nitrogen in the lungs, with oxygen, thereby prolonging the *safe apnoea time*. Note: a pregnant patient has a reduced Functional Residual Capacity, so will de-saturate quicker.

Prefixes

Ecto=outside, Endo=inside, Enter=intestines, Epi=over/near, Exo=external, Gastro=stomach, Hist=tissue, Hyper=beyond, Hypo=under, Infra=below, Inter=amongst, Intra=within, Isch=too little, Iso=equal, Juxta=adjacent to, Myo=muscle, Ren=kidneys, Soma=, Supra=above, Sym=jointly, Syn=together.

Pregnancy Complications

Includes: dehydration, oedema, gastroesophageal reflux disease, DVT, anaemia, venacava compression, abdominal separation.

Preload

Aka *end diastolic pressure*: The amount of myocyte (cardiac muscle) stretching, at the end of diastole, prior to contraction. Preload stretching is reduced by hypovolaemia.

Preload Reserve

The amount that cardiac muscle can stretch if stroke volume is to be increased. If the heart is already at its maximum preload point, stroke volume cannot be increased, so any increase in output will be determined by an increased heart rate.

Preoperative Assessment

Safety protocol, before regional or general anaesthesia, for the anaesthetist to identify anomalies in the patient's anatomy, physiology, or pathophysiology, that might adversely affect the optimum anaesthetic regime. See Appendix A84 (495).

Pressure

A scalar value (magnitude, not direction) of force per unit area. The S.I. derived unit of pressure is the pascal, which describes one newton of force, applied over one square metre. Gas pressure differentials are what constitute the concentration gradients governing the direction and force of the movement of gases.

There are three types of description for pressure:

GAUGE pressure is relative to ambient (atmospheric) pressure. For example, systolic blood pressure is the amount of pressure which exceeds ambient pressure.

RELATIVE pressure is the difference between any two pressures.

ABSOLUTE pressure is the sum of gauge and ambient pressures.

Example: if a spirometer indicates patient airway pressure of 20 cmH_2O, then that is the gauge pressure, because it is 20 cmH_2O above ambient (atmospheric) pressure. The patient's absolute airway pressure, on the other hand, is 20 + 1,033 (ambient) = 1,053 cmH_2O (assuming atmospheric pressure of 1,033 cmH_2O).

Pressure Controlled Ventilation (PCV)

Pre-set inspiratory and PEEP pressures, with variable tidal volumes, determined by patient characteristics, such as lung compliance. Prevents barotrauma.

Pressure Regulator

A pressure reducing valve, from a high pressure gas supply (up to 200 bar), to a low pressure device, such as a gas cylinder on an anaesthetic machine (4 bar). When an anaesthetic machine cylinder is switched on, the regulated delivery pressure should be lower than that delivered by the low pressure pipeline supply, so that the resultant higher pipeline pressure prevents the cylinder from being drained, should it be accidentally left on. On an anaesthetic machine, the regulator is of the *Adams* type.

Pressure Sore/Ulcer (Bed Sore)

See Decubitus Ulcer.

Pressure Support

A pressure ventilation mode, in spontaneously breathing patients, which supplements and synchronises with the patient's own breathing efforts.

Pressure (Decubitus) Ulcers

Aka Bed Sores: The breakdown of an area of skin and underlying tissue, caused by prolonged pressure to a body part, particularly boney prominences, caused when the skin is placed under a persistent pressure. The extra pressure leads to a disruption of the flow of blood through the skin, resulting in reduced perfusion of oxygen and nutrients. The ulcers/sores can range from patches of discoloured skin, to open wounds which expose the underlying bone or muscle. Stage **1**: reddened but unbroken skin; Stage **2**: broken skin and shallow ulcer; Stage **3**: a deep ulcer; Stage **4**: multiple tissue layers broken, down to bone. On operating tables, gel padding is used to protect vulnerable areas.

Intrinsic risk factors...

- Reduced mobility
- Sensory impairment
- Very young or old
- Level of consciousness
- Malnutrition
- Previous pressure damage
- Vascular disease
- Dehydration
- Illness

Pressure Volume Loop

Relationship between airway pressures and volumes can be graphically illustrated as a Pressure:Volume loop, using values taken from circuit spirometry. The anaesthetist may discern different conditions from the different shaped loops, particularly with respect to lung compliance and state of surfactant.

Primary Alveolar Hypoventilation

Condition where hypoventilation is caused by failure of the brain and nervous system to recognise low blood oxygen and high CO_2 levels, or to properly respond by increasing minute volume, in a patient with an otherwise healthy respiratory system.

Prodrug

An agent that is a pharmacologically inactive derivation of an active drug, which is transformed, after administration, into the active form, by biochemical or enzymatic processes.

Pro Re Nata (PRN)

In pharmacology, an instruction to take “when needed”.

Procalcitonin Test (PCT)

A quick blood test that helps diagnose bacterial sepsis. Most procalcitonin is produced by the thyroid gland (C cells) but, in the presence of sepsis, many other organs produce procalcitonin, and the high count is the biomarker for sepsis.

Procedural Sedation

The technique of invoking conscious sedation, either for a minor procedure, or to facilitate Delayed Sequence Intubation.

Prognosis

Predicted outcome of an illness.

Prolapse

An organ which has moved out of position - downwards.

Propofol

Fast onset (30 sec, due to fast distribution from plasma to CNS) sedative-hypnotic injectable emulsion induction agent, causing: loss of cough reflex, reduced arterial resistance, vasodilation, with drop in venous return and blood pressure, and more respiratory depression than other induction agents. Adult dose: 2-3 mg/kg, ~ 30 mg every 10 seconds (lidocaine can be added to reduce the pain of injection). Duration 5-10 minutes. 2% (red cap) propofol is for infusions. Flush cannula before going to Recovery.

Propofol Related Infusion Syndrome (PRIS)

A rare but life threatening reaction to prolonged propofol infusion, signified by refractory (uncontrollable) bradycardia, leading to asystole, and death. Signified by any/all of: hyperlipidaemia, enlarged/fatty liver, severe metabolic acidosis, hyperkalaemia, kidney failure, arrhythmias, and rhabdomyolysis. Maximum safe dose is deemed 4 mg/kg/hour. Treatment is cessation of propofol; maybe extracorporeal oxygenation.

Proseal

A reusable (after autoclave) laryngeal mask airway, with a

reinforced airway tube, bite block, and a drain tube which opens at the upper oesophageal sphincter, allowing drainage of gastric secretions, and access to the alimentary tract.

Protamine Sulfate

An intravenously administered agent to reverse the anticoagulant effects of heparin. Protamines are derived from the sperm of fish, especially salmon. 1 mg of protamine sulfate will counter approximately 100 international units of heparin.

Prothrombin Complex Concentrate (Factor IX Complex)

A combination of blood clotting factors II, VII, IX, and X. Used to counteract heavy bleeding, or to reverse the effects of Warfarin.

Prothrombin Time

Time, in seconds, for an anticoagulated sample of plasma or whole blood to clot, after it has been added to a thromboplastin reagent. Normal time is 11-13 seconds. The test is the central feature for determining a patient's *International Normalised Ratio*.

Prothrombotic

Something which leads to thrombosis.

Pseudocholinesterase

Another name for *Butrylcholinesterase*.

Pulmonary Acinus (“asinus”)

Functional parts of the lung that are distal to terminal bronchioles.

Pulmonary Aspiration

Respiratory tract and lung pollution by pathogens, saliva, drink, or food, from the pharynx or stomach. If infection occurs, *Aspiration Pneumonia* develops.

Symptoms: Fever, cough (yellow/green phlegm), vomiting, headache, tachycardia.

Treatment: Trendelenburg, suction trachea and pharynx, give PEEP (positive end expiratory pressure), intubate.

Pulmonary Circulation

Takes de-oxygenated blood from the right side of the heart, to the lungs, via the pulmonary arteries. The blood then picks up a fresh supply of oxygen from the alveoli, and then transports the oxygenated blood to the left atrium, via the pulmonary veins.

Pulmonary Consolidation

Alveoli that are blocked by fluid or solids, making the tissue less flexible, and preventing normal gas exchange. The sufferer may expectorate green phlegm or blood, have a painful cough, fatigue or fever, and suffer noisy and rapid breathing. **Causes** include: Aspiration, pneumonia, congestive heart failure, cancer, bleeding in the lungs. Lung volume usually remains normal.

Pulmonary Embolism (PE)

An embolism (clot, gas bubble, etc) in a blood vessel of a lung, which usually originates from the proximal veins of the thigh and pelvis. See Appendix A86 (pg 496).

Pulmonary Fibrosis

Scarring between the alveoli, causing them to stiffen and lose elasticity, impairing diffusion of oxygen to the bloodstream, and so degrade respiration. **Symptoms**: Fatigue, dry cough, muscle/joint aches, shortness of breath, finger and toe clubbing.

Pulmonary Hypertension (PH)

Excessive pressure (> 25 mmHg) in the pulmonary arteries, which can damage the right heart, and can escalate to heart failure.

Pulmonary Oedema

Excess transudate (filtrate leaked out of blood vessels) fluid in the lungs, which collects in the alveoli, making it difficult to breathe. Most often caused by heart problems, such as *Congestive Heart Failure*, but it may be caused by other conditions, which do not directly affect the heart (non-cardiogenic pulmonary oedema).

Symptoms include:

- Wheezing
- Difficult breathing, esp when lying down
- Fatigue
- Weight gain, and swelling in legs

Immediate treatment is 100% oxygen, in a sitting position.

Pulmonary Shunt

See Intra Pulmonary Shunt.

Pulmonary Thrombosis

A blocked artery, in the lung, caused by an embolism.

Pulmonary Trunk

The main pulmonary artery, from the heart, that bifurcates (divides) into the left and right pulmonary arteries, where deoxygenated blood is taken to the lungs.

Pulmonary Ventilation

The process of breathing. Mechanical process of changing pressure gradients (following Boyle's Law), in the lungs, to alllow movement of air between lungs and atmosphere, determined by atmospheric, intra-alveolar, and intrapleural pressures.

Pulsatile

A pulsing motion, as occurs with blood flow through an artery.

Pulse Flow Oxygenation

The patient receives a pulse (bolus) of oxygen when the breathing machine detects the start of an inspiration, or if the patient needs an extra amount of oxygen, as opposed to a "continuous flow".

Pulse Oximeter

A non-invasive sensor for finger, toe, or ear lobe, that measures peripheral capillary haemoglobin oxygen saturation % (SpO_2) (and pulse rate), of oxygenated Hb as a fraction of total Hb that is capable of binding with oxygen, using infrared light absorption rates to gauge oxygen levels. See *Oximetry, CO-Oximetry*.

Pulse Pressure

The difference between diastolic and systolic pressures – a normal value being 40 mmHg. Greater than 60 mmHg (wide) suggests cardiovascular problems, such as hypertension or atherosclerosis; less than 40 mmHg (narrow) means decreased cardiac output, possibly due to heart failure.

Pulseless Electrical Activity (PEA)

A cardiac arrest where the patient has cardiac electrical activity, which would otherwise produce cardiac output and an obvious pulse. PEA usually has an underlying treatable **cause** which, in emergency situations, is most often hypovolaemia or hypoxaemia; other causes include tension pneumothorax, cardiac tamponade, pulmonary embolism, coronary thrombosis, and hypoglycaemia. Performing a pulse check, after a rhythm/monitor check, will ensure that PEA is identified. See Appendix A87 (pg 498).

Pulsus Alternans

An arterial waveform with an alternating pattern of high and smaller pulses, but with a uniform cycle length. Typically due to heart failure, where the left ventricle fails to properly eject blood into the aorta. **Causes** include hypertension, coronary atherosclerosis, aortic stenosis, and other cardiac myopathies.

Pulsus Paradoxus

A larger than normal decrease in stroke volume on inspiration, during spontaneous quiet breathing, resulting in a drop in systolic blood pressure of at least 10 mmHg. **Causes** include cardiac tamponade, hypovolaemia, asthma, and pulmonary embolism.

Purpura (Blood Spots)

Purple coloured patches on the skin and mucus membranes, caused by bleeding under the skin.

Pyothorax

A type of pleural effusion, where the fluid is pus.

Pyrexia

Body temperature, above the normal 37° C. The hypothalamus initiates pyrexia, as a response to virus or bacterial infection.

Pyrogenic

Something that produces, or is produced by, heat or fever.

qSOFA

A "quick" version of SOFA, identifies infected patients at greater risk of poor outcomes, from a score of 2 or 3. The three criteria are: ☠ Systolic BP $<$ 100 mmHg ☠ Respiratory rate $>$ 21/minute

☠ Altered mental state.

Quater Die Sumendus (QDS)

Aka *Quater In Sumendus*. Instruction to take drug 4 times a day.

Queckenstedt Test

Test to see if cerebrospinal fluid is flowing correctly, by applying pressure to the jugular veins, during a lumbar puncture.

QuickTrach Cricothyrotomy Kit

Equipment to make an emergency *front of neck airway* opening during a "can't intubate can't oxygenate" emergency.

Quiet Breathing (Eupnea)

A passive and relaxed mode of breathing that does not require extra effort, expiration only requires the natural elastic recoiling of the lungs, and exhalations are 3-4 times inspiration time. The muscles involved are the diaphragm and external intercostals.

QT Interval

Start of Q wave to end of T wave: time for ventricular depolarisation and repolarisation (ventricular systole). Fast heart rate means a short interval, and vice versa. A long interval increases risk of arrhythmias.

Radiolucent

Something which is transparent to X-rays.

Radiopaque

A property of absorbing X-rays, making radiopaque substances visible on X-rays. Seen on gauze swabs, ET and NG tubes.

Radius

The shorter of the two forearm bones, on the thumb side.

RAE Endotracheal Tube

Preformed ET tube, cuffed and uncuffed types, named after their creators - *Ring, Adair, Edwin*. South and North facing tubes are available, designed to facilitate ear, nose, & throat surgery. A RAE tube can be straightened to accommodate a bougie.

Rales

Aka *Crackles*: Abnormal lung sounds, on auscultation, which can be described as sounding like opening a velcro strap, sloshing, or a crackling, caused by the lower airways and alveoli opening during inspiration, and closing during expiration. Rales can be a sign of asthma, pulmonary oedema, or congestive heart failure.

Ramping

Placement of a wedged structure under a bariatric patient, with the aim of creating an optimal position for intubation.

Ranitidine

An antacid, given intravenously, to treat gastro-oesophageal reflux disease, or before caesarian sections, to raise gastric pH. Banned in 2020, due to cancer (GI, bladder, nasopharynx) risk.

Rapid Infuser

A device that enables quick infusion of warmed fluids through an RIC or large venous cannula. Indications: to counter hypovolaemia and surgical blood loss, warming of the hypothermic patient, and warmed irrigation during urology procedures. Example devices: Belmont, Smiths Medical (Level 1), and Mequ.

Rapid Sequence Induction (RSI)

For patients who are at risk of gastric aspiration, particularly non-fasted and obstetric patients (avoid positive pressure ventilation). See Appendix A88 (pg 499).

Rash (Exanthem)

Skin that may be dis-coloured, itchy, painful, or swollen; caused by a sting, allergy, hormones, heat, or infection/virus. Bleeding under the skin can also give the appearance of a rash. A **petechial** rash is non-blanching (glass test), with red, brown, or purple round spots, 2 mm wide. A **purpuric** rash has red/purple spots of 1-2 mm wide, is caused by bleeding under the skin, and is non-blanching. Rashes can be caused by antibiotics, chlorhexidine, and NMBAs (eg atracurium). A nurse/ODP must be able to identify these non-blanching rashes, particularly in children, because they may indicate serious conditions, such as meningitis.

RBCs

See *Red Blood Cells.*

Reactive Airway Disease

Any condition, temporary or otherwise, where the airway responds, negatively (bronchoconstriction), to an external stimulus which might be chemical, bacterial, environmental, or pharmacological. Symptoms include wheezing, coughing, and fatigue. Underlying causes might be COPD, asthma, or hay fever.

Rebreathing Circuit

A circuit where expired gases remain within the circuit, after carbon dioxide has been removed by soda lime, and the used oxygen is replaced by a fresh supply from the anaesthetic machine.

Receptor

A special cell or nerve ending which detects external stimuli, such as heat or touch, and passes the information to the central nervous system, in the form of an impulse. In anaesthesia, notable receptors are muscarinic and nicotinic.

Receptor Selectivity

The extent to which a drug binds to target receptors, compared with other receptors; if the drug binds with many receptor types, in addition to the type it is intended for, it has low selectivity. Ideally, a drug will only bind to the receptors that produce an intended effect but, if it has low selectivity, it will bind to other receptor types and sub-types, and so produce side-effects.

Reconstitution

The combining of a powdered drug with a solvent, such as Water For Injections, to form a solution.

Recovery

Provision of evaluation and stabilisation of the postoperative patient, and to anticipate and prevent complications resulting from anaesthesia and surgery. See Appendix A89 (pg 501).

Recrudescence

A resumption of a condition, or symptoms, some days after a remission period.

Recruitment Manouevres

Techniques of increasing lung pressure (40 cmH_2O, 30 seconds), to inflate collapsed alveoli, then using PEEP to keep the alveoli open, with the aim of increasing oxygenation. Care must be taken to avoid over distension of the lungs, which could occur when too much PEEP is applied. Used for ARDS.

Red Blood Cells (RBCs)

Aka *Packed Cells*: The residue of RBCs when plasma is removed, by centrifugation, from whole blood. RBCs are given: to correct a low haemoglobin (Hb) level (< 70 g/litre), significant haemorrhage, to provide the Hb required for oxygen and CO_2 transport, iron deficiency, bleeding, and low vitamin B12. Should be given by blood giving set with 10-200 micron filter, and through a blood warmer - 1 unit over 2 hours, and finished max 4 hours from fridge removal. An RBC count for (adult) males is 4.7-6 million cells per microlitre; For females: 4.2-5.3 million cells/microlitre. RBCs are normally packaged with sodium citrate, to provide anticoagulation.

Reflex Bradycardia

Bradycardia induced by the Baroreceptor Reflex: the body's response to increased blood pressure, by reducing cardiac output.

Refractory

Unmanageable, or resistant to a treatment, drug, or process.

Reflux

See Acid Reflux.

Refractory Hypoxaemia

Occurrence of hypoxaemia in the presence of 100% inspired oxygen (FiO_2). Causes: Pulmonary right-to-left shunt, pulmonary oedema, ARDS, atelectasis, burns, radiation, toxins, smoke inhalation, aspiration, and pulmonary embolism, pneumonia, sepsis, drowning. Common treatments include: high frequency oscillatory ventilation, airway pressure release ventilation, inhaled vasodilator agents, and putting the patient in the prone position.

Regional Anaesthesia

Anaesthesia affecting only part of the body, typically a limb, using local anaesthetic to block the nerve supply to a part of the body. Unlike general anaesthesia, patients may remain awake, resulting in reduced side-effects, and enabling the surgeon to converse with the patient during the procedure. See Appendix A90 (pg 503).

Relative Molecular Mass (MR)

Formal term for "Molecular Mass".

Remifentanil

A short acting synthetic opioid, often administered by continuous infusion, which takes ~8 minutes to effect. Adult bolus: 0.25-1 microgram/kg, over 30-60 seconds.

Ren-

Referring to the kidneys.

Renal System

Main kidney functions are: Acid-base balance, Water balance, Electrolyte balance, Toxin removal, Blood pressure regulation, Erythropoietin (hormone) production, and vitamin D metabolism.

Reperfusion

Restoring blood flow to an organ after, eg., a heart attack or stroke, with the aim of oxygenating tissues before necrosis sets in.

Residual Volume

Volume of air remaining in the lungs after maximum expiration.

Respiration

Refers to **(1)**: pulmonary ventilation – getting air into the lungs **(2)** external respiration – oxygen diffusion from alveoli to blood, and CO_2 from blood to alveoli **(3)** transport of oxygen through the body **(4)** internal respiration – oxygen from blood to tissues, CO_2 in the other direction **(5)** CO_2 is returned to the lungs. Once in the cells, the chemical reaction of glucose with oxygen produces an energy source, in the form of adenosine triphosphate, and gives water and carbon dioxide as a by-product. **Aerobic** respiration means in the presence of adequate levels of oxygen.

Respiratory Acidosis

The process that leads to acidaemia (pH < 7.35), where $paCO_2$ would climb above 6 kPa (45 mmHg). **Acute causes**: CO_2 retention (due to hypoventilation, atelectasis, pneumothorax, anaesthetics, alcohol, asthma, or toxins), or CNS problems affecting respiratory drive (eg, infection), airway inflammation/obstruction, opiate induced respiratory depression, chest trauma. **Signs**: breathing difficulty, tachycardia, confusion, headache. **Chronic causes**: COPD, pneumonia, obesity. Note: chronic cases may have few or no signs. **Treatment**: determined by cause, and may include CPAP, intubation, increased minute volume, bronchodilators, oxygen. Chronic respiratory acidosis and metabolic compensation seem similar to mixed respiratory acidosis and metabolic alkalosis, so the mixed case may be identified by vomiting. Respiratory acidosis and respiratory alkalosis can not occur together.

Respiratory Acidosis: Metabolic (Renal) Compensation

The body's attempt to normalise pH in respiratory acidosis, by early buffering of H+ ions, which is mostly intracellular, by phosphates, proteins, and haemoglobin. Metabolic buffering with bicarbonate (HCO_3^-), by the kidneys, takes 12-24 hours to take effect, with HCO_3^- levels estimated as: for every 10 mmHg increase of blood gas $paCO_2$ above 40 mmHg, the expected compensatory increase in HCO_3^-, above 24, is approximately ~1 mmol, and is calculated by **$HCO_3^- = 0.1 * [pCO_2 - 40] + 24$** mmol/L. In a **chronic** condition, expected increase of HCO_3 is slightly different: expected $HCO_3^- = 0.4 * [pCO_2 - 40] + 24$ mmol/L. If the blood gas HCO_3^- value is lower than expected, there may be a mixed respiratory/metabolic acidosis. Conversely, if blood gas HCO_3^- is higher than expected, there may be a mixed respiratory acidosis/metabolic alkalosis.

Respiratory Acidosis/Alkalosis -> pH Balance

In **acute** respiratory acidosis, for every 10 mmHg increase in pCO_2, there will be a decrease in pH of 0.08. In **acute** respiratory alkalosis, for every 10 mmHg decrease in pCO_2, there will be an increase in pH of 0.08. In **chronic** acidosis or alkalosis, the figure of 0.08 is replaced by 0.03. The calculated value will be modified by compensation mechanisms, and mixed acid-base conditions.

Respiratory Alkalosis

The process that can lead to alkalaemia ($pH > 7.45$), where $paCO_2$ would fall below 4.7 kPa (35 mmHg). Sedation or reducing minute volume may lower pH to a more normal value. **Causes**: hyperventilation, anxiety, liver failure, pain, sepsis, pregnancy, drugs (esp salicylates) asthma, stroke, head injury, hyperthyroidism, toxins, stroke, myocardial infarction, COPD, pulmonary embolism, meningitis, doxapram. Can produce myasthenia gravis and CNS depression. **Signs** (acute cases): blurred vision, palpitations, sweating, dry mucous membranes.

Respiratory Alkalosis: Metabolic (Renal) Compensation

With respiratory alkalosis, it takes > 12 hours before metabolic compensation starts to have an effect, after that, in **acute** respiratory alkalosis, for every 10 mmHg decrease in blood gas $paCO_2$ below 40 mmHg, the expected decrease in HCO_3^-, below 24 is ~ 2 mmol, calculated by **HCO_3^- = 24 - {0.2 * [40 – pCO_2]}** mmol/L. In a **chronic** condition, expected **HCO_3^- = 24 - {0.5 * [40 – pCO_2]}** mmol/L. If the HCO_3 fall is greater than expected, there may be mixed respiratory alkalosis/metabolic acidosis. Or, if HCO_3^- does not fall as far as expected, it may be mixed respiratory AND metabolic alkalosis.

Respiratory Arrest

The patient is apnoeic although they will still have a pulse. The patient's airway should be checked for patency and, if necessary, supported by the use of an oral/nasal airway device, chin lift, or jaw thrust. Additionally, the patient's ventilatory function might have to be managed with oxygen, plus a bag/valve/mask or Mapleson C circuit. If not corrected, cardiac arrest may ensue.

Respiratory Bronchioles

The smallest bronchioles, between a terminal bronchiole and alveolar ducts. They contain alveoli, so take part in gas exchange.

Respiratory Control Centre

The brainstem contains the medulla oblongata and pons, which provide the respiratory system with a control centre, using signals from various receptors, to control respiratory behaviour.

Central chemoreceptors (central nervous system) monitor CO_2 and acidity of cerebrospinal fluid. When CO_2 enters the cerebrospinal fluid, the pH drops, and the chemoreceptors stimulate the respiratory centre to increase the inspiratory rate, in order to flush out the CO_2 that has caused the acidity.

Peripheral chemoreceptors (peripheral nervous system), in aortic and carotid bodies, monitor the levels of CO_2 and oxygen in the aorta and carotid arteries. Any decrease in oxygen, or increase in CO_2, results in an increase in respiratory rate, or a corresponding decrease, if oxygen levels rise, or CO_2 levels fall.

Stretch receptors in the walls of bronchi and bronchioles signal the respiratory centre to halt the inspiration phase of the breathing cycle, and trigger expiration (inflation reflex).

Respiratory Cycle

The phases of respiration, which can be pre-set on a ventilator, according to patient specific needs:

√ **Inspiratory flow**: Breathing in fresh gas.

√ **Inspiratory pause**: Gas flow stops, and circuit pressure matches alveoli pressure.

√ **Expiratory flow**: Expiration, and "deflation" of alveoli – unless PEEP is applied.

√ **Expiratory pause**: Pause before inspiration.

Note: Inspiration time is usually half that of expiration time (1:2), and can be modified on ventilators.

Respiratory Distress

A term to describe the extra effort required to breathe. **Signs** include: increased respiratory rate, nasal flaring, bending forward, cyanosis, grunting on exhalation, sweating, wheezing, sunken chest, intercostal retractions, and tachypnoea.

Respiratory Drive

The regulation of minute volume, in response to the level of pH and CO_2 in the blood and cerebrospinal fluid, detected by peripheral and (mostly) central chemoreceptors, and which results in a change in the ventilation depth or rate (signals sent to the medulla), until a more normal pH level is reached.

Respiratory Exchange Ratio

Similar to the *Respiratory Quotient*, but measured externally to the body. The volume of CO_2 produced compared with the volume of oxygen consumed, measured in expirations at nose or mouth. Typically used in sports training.

Respiratory Failure (RF)

Cardiac or respiratory dysfunction, where the lungs cannot supply sufficient oxygen to the circulation, resulting in low paO_2 (arterial oxygen pressure) and inability to maintain normal metabolism. **Type I** (hypoxaemic) RF is signified by paO_2 < 8 kPa (60 mmHg) and SaO_2 < 91%. If low paO_2 is accompanied by high arterial CO_2 partial pressure ($paCO_2$) > 6 kPa (45 mmHg), it is **Type II** (hypercapnic) RF, with typical causes of COPD, infection, myasthenis gravis, asthma, deformed chest wall, or hypothyroidism. A large *pAO_2 – paO_2 gradient* suggests lung problems; otherwise the cause is more likely extra-pulmonary (not lungs). Target O_2 sats: 88-92%. See Appendix A91 (pg 505).

Respiratory Quotient (RQ)

Calculation of basal metabolic rate, to indicate which macronutrients are being metabolised, using the ratio of the volume of CO_2 to the volume of oxygen absorbed, measured by respirometer. When using carbohydrates for energy, one CO_2

molecule is created for every O_2 molecule consumed, so RQ = 1. If fatty acids (lipids) are used for energy, for every ten O_2 molecules consumed, only seven CO_2 molecules are created, which gives RQ = 0.7, a value of 0.8 for proteins. Normally, a combination of carbohydrates and fatty acids is used for energy, giving 0.8 as the mean RQ. See also *Respiratory Exchange Ratio*.

Respiratory Splinting

The tendency to make reduced breathing effort, due to pain on inspiration, and which can lead to atelectasis.

Respiratory System

The nose, mouth, pharynx, larynx, trachea, and lungs. Ventilation moves air in and out of the lungs. Gas exchange occurs at alveoli (external respiration) and tissues (internal respiration).

Respiratory Tract

The combination of the upper and lower respiratory tracts.

Upper respiratory tract: The passages of the mouth, nose, pharynx, and larynx.

Lower respiratory tract: The trachea, bronchi (main, lobar, segmental), segmental, terminal, respiratory bronchioles, alveolar ducts, alveolar sacs, and alveoli.

Respiratory Tree

The trachea, bronchi, multi-branched bronchioles, leading to the alveolar ducts/alveoli.

Anatomy

- Ω Left and right **primary bronchi** branch into secondary (lobar or intermediate) bronchi to the main lung lobes (left 2, right 3).
- Ω A **lobar bronchus** divides into tertiary (segmental) bronchi.

Ω A **segmental bronchus** divides into sub-segmental bronchi.

Ω A **sub-segmental bronchus** divide into terminal bronchioles.

Ω **Terminal bronchioles** divide into respiratory bronchioles.

(Gas exchange starts in the respiratory bronchioles)

Ω **Respiratory bronchioles** divide into alveolar ducts.

Ω **Alveolar ducts** branch into alveolar sacs, containing alveoli.

Respirometer

Device to measure tidal and minute volume, and the rate of exchange between oxygen and CO_2. Typically used to check that an anaesthetic machine is delivering what it is set to deliver.

Restrictive Pulmonary Disease

When breathing, inspiration is degraded, due to poor lung compliance, characterised by chest pain, weight loss, wheezing, and shortness of breath. Examples include: lung cancer/disease, rheumatoid arthritis, pneumonia, and tuberculosis.

Retrognathia

A condition where the lower jaw is set back from the upper jaw – seen as an "overbite", such as with Pierre Robin Syndrome.

Retrograde Intubation

For difficult intubations where, for example, secretions or trauma prevent visualisation of the vocal cords, or when fibreoptic equipment is unavailable. The cricothyroid membrane is punctured with a 16g needle, cephalic (towards the head), and a Central Venous Cannulation guide wire is passed through the needle, into the trachea and oropharynx, and out through the mouth or nose, using Magill forceps. An ET tube is railroaded over the guide wire (or tube exchanger first), and pulled into position.

Retromolar Intubation

In maxillofacial procedures - where normal oral or nasal intubation is inappropriate - a non-invasive and simpler alternative to submental intubation and, in the short term, tracheotomy. After oral intubation with an armoured ET tube, the tube is wired (ligature) to a molar/premolar tooth, giving room for the surgeon to operate.

Reversal Agent

A drug that reverses (antagonises) the effects of another drug, e.g., Neostigmine reverses the effect of a competitive blocking agent, such as Atracurium; Flumazenil reverses benzodiazepines; Naloxone reverses effects of opioids.

Rhonchi

A persistent low pitched wheezing or gurgling sound, heard on auscultation, and commonly caused by secretions in the upper airways, which might be cleared by coughing.

RIC (Rapid Infusion Catheter)

A large bore intravenous catheter, specifically for use with rapid infusion devices. See also *Rapid Infusion*.

Right Heart Failure

Backward Heart Failure where the right ventricle fails to pump sufficient blood into the pulmonary circulation (via pulmonary artery). As a result, blood backs up in the veins (congestion), with oedema in the abdomen (ascites), ankles, and legs. **Symptoms**: enlarged liver or spleen, ascites, fatigue, jaundice, pleural effusion, distended jugular veins.

Right to Left Shunt

Normally, de-oxygenated blood reaches the right side of the heart, via the vena cavae, is sent to the lungs to be oxygenated, travels to the left side of the heart, and is then ejected into the systemic circulation. In a right to left shunt, some of the deoxygenated blood fails to travel to the lungs and, instead, takes a short cut (shunt) from right to left sides of the heart. Consequently, deoxygenated blood enters the systemic circulation and, thereby, dilutes the amount of oxygen in the arterial circulation.

Ring Block (Field Block)

Local anaesthetic infiltration circling the surgical site, without injection into the site itself. The block prevents nerve impulses from leaving the site when, for example, it is undesirable to 'pollute' surrounding tissue with the anaesthetic agent.

Robert Shaw Endotracheal/Endobronchial Tube

See Double Lumen Endotracheal/Endobronchial Tube.

Rocuronium

A quick (2 min) acting neuromuscular blocking agent (refrigerated) with 30-40 minute duration. Antagonised by Neostigmine or Sugammadex. Dose is 0.6 mg/kg from 10 mg/ml.

Ropivacaine

A longer lasting local anaesthetic than marcaine (bupivacaine), with less CNS and cardiovascular toxicity.

ROSIER Score

Recognition Of Stroke In the Emergency Room: A seven point scoring system to aid in recognising Stroke. See *Stroke* and Appendix A101 (pg 522).

RSI

Rapid Sequence Induction.

RSV, Respiratory Syncytial Virus

A virus that produces respiratory tract infections, particularly pneumonia and bronchiolitis, especially in Winter months. Usually spread by droplets from coughs and sneezes.

Rule of Ten

In a healthy patient, pAO_2 (alveolar oxygen partial pressure) should be 10 kPa higher than paO_2 (arterial oxygen partial pressure). If the inspired difference is greater than 10 kPa, the patient may be suffering from pulmonary disease. Normal pAO_2 is ~100 mmHg (13.3 kPa); paO_2 is 75 - 100 mmHg (10-13.3 kPa).

Saddle Block

A *spinal block* that is used, for example, where childbirth produces perineum lacerations and 3rd degree tears. Method: 1.5 ml of standard 0.5% hyperbaric marcain is injected when the patient is in the sitting position.

Saddle Embolus

A blood clot in the main pulmonary artery (pulmonary trunk). See Appendix A86 (pg 496).

Safe Apnoea Time

The period between when the patient stops breathing (or ventilation stopped), and when oxygen saturation (SaO_2) drops below 90%. Before induction, pre-oxygenation prolongs safe apnoea time.

Salbutamol

An inhaled bronchodilator which helps to open airways in cases of asthma or bronchospasm.

Saline Solution

Sodium chloride dissolved in water, used for fluid replenishment and wound cleaning. The type of saline solution used has a weight/volume concentration of 0.9%, so is isotonic with body fluids. A lower concentration of saline solution, if ingested, would cause excess fluid to enter the cells, by osmosis. Conversely, a higher concentration would result in cells losing fluid.

Salt

An electrically neutral compound of cations (positive ions from a metal) and anions (negative ions from non-metal) that results from a neutralisation reaction between two groups - acids and bases. When in solution, such as in water, the ions separate (ionisation) and are electrically conductive (electrolytes). Examples: calcium chloride, sodium chloride, and magnesium sulphate.

SaO_2

Direct measurement of **oxygen saturation** (%) of healthy arterial Hb (haemoglobin) that is saturated with oxygen, as a fraction of total Hb, using blood gas analysis. $SaO_2 = 100 * O_2Hb / (O_2Hb + HHb)\ \%$ where O_2Hb is the concentration of oxygenated Hb in arterial blood, and HHb is the concentration of deoxygenated Hb in arterial blood. Some blood gas machines measure the SaO_2 directly (spectrophotometric), giving an accurate figure, but other machine ("Point-of-care") types calculate the % from oxygen tension (paO_2), using values from the oxygen dissociation curve. Co-Oximeters also exclude mathaemoglobin type Hb from readings, which would otherwise give a less accurate measure of "Sats". SaO_2 is unaffected by Hb levels, so is not a check for anaemia. See *CO-Oximetery, Oxygen Saturation, SpO_2.*

Saphenous

The nerve connecting the femoral nerve with sensory nerves in the skin of the lower leg, and the 2 veins draining blood from the foot.

SARS

See Severe Acute Respiratory Syndrome.

Sats

See Oxygen Saturation.

Scavenging

See Gas Scavenging.

Schrader Socket Valve

Colour coded push-fit connector between low pressure gas supply (wall or ceiling) and anaesthetic machine.

Sclerosis

A hardening (scler) of skin, internal tissue, or organ.

Second Gas Effect

Adding high flow nitrous oxide (1st gas) to a gas induction scheme tends to reduce induction time, because the nitrous oxide (N_2O) enters capillaries faster than the other gases, and so produces increased alveolar concentration of a second gas, such as sevoflurane. See Appendix A93 (pg 507).

Secondary Infusion

Intravenous infusion of an agent from a source that is additional to the primary infusion source, which may be either gravity fed, or of the pumped (volumetric) type. The secondary infusion connects to the primary infusion line by means of a tapped port on the primary line, or to a spare lumen of an "octopus" type iv extension tube. Also known as a "piggyback" system.

Secondary Survey

More in depth than *primary* survey. See Appendix A94 (pg 509).

Sedation

The patient is given drugs, such as Midazolam or Propofol, to depress the central nervous system, producing a calming effect.

Sedation score

Measurement scheme to describe a patient's level of sedation.

Score	*Meaning*
S	Normal sleep
0	Awake and alert
1	Drowsy
2	Sedated/difficult to rouse
3	Unrousable

Sedative

An agent that relieves tension and anxiety. Commonly used sedatives are the Benzodiazepine anxiolytic agents:

Benzodiazepine Sedatives...

☺ Diazepam ☺ Lorazepam ☺ Midazolam

☺ Oxazepram ☺ Nitrazepam ☺ Temazepam

These agents are antagonised by Flumazenil.

Sedation Scores

Sedated patient monitoring schemes. Examples: Riker Sedation-Agitation Scale, Richmond Agitation-Sedation Scale, and the Ramsay Sedation Scale.

See-Saw Breathing

Breathing pattern, seen in airway obstruction, where the chest and abdomen move in opposite (paradoxical) directions: when **attempting** to breathe in, the abdomen raises, and the chest tends to sink. Attempting to breathe out has the opposite effect.

Seldinger technique

A method of introducing catheters and probes into vessels.

- Puncture the vessel with a percutaneous needle.
- Insert the Seldinger wire through the needle into the vessel.
- Remove the needle.
- Use the Seldinger wire as means of access to the vessel.

Sensible Fluid Loss

Loss of fluid (blood and urine) that can be seen and measured.

Sepsis

Sepsis is an immune system dysregulated or over-reactive inflammatory response to infection (usually bacterial), resulting in hypoxia and possible life threatening organ damage, sometimes indicated by high WBC or lactate levels. The term “severe sepsis” is no longer used, and recognition no longer uses criteria from Systemic Inflammatory Response Syndrome. Instead, **identification** and severity are gauged by SOFA (Sequential Organ Failure Assessment). The sepsis-3 definition is, therefore: **infection + 2 or more SOFA points, as a consequence of infection**. See *Septic Shock* and Appendix A95 (pg 511).

Sepsis Monitoring (minimum)

Adults and Children over 12+ years ...

- Blood pressure
- Heart rate
- Respiratory rate
- Temperature
- Level of consciousness
- Oxygen sats
- Changed mental state

Children Under 12 years ...

Same as above, plus capillary refill time. Only check blood pressure if finger capillary refill time is more than 2 seconds, or more than 4 seconds for foot or chest.

Sepsis Six

The UK Sepsis Trust protocol for managing sepsis, produced from the International Surviving Sepsis Campaign guidelines, to ensure rapid response, with senior clinician attendance and:

- Oxygen, to maintain sats > 94%, or 88-92% if hypercapnic
- Take bloods + CSF, sputum, urine
- Give 500 ml IV fluid if low BP or lactate > 2 mmol/L
- Give intravenous antibiotics
- Check lactates (if > 4 mmol/L, admit to ICU)
- Measure urine output

Septic Shock

Deterioration of sepsis to distributive shock, with organ failure, and culminating in cardiac arrest. Characterised by serum lactate >= 2 mmol/L and hypotension (not responsive to fluid resuscitation) that requires vasopressors to maintain MAP above 64 mmHg. High risk of mortality is due to metabolic, circulatory, and cellular irregulatories. If persistent, despite volume resuscitation and inotropes or vasopressors, it is deemed "refractory". See Appendices A95 (pg 511), A96 (pg 513).

Septicaemia

Blood poisoning caused by bacteria infection, from another part of the body (lungs etc), entering the bloodstream. Can lead to sepsis.

Sequela

A morbid condition resulting from a previous disease or trauma. For example, vision disturbance resulting from a head injury.

Sequential Organ Failure Assessment (SOFA)

A scoring system which describes the severity of sepsis, where six body systems are used as references, with each system being ascribed a score of 1-4. See Appendix A97 (pg 514).

Serous

Something which contains or secretes serum.

Serous Membrane (Serosa)

Folded layer of cells that line a cavity (parietal) and surrounds an organ (visceral), with serous lubricating fluid between the folds. Locations: ① Visceral and parietal pleura (lungs) ② Inner pericardium (heart) ③ Peritoneum (abdominal cavity).

Serum

Fluid component of blood, after cells and clotting agents are removed (or plasma without clotting factors). Serum includes all proteins not used in blood clotting, electrolytes, antibodies, antigens, hormones, and any exogenous substances (e.g., drugs and microorganisms). Also described as the liquid remaining after a clot has formed. The main difference between serum and plasma is that plasma contains fibrinogen.

Severe Acute Respiratory Syndrome (SARS)

An airborne infectious disease, SARS-CoV. Spread by touch, faeces, coughing, or sneezing droplets that others inhale. **Caused** by a coronavirus originating in China (2002). **Symptoms**: headache, fever, shivering, coughing, diarrhoea, fatigue.

Sevoflurane

A volatile (evaporates easily) inhalational agent, used for induction and maintenance phases (with oxygen) of anaesthesia. Sevoflurane can cause increased intracranial pressure, but does not increase heart rate as much as other inhalation agents. It is the only volatile agent that is suitable for gas induction. Minimum Alveolar Concentration ranges from 1.4%, for patients over the age of 80, to 3.4%, for new born babies. With an oil:gas partition coefficient of 47, Sevoflurane has a potency between Isoflurane and Desflurane. See also *Volatile Anaesthetic Agents*.

Sharps Management

A set of actions intended to prevent injury or poisoning by accidental skin/venal puncture from sharp instruments, such as needles, sutures, trocars, and blades.

Specific Management Techniques

- Do not break needles prior to use or disposal.
- Do not disassemble.
- Do not re-sheath needles.

- Dispose as a single unit.
- Do not over fill sharps bins.
- Never leave sharps lying around.
- Full bins must be sealed and labelled before disposal.
- A sharps bin should be within arms reach.

Shock (Acute Stress Disorder)

Failure of the cardiovascular system to deliver perfusion to supply oxygen and nutrients to vital organs, particularly the kidneys and brain. The reduced cardiac output causes an accumulation of lactate, producing lactic acidosis. If untreated, shock can lead to multiple organ failure. The main shock criterion is **Hypotension** after giving 30 ml/kg (20 ml, paeds) iv fluid, with systolic < 90 mmHg, and mean BP < 65 mmHg, or a fall of 40 mmHg from systolic. Other early **signs** are hypoxaemia, tachycardia, and tachypnoea. Other signs: fever, metabolic acidosis, tachycardia, tachypnoea, clammy peripheries, low pH, paO_2, oliguria, lactate > 2 mmol/L, confusion. Shock types: Appendix A98 (pg 516).

Shunt

Mixing of venous and arterial blood, due to low lung oxygenation (intra-pulmonary shunt), or blood bypassing the lungs (cardiac shunt). See *V/Q Mismatch; Cardiac* and *Intra Pulmonary Shunt*.

SIMV

Synchronised Intermittent Mandatory Ventilation.

Sinoatrial Node (SA Node, Sinoatrial Node)

The heart's natural pacemaker. A cell (myocytes) cluster in the right atrium, inferior to the Vena Cava opening.

Sinus Arrhythmia

An abnormal pulse rhythm caused by sinus node disturbance, causing tachycardia on inspiration, and bradycardia on expiration. A slight arrhythmia is normal.

Sinus Bradycardia

Bradycardia due to the Sinus Node firing at a low rate – giving a resting heart rate < 60 beats/minute.

Sinus Node

See Sinoatrial Node.

Sinus Rhythm

Describes normal heart rhythm, governed by the sinus node...

- Sinus node creates electrical stimuli (action potential).
- Stimuli travel through the atrioventricular node.
- Stimuli continue through Bundle of Hiss and branches.
- Stimuli reach Purkinje Fibres.
- Atria and ventricles depolarise.

Sinus Tachycardia

An increase in heart rate which occurs when the sinus node triggers electrical signals at a faster than normal rate.

Causes include...

- Exercise
- Anxiety
- Pregnancy
- Hyperthyroidism
- Anaemia
- Alcohol
- Caffeine
- Hypoxaemia
- Nicotine
- Infection
- Pain
- Hypovolaemia
- Salbutamol
- Recreational drugs

Treatment is aimed at the underlying cause.

SIRS

Systemic Inflammatory Response Syndrome.

Sleep Apnoea

Sleep Apnoea is the cessation (10 seconds) of normal breathing, during sleep, there being three types...

Obstructive Sleep Apnoea: During sleep, the larynx relaxes and constricts, and interrupts normal breathing.

Central Sleep Apnoea: A less common type of sleep apnoea, when the brain fails to signal the muscles which control breathing.

Complex Sleep Apnoea: A combination of obstructive and central sleep apnoea.

Sliding Scale Insulin Administration

Regime for short-term intravenous administration of insulin, according to blood glucose levels (e.g., 5 mmol/litre), sometimes to supplement long acting insulin. A *sliding scale* is used when the diabetic mellitus patient is ill, or hospitalised. Finger prick capillary glucose levels are monitored every 1-2 hours, and insulin dose is titrated according to those readings. Because sliding scale insulin injections are given in reaction to glucose levels, it is not necessary for a doctor to be consulted each time. The sliding scale method can result in large swings in glucose, because it is not a proactive way of managing blood glucose levels.

Slough (Sluf)

Dead tissue resulting from inflammation or injury, which is washed away by serum exudate.

Sniffing The Morning Air

The patient position which best facilitates endotracheal

intubation. For a typical adult patient – not obese – the mouth will be horizontally aligned with the trachea. A pillow is used to raise the patient's head (not the shoulders) 3-4 inches (8-10 cm).

(1) For bariatric patients, it may be necessary to create a ramp under the patient's upper body, so that the ear canal is horizontally inline with the sternum, by using, for example, an Oxford HELP pillow, thereby creating the "Sniffing" position.

(2) For small children, the optimal position may be achieved by not using a pillow.

Sodium (Na)

The main extracellular cation, which takes part in muscle contraction, transmission of nerve impulses, helps maintain blood pressure. and fluid balance. A low Na serum level (hyponatraemia) may be due to oedema. A high level might be caused by dehydration, diarrhoea, diuretics, or vomiting. Normal plasma range is 135 – 145 mmol/litre. Note: Sodium is the body's main cation and, with potassium, constitutes 95% of the total cations.

Sodium Bicarbonate ($NaHCO_3$), Bicarbonate of Soda

A salt compound of a sodium cation and bicarbonate anion, used as a buffer in cases of severe acidosis, with typical dose being 1 ml/kg 8·4% w/v. (Use is controversial) Given orally or IV, buffers (mops up) hydrogen ions, so raising pH. Also drives potassium from the extracellular space, into the cells. For cardiac arrest with hyperkalaemia, give 50 mmol (50 ml of 8.4%).

Sodium Chloride (NaCl)

A halide (binary) ionic compound, commonly used as a dissolution in water, to form an electrolyte solution which is isotonic with blood and other body fluids – Normal Saline (0.9%).

Sodium Citrate

A prophylactic antacid compound, 30 ml of which is usually given, orally, immediately before intubation in caesarian section cases, in case of acid aspiration. Side-effect can be nausea/vomitng.

Sodium Nitrite

To treat cyanide poisoning. Given with sodium thiosulphate.

SOFA

See Sequential Organ Failure Assessment.

Solubility

The tendency for a substance (the solute), which might be solid, liquid, or gas, to dissolve in a solvent (blood etc), and form a solution, rather than a mixture or suspension.

Solute

The minor component ions or molecules of a mixture, which are dissolved in the solvent, forming a solution. In normal saline, water is the solvent, sodium and chloride ions are the solutes.

Solution

A homogeneous mixture of two or more types of molecule, where the most abundant molecule type is the solvent, and which decomposes the other molecules, known as the solutes. To form a solution, the solvent molecules surround ("solvation", or "hydration" if the solvent is water) the solute molecules, and the formed components tend to evenly diffuse through the solvent. The even diffusion of the solutes, in the solvent, results in the solution. Solutions can contain a combination of solid, liquid, or gas phases. The small particles, which have been dissolved into the solvent, have a diameter smaller than one nanometre, so they will not “settle”, otherwise, the mixture will not be a true solution. The solvent will only be able to dissolve a specific maximum amount of solute, known as its saturation point, after which, more solute will be mixed with, but not absorbed by, the solvent.

Solvent

The component of a solution which dissolves the solute, and which is present in the greatest amount.

Soma-

Referring to the body of something, rather than the mind.

Somatic

Pertaining to the physical body, rather than the viscera or mind. Somatic pain is localised to muscles, skin, joints, and bones, such as that caused by superficial injury.

Somatic Nervous System

The part of the peripheral nervous system that deals with the voluntary (not automatic) control of muscles and movement, using afferent (sensory) and efferent (motor) nerves.

Soporific

Producing sleep.

Spasm

Sudden involuntary muscle contraction.

Specificity

If a drug only acts on its intended target receptors, the drug is classed as having good *specificity*. In most cases, drugs act on more than just their intended receptors, and the degree to which they target other receptors describes their *selectivity*.

Speed Shock

A sudden reaction to an intravenous drug that has been administered too quickly. Signs include headache, flushing, chest tightness, irregular pulse, and cardiac arrest. Speed shock may be prevented by use of an infusion device.

Spinal Anaesthesia

Aka: Spinal, intradural, subarachnoid, or intrathecal block. A quick acting neuro-axial regional block of peripheral nociceptors, suitable for caesarian sections and some below umbilicus procedures, where anaesthetic agents are injected into the CSF of the subarachnoid space (needle pierces dura mater with a "pop"), and effectively spreads the anaesthetic, so that the agent acts directly on the spinal cord. Onset is a few minutes, and duration is 2-3 hours. Note: a "spinal" is usually given with the patient in a sitting position but, if the patient is sedated, this might cause a vasovagal syncope (fainting). See Appendix A99 (pg 519).

Spinal Needle

A 2-6 inch (5-15 cm) 22g hollow needle for spinal injections. Three most popular types:

Whitacre: Blunt pencil point (atraumatic) needle that spreads rather than cuts dura fibres, making a smaller "hole" than with Quincke, giving less CSF leakage and PDPH than other needles.

Sprotte: An atraumatic ogive (bullet) shaped pencil point needle, that also spreads rather than cuts dura mater fibres.

Quincke: A cutting tip, and short bevel, uses introducer - more likely to cause PDPH than other needle types.

See Appendix A100 (pg 521).

Spirometry

Measurement of lung volume and flow rate, using a spirometer, with the view to help identify restrictive and obstructive ventilation, and diagnosing, for example, asthma, bronchitis, and COPD. Spirometry is integral to anaesthetic machines. A graphical representation is given by a *flow-volume loop.*

Splanchnic

Referring to abdominal cavity (visceral) organs.

Splinting

The tendency to stop moving a part of the body because the movement causes pain.

Splitting Ratio

The ratio between the volume of gas flow through a vapouriser agent (fluid) chamber, against what flows through the bypass pipe. If the flow dial is set to "0", all of the gas will bypass the chamber.

SpO2, SPO2

The percentage of arterial haemoglobin that is bound with oxygen, measured by pulse oximetry. Anaemia (low Hb) does not affect SpO2, so the patient may have normal sats, but may be hypoxic. See also SaO2, *Oxygen Saturation.*

Spodick Sign

An ECG trace with a downward sloping SP segment (base line), indicating possible Stage I pericarditis, seen in 80-90% of cases.

Spondyl-

Referring to the spine.

Spontaneous Breathing

The natural action of ventilation, through the autonomous vacuum like action of the lungs, which creates the over and under pressure differentials, with respect to ambient pressure, which governs the movement of respiratory gas in and out of the lungs.

Staggered Overdose

Where repeated doses of some drugs, such as Paracetamol, can accumulate and cause illness or death.

Standard Precautions

Previously referred to as *Universal Precautions*, are the non-exclusive set of actions that contribute to infection control and the prevention of contamination of people, surfaces, equipment, fittings, and atmosphere. See Appendix A108 (pg 532).

Standard Temperature and Pressure (STP)

STP is less than *mean atmospheric pressure*, and was defined so that scientific measurements would be easier, and provide consistency. In 1982, the International Union of Pure and Applied Chemistry defined air *Standard Temperature* to be 0° C, with molar volume of 22.711 litre, and *Standard Pressure*:

Φ 1 bar Φ 100 kPa Φ 750 mmHg

The lower pressure at higher altitudes means vapourisers have to provide more vapour to maintain the agent's required absolute partial pressure, so must be calibrated to ambient pressure.

Steady State

When the amount of drug absorbed is equal to the amount eliminated. This is an important factor in TIVA.

Steerable Bougie

Flexible tipped bougie, controlled by a slider at the controlling end.

STEMI (ST Elevation Myocardial Infarction)

The most serious form of heart attack, where the ECG trace shows a distinct elevation of the ST segment, which represents a major blockage of a coronary artery.

Stenosis (Stricture)

Narrowing (sten) of an opening or vessel, such as an artery.

Stent

Mesh inserted into an artery to support or widen it.

Step Down Recovery Unit

After recovering from a general anaesthetic, in a Recovery Unit, the spontaneously breathing and fully conscious patient may be moved to an intermediate room, prior to discharge, for a short period of final adjustment to normality.

Sternomental Distance

The distance between the suprasternal notch (connects clavicles with sternum) and the point of the chin (mouth closed and head fully extended). For an adult, intubation difficulty is anticipated if the distance is measured at less than 5 inches (12.5 cm).

-stomy

Procedure to make an opening, such as in tracheostomy.

STP

See Standard Temperature and Pressure.

Stretta

Minimally invasive endoscopic technique to treat gastroesophageal reflux disease, by strengthening the Lower Oesophageal Sphincter, without the need for a general anaesthetic; a radio frequency catheter is passed through the endoscope, then radio frequency energy creates lesions, which heal to strengthen the tissue.

Stridor

A harsh vibrating sound (crowing), caused by tumour, infection, or partial obstruction of the larynx or trachea. Stridor, on inspiration, suggests upper airway obstruction; on expiration, the lower airway obstruction. Biphasic (inspiration and expiration) stridor suggests obstruction in the vicinity of the cricoid cartilage.

Treatment:

- Oxygen and positioning the head of the bed up 45-90 degrees.
- Nebulised racemic Adrenaline (0.5 to 0.75 ml of 2.25% racemic Adrenaline added to 2.5 to 3 ml of normal saline) in cases where airway oedema may be the cause of the stridor.
- Dexamethasone 4-8 mg IV, in cases where airway oedema may be the cause of the stridor; note that some time (hours) may be needed for dexamethasone to work fully.
- Inhaled Heliox (70% helium, 30% oxygen); the effect is almost instantaneous. Helium, being a less dense gas than nitrogen,

reduces turbulent flow through the airways.

Stroke

Serious condition which occurs when the blood supply to part of the brain is cut off, due to bleeding (haemorrhagic) or blockage (ischaemic, 80%). See ROSIER and Appendix A101 (pg 522).

Stroke Volume (SV)

The amount of blood expelled by the left ventricle, during each beat. For a typical adult, 50-100 ml, or 1 ml/kg body mass.

Stroke Volume Variation (SVV)

Differences between min and max stroke volumes during different phases of a respiratory cycle, in a ventilated patient. Large variations suggest the patient will be more fluid responsive.

Stylet

A device for pre-forming and giving rigidity to an endotracheal tube, or flexible laryngeal mask airway, prior to insertion.

Subarachnoid (Intrathecal) Space

The “spider web” like space between pia and subarachnoid maters, containing cerebrospinal fluid (CSF), and the target for spinal injection and lumbar puncture.

Subcutaneous Injection

Injection (12 mm) of a water soluble agent into fatty tissue, between skin and muscle. With few subcutaneous blood vessels, a substance is absorbed more slowly, giving a low dose sustained release, suitable for slow infusion of insulin, vaccines, Growth Hormone, and Adrenaline. See Appendix A102 (pg 524).

Subdural Space

Between the arachnoid and dura maters, which are normally pressed together, with a tiny amount of serous fluid between them, but spine or brain trauma can cause a space to open up.

Sublimation

The process whereby a substance changes from solid to vapour.

Sublingual

Under the tongue.

Submental Intubation

{Submental: *below chin*} A ventilation/intubation technique which allows full surgical access to the oral and nasal cavities, used in cases of facial trauma, and when dental occlusion (closing the jaw) is required. See Appendix A103 (pg 526).

Sugammadex

Quick acting reversal agent for neuromuscular blockade caused by rocuronium or vecuronium. Intravenous dose is 2-4 mg/kg.

Supraventricular Tachycardia (SVT)

Tachycardia (150-230 beats/min), where impulses originate at the atria – not the ventricles. Aka *Paroxysmal SVT.*

Surety

Alternative to the Luer connector type, no longer manufactured, and superseded by the NRFit connector system.

Surfactant

A compound which reduces the surface tension between two liquids, or a liquid and a solid. In the lungs, surfactants reduce surface tension of fluid, prevents alveoli from collapsing during exhalation, and increases pulmonary compliance.

Surgical Airway

An intervention to make a patient's airway artificially patent, during a CICO (Can't Intubate Can't Oxygenate) situation, by means of cricothyroidotomy, or a planned surgical airway access, by tracheostomy or laryngotomy.

Suspension

Particles, with a diameter larger than one micrometre, mixed, rather than dissolved, into another medium, such as a liquid. The size of the particles means that they will tend to settle.

Suxamethonium Apnoea (Scoline Apnoea)

Apnoea caused by an inability to metabolise Suxamethonium, due to insufficient *pseudocholinesterase* in the blood. The prolonged paralysing effect of Suxamethonium means a patient may reverse from anaesthesia, but remain paralysed. As the patient becomes aware, blood pressure and heart rate increase, the patient may sweat, and the pupils may dilate. A nerve stimulator can show whether the patient is still paralysed and, if so, the patient should be re-anaesthetised and ventilated.
Treatment: Anaesthetise, ventilate, and monitor *Train of Four*.

Suxamethonium Chloride (Succinylcholine, Anectine)

A non-reversible rapid acting and short duration (5 min, quickly broken down by plasma cholinesterase) **depolarising** neuromuscular blocking agent, used in rapid sequence induction; 1-2 mg/kg from 50 mg/ml supply. Paralysis is marked by fasciculations (muscle twitches), and bradycardia may occur, so prophylactic atropine may be given prior to administration. Can be a trigger for malignant hyperthermia. Keep refrigerated.

SVT

Supra Ventricular Tachycardia.

Swiss Staging System

Method to gauge hypothermia, when temperature measurements are inaccurate or not possible. See Appendix 57 (pg 457).

Sym/Syn-

Together.

Sympathetic Nervous System

The division of the autonomic nervous system that helps maintain homoeostasis (sweating etc). It is also responsible for the fight or flight response to danger, by increasing heart rate and cardiac output, and dilating the pupils and bronchioles. The primary neurotransmitter of the SNS is noradrenaline.

Sympathomimetic (Adrenergic)

Drugs that emulate the effect of stimulating adrenergic receptors of sympathetic nervous system nerves (either directly or indirectly), matching the effects of, for example, adrenaline. Example direct (act at postsynaptic receptors) sympathomimetics: adrenaline, dopamine, metaraminol, noradrenaline, phenylephrine,. Cocaine and ephedrine are indirect (release neurotransmitters from presynaptic receptors) sympathomimetics. Side effects are hypertension, muscle spasm, and tachycardia.

Synapse

A junction between two nerve cells, consisting of a minute gap across which impulses pass by diffusion of a neurotransmitter (chemical messenger), which serves to allow information to pass from one neuron (pre-synaptic) to another neuron (post-synaptic). A synapse is necessary because neurons are not connected.

Synchronised Intermittent Mandatory Ventilation (SIMV)

Ventilation mode where the ventilator delivers a set number of breaths per minute, whilst allowing the patient to make spontaneous breaths. The ventilator detects respiratory effort (triggered when airway pressure falls below end expiratory pressure), and assists that effort by completing the "breath" to the maximum inspiratory pressure, plus PEEP. If the patient does not make a sufficient number of efforts to breathe (per min), the ventilator makes the breaths for them. SIMV is used when weaning patients off intubation, or if they just need help in breathing.

Syncope (Fainting)

A brief period of unconsciousness, due to reduced blood pressure.

Syndrome

An identifiable condition that is characterised by a particular set of symptoms, often without an understanding of the causes.

Synostosis

The fusing of bones by formation of new bony tissue.

Syntocinon (trade name)

An oxytocic: A synthetic form of oxytocin, used to induce labour, given immediately after caesarian section delivery, to minimise postpartum bleeding, and to stimulate contractions to push out the placenta. The anaesthetic assistant should ensure that the obstetric theatre fridge contains a supply of syntocin, and is immediately available. Additionally, the syntocin infusion should be set up, by the assistant, well in advance of use. Note also: a syntocinon infusion should **never** be connected to, or disconnected from, a patient unless it is administered via an infusion pump. For details, see Appendix A29 (pg 391).

Système International d'Unités (SI)

The group of seven integrated measurement systems, from which, other systems, such as pressure (pascal), are derived.

Length	Metre
Mass	Kilogram
Time	Second
Electrical current	Ampere
Temperature	Kelvin
Amount of a substance	Mole
Light intensity	Candela

Systemic Circulation

Carries oxygenated blood from the left ventricle to the aorta, to supply body tissues with oxygen, and gather carbon dioxide and waste material, from the tissues, for return to the right heart.

Systemic Inflammatory Response Syndrome (SIRS)

Body wide inflammation, leading to organ damage. Symptoms are any two of hypothermia, fever, tachycardia, and tachypnoea.

Systemic Vascular Resistance (SVR)

Resistance to blood flow offered by all of the systemic vasculature, and which gives blood pressure. Constricting blood vessels increase SVR and blood pressure; dilating vessels do the opposite.

Systole

Greek "to squeeze": Heart cycle phase when cardiac muscle contracts, the aortic valve opens, blood is ejected into the aorta, and BP is at its peak. On the ECG trace, atrial systole is indicated by the "P" wave, and ventricular systole by the "QRS" complex.

Tachycardia

A faster than normal heart rate (> 100 beats/minute), for at least 3 consecutive beats, due to a fast rate of electrical impulses, which can prevent proper filling of the ventricles.

Three main tachycardia classifications:

- Atrial: Impulses are supraventricular
- Sinus: *S*inus node produces high rate of impulses
- Ventricular: Impulses originate in the ventricles

The main cause of persistent tachycardia is heart disease. Treatment depends on the type of tachycardia, and the patient's specific condition and circumstances.

Tachycardia Syndrome

The Sinus Node (heart pacemaker) is dysfunctional.

Tachypnoea

Shallow and fast (> 20 breaths/min) breathing rate.

Target Controlled Infusion (TCI)

Programmable infusion pumped version of TIVA, that uses patient characteristics and pharmacokinetic models to calculate the optimum and steady state plasma concentration, with a **loading dose** to reach the target concentration, and a **maintenance dose** to maintain plasma concentration. Commonly used with propofol and remifentanil. See Appendix A105 (pg 529).

TEE

See Trans Thoracic Echocardiogram.

TEG

See Thromboelastogram.

Teicoplanin

Antibiotic against aerobic and anaerobic Gram+ bacteria, such as MRSA. Similar to vancomycin, but longer duration of action.

Temperature

A normal body temperature range is 36 - 37.6° C (96.8 - 99.7° F). A high temperature may rise to 40° C (104° F), and may be a response to infection.

Tension Pneumothorax

Pressure on intrathoracic structures due to pneumothorax that involves a progressive build up of air (and pressure) in the pleural cavity, often as a consequence of a penetrating injury. A reversible cause of cardiac arrest. See Appendix A104 (pg 528).

Ter Die Sumendum (TDS, TID)

Pharmacology: take three times a day.

Tetracycline

A broad spectrum polyketide antibiotic, typically used to treat urinary and respiratory tract infections.

Thalassaemia

Inherited problem of not producing enough haemoglobin, with consequent anaemia. Main victims are from: S Asia, Mediterranean, Middle East.

Therapeutic Index (TI)

A value to describe how close a safe drug dose is to a lethal dose, where safety is suggested by a higher TI, given by **Median Lethal Dose** (TD_{50}) divided by **Median Effective Dose** (ED_{50}). A small TI (gentamicin, amikacin, vancomycin, phenytoin, warfarin, digoxin) means safety can only be served by precise dosing, in a narrow range. A large TI (clarithromycin, erithromycin, penicillin) means larger fluctuations in plasma concentrations might remain safe.

Therapeutic Range

The range of plasma drug concentrations that will produce the desired effect, without also producing unwanted side-effects.

Thiopentone (Sodium Pentothal, Thiopental Sodium)

Quick acting (30 sec) and 5-10 minute duration barbiturate which depresses the CNS, for induction of hypnosis and anaesthesia, without analgesia. Reconstituted into 20 ml of a 2.5% w/v concentration, suitable for rapid sequence induction, at a dose of 3–5 mg/kg. See Appendix A106 (pg 530).

Third Gas Effect

See Diffusion Hypoxia.

Third Spacing

The shift of intravascular fluid into the interstitial space, especially in the bowel, peritoneum, and pleura. Causes include trauma, inflammation, obstructions, and infection.

Thoracocentesis

Pleural Tap: A process to reduce pleural effusion, i.e., to aspirate liquid or gas from the pleural space.

Thoracotomy

An incision into the thorax, to access chest organs or upper aorta.

Thorax

The chest cavity and structures; containing the heart, lungs, bronchi, and oesophagus.

Thorpe Tube

A vertically calibrated type of flow meter, or *rotameter* - a device which governs the flow rate (litres per minute) of a medical gas, at a constant pressure, and has a "bobbin" which floats up to a mark on the tube, corresponding with the particular flow rate, set by a rotary dial. The tube diameter increases, from bottom to top, so that more gas flow is provided for pressure to support the bobbin, reflecting the flow rate, which is calibrated on the side of the tube.

Three-Way Tap

Access device for intravenous lines, with an access port for a syringe, and valve to isolate the port, fluid supply, and line to the iv connection. Disadvantages: does not allow full fluid flow rate of large bore cannula, and adds to infection risk.

THRIVE

Transnasal Humidified Rapid-Insufflation Ventilatory Exchange is a method of increasing safe apnoea time, by fitting the patient with a trans-nasal oxygen device, with a flow rate of 70 litres of oxygen per minute, producing a CPAP delivery method. The intention is to passively oxygenate the patient until a definitive airway is established. One example system is the Optiflow product, which is designed to be used in rapid sequence induction.

Thrombectomy

Surgery to remove a blood clot.

Thrombin

An enzyme that converts fibrinogen into fibrin, and forms a mesh at a haemorrhage site, during the later stages of blood clotting.

Thrombin Time (TT)

Aka *Thrombin Clotting Time*: An assay (screening test) to determine how long it takes thrombin to catalyse fibrinogen into fibrin (clot formation), in the plasma – usually 15-20 seconds.

Thrombocyte

See Platelets.

Thrombocytopenia

A low platelet count, below $150 * 10^9$/litre. Symptoms: purpura, excessive bleeding, blood in stools/urine, fatigue, enlarged spleen.

Thrombocytosis

A high platelet count, over $450 * 10^9$/litre. Symptoms: weakness, headaches, chest pain, dizziness.

Thromboelastogram (TEG)

Thromboelastography tests speed of blood coagulation, platelet function, clot strength, thrombin and prothrombin times, and fibrinolysis, by measuring the physical properties of a clot. The test shows how platelets interact with the coagulation cascade, and helps to indicate whether or not a transfusion is needed.

Thromboembolism

A blocked blood vessel, caused by a clot. An example venous thromboembolism is Deep Vein Thrombosis, formed in the femoral vein. When a thrombus breaks away, it becomes an embolus, and travels through the bloodstream until it reaches a choke point, where it blocks circulation. An embolus in pulmonary circulation is a *Pulmonary Embolism*. Venous thromboembolism is a risk in surgery of long duration, for abdominal procedures, and with obese patients. Prophylactic treatment is by compression stockings or intermittent pressure cuffs.

Thrombolysis

Administration of drugs (eg, alteplase, streptokinase, eminase, activase) to dissolve blood clots, and prevent deep vein thrombosis, particularly in cases of STEMI (heart attack).

Thrombolytic Therapy

See Thrombolysis.

Thromboplastin

A plasma protein which aids blood coagulation.

Thrombophlebitis

Phlebitis (inflamed veins) caused by a thrombus (blood clot).

Thrombosis

Formation of a thrombus.

Thrombus

A stationery blood clot, made of platelets, cells, and proteins, that clump in a blood vessel, impeding blood flow.

Thyromental Distance

The distance between the thyroid notch and the tip of the mentum (chin), when the head is extended (mouth closed). If it is less than 7 cm (2.8 inch), it suggests difficult intubation.

Tidal Volume (V_T)

The volume of air displaced between inspiration and expiration, when extra effort is not applied. Typical adult resting values are 400 - 500 ml, or 6-8 ml/kg bodyweight.

Tissuing

See Infiltration.

Titrate

Administering a dose of a fluid or drug, which is optimal for a particular patient, and with minimal side-effects, rather than giving a pre-determined dose.

TIVA

See Total IntraVenous Anaesthesia.

TOE (TEE)

See Trans Oesophageal Echocardiagram.

Tonic Clonic Seizure

Old name *Grand Mal* seizure, a convulsion experienced by epileptics, in two stages: ① The **tonic** phase: the sufferer experiences muscle stiffness and unconsciousness. ② The **clonic** phase: the legs and arms jerk in rapid movements. When seizures stop, place the unconscious patient in the recovery position.

Tonicity

Describes the difference in osmolarity between two systems: if, for example, extracellular fluid has higher concentration of a solute (and higher osmolarity) than intracellular fluid, the extracellular fluid is **hypertonic** to the cells, and so fluid will flow from cells to the extracellular space. Alternatively, if the intracellular fluid has a higher solute concentration than extracellular fluid, the extracellular fluid is **hypotonic** to the cells, and extracellular fluid flows into the cells. If the intracellular and extracellular fluids have equal osmolarity, they are are termed **isotonic**.

Torsades de Pointes

A specific form of PVT (polymorphic ventricular tachycardia) in patients with a long QT interval on their ECG trace. It is characterized by rapid, irregular QRS complexes, which appear to be twisting around the ECG baseline. The arrhythmia may degenerate into ventricular fibrillation.

Total IntraVenous Anaesthesia (TIVA)

General anaesthesia, using intravenous agents, but no inhalational gases. TIVA can be delivered manually (EEG monitors depth), by setting infusion rates, or programmatically, by using a pump, to maintain a steady-state drug concentration (see also *Target Controlled Infusion*). Indications include risk of malignant hyperthermia, severe PONV, neuromuscular disorders, anticipated difficult intubation, patient preference. TIVA does not affect HPV (Hypoxic Pulmonary Vasoconstriction).

Total Lung Capacity

The maximum volume the lungs can hold; the sum of Vital Capacity and Reserve Volume.

Total Parenteral Nutrition (TPN)

Method of providing nutrition to a patient, who is unable to eat in the normal way, because of digestive system pathology or surgery. TPN bypasses the gastrointestinal tract, by administration via a central or peripheral catheter, with the subclavian vein being the preferred route. TPN provides patients with the necessary protein, fat, glucose, electrolytes (calcium, chloride, magnesium, phosphate, potassium, potassium, sodium), vitamins, minerals, and trace elements (chromium, cobalt, copper, iodine, manganese, molybdenum, selenium, zinc). If parenteral nutrition is not the sole means of nourishing the patient, it is termed *Supplementary Parenteral Nutrition*. A safe adult dosage is somewhere below 2.5 ml/kg/hour, otherwise there could be unpleasant side-effects, such as thrombophlebitis, headaches, and pyrexia.

Total Spinal Block

A high spinal block that has progressed to interference with brain stem and cervical spine nerve function, causing respiratory paralysis and unconsciousness. See Appendix A56 (pg 452).

Tourniquet

A device which compresses a limb, so that blood flow is occluded to/from a surgical field, making the surgery easier, and reducing blood loss. For adults, the pressure to which the cuff is inflated is largely determined by the patient's personal attributes, such as age, BMI, blood pressure, and medical condition but, typically, will be between 200 and 300 mmHg (26-40 kPa). Similarly, the duration of the tourniquet pressure is influenced by the particular patient, with two to three hours being a typical inflation time range. If the patient needs antibiotics, they should be given **before** the tourniquet cuff is inflated.

Trachea (Windpipe)

A 4-5 inch (10-12 cm) hollow passageway, protected by hyaline cartilage (16-20 rings), that connects the larynx with the carina, to facilitate movement of respiratory gases between the atmosphere and lungs. The trachea also traps debris, and stimulates the cough reflex, via irritant receptors, so that the debris is expelled. The first (superior) ring, the cricoid, is the only complete ring.

Tracheal Deviation

Lateral inclination of the trachea, caused by asymmetrical chest or throat pressures. The deviation is to the low pressure side, as seen in pneumothorax, pleural fibrosis (stiffening of pleura), atelectasis, or pneumonectomy (part of lung missing/removed).

Tracheal Stenosis

Narrowing of the trachea, either congenital, or due to illness or injury. Intubation and tracheotomy can cause tracheal stenosis, particularly in paediatric patients. **Symptoms**: noisy/difficult breathing, respiratory infections, asthma, central cyanosis.

Tracheal Suction

Removal of secretions from the tracheal part of the airway, especially at time of extubation.

Tracheal Tube Introducer

See Bougie.

Tracheal Tug

Inward movement of the trachea, during inspiration, indicating airway obstruction. Often seen in children, during induction.

Trachealis Muscle

The trachea is supported by hyaline cartilage, the ends of which are supported by the trachealis muscle, which serves to constrict the trachea, in an attempt to increase the force of coughing.

Tracheobronchial Generations

The different components of the respiratory pathway, from the trachea (generation 0) to the terminal bronchioles (generation 23).

Tracheostomy

The opening in the anterior trachea, below the vocal cords, between the 2nd and 3rd tracheal rings (cartilages), produced by tracheotomy, to facilitate ventilation with a secure airway, using a tube to bypass a tracheal blockage caused by, for example: trauma, swelling, tumour, throat muscle paralysis. Also for long term assisted ventilation of comatose patients, and those at risk of aspiration. Specialist nurses must ensure the tracheostomy tube remains patent, by keeping the airway properly humidified, and secretions suctioned out.

Tracheotomy

A procedure to create a *front of neck opening* of the trachea (tracheostomy). The opening can be made surgically (cut) or percutaneously (needle), under local or general anaesthetic. See also *Cricothyrotomy*.

Track and Trigger

A system that uses physiological parameters to detect patient deterioration, and initiate clinical interventions as a response. An example system is NEWS2.

Train of Four

A technique, using a nerve stimulator, to determine the level of neuromuscular blockade.

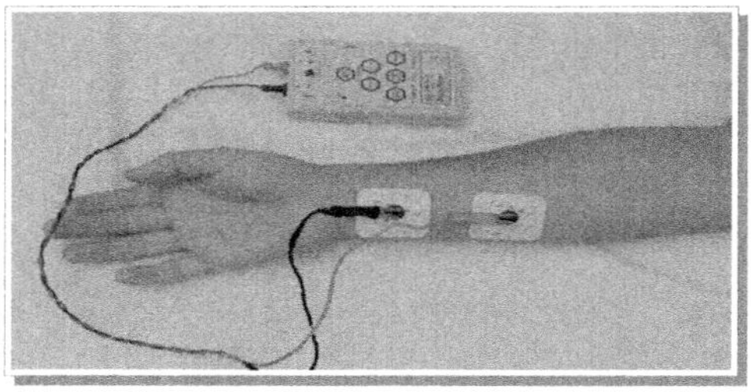

2 twitches: Indicates the correct level of blockade.

4 twitches: Suggests no blockade.

3-4 twitches are necessary before reversing the blockade, otherwise, the reversal agent (Neostigmine) might wear off before the blockade, and the patient could awaken, whilst still paralysed.

Tramadol

A long lasting (3-6 hours) strong analgesic given, intravenously, as a 50-100 mg dose, administered over three minutes. Contra-indicated for alcoholics, drug addicts, renal or liver disease, and brain injury. Usual side-effects include dizziness and nausea.

Tranexamic Acid

A manufactured version of the amino acid, Lysine, used as an antifibrinolytic – it reduces the breakdown of clots. Often given when blood loss is greater than 500 ml. Initial dose is 1 g, within 3 hours of injury.

Trans Oesophageal Echocardiagram

Real-time ultrasound image of the heart valves and chambers, using a probe that is passed down the oesophagus. TOE images are more detailed than Trans Thoracic Echocardiogram (TEE).

Trans Thoracic Echocardiogram (TEE)

Similar to a TOEG, but non-invasive, with the probe on the chest.

Transcellular Fluid

Extracellular fluid (2% total body fluid) within epithelial lined spaces, e.g., intrapleural, synovial, pericardial, CSF, urine, aqueous humour, bile, respiratory and glandular secretions, tears, sweat, bile, mucous, serum, saliva, pleural fluid, vitreous humour.

Transcutaneous Pacing

An emergency and temporary method of correcting the abnormal electrical conduction of a patient's heart, by passing a current through the patient's chest.

Transducer

A device which converts energy from one type to another. An arterial line transducer converts pulsatile pressure changes into electrical voltage, using strain gauges (Wheatstone Bridge), allowing a pressure waveform of arterial pressure to be displayed.

Transfusion Associated Circulatory Overload (TACO)

Too much of a transfused volume, causing hypertension, pulmonary oedema, and respiratory distress.

Transfusion Related Acute Lung Injury (TRALI)

Respiratory distress and severe reaction within 6 hours of transfusion, when donor antibodies react with recipient antigens, causing alveolar capillary leak. **Signs**: Pulmonary oedema, hypoxia (sats < 90%), fever, and hypo/hypertension, with frothy pink or yellow tracheal secretions. Treat as for ARDS.

Transmural Pressure

Aka Transpulmonary Pressure.

Transpulmonary Pressure (P_{tp})

The difference between alveolar (P_{alv}) and intrapleural (P_{ip}) pressures, with alveolar pressure being higher; $P_{tp} = P_{alv} - P_{ip}$. If alveolar and intrapleural pressures are equal, such as during pneumothorax, the lung will recoil/collapse.

Transudate

A filtrated fluid that is forced, by hydrostatic pressure or osmosis, through a membrane, such as a blood vessel wall. Transudate from blood, which does not contain much protein, cells, or other cell matter, collects in tissues surrounding blood vessels, causing oedema. Compare with *exudate*.

Transversus Abdominis Plane (TAP) Block

A peripheral nerve block, where the anaesthetic is injected into the plane between the internal oblique and transversus abdominis muscles, with the object of anaesthetising the anterior and lateral abdominal wall (T6 to L1) which numbs the muscles, skin, and parietal peritoneum. The block does not reduce visceral (inner organs) pain. Usage: after lower abdominal wall surgery.

Trauma Lethal Triad

The three main factors that must be managed to prevent death: hypotension, coagulopathy, and acidosis.

Trendelenburg Position

The patient lies flat on the trolley or operating table, with a head down inclination. Care must be taken to ensure that the patient does not slip off the table, especially when using slide sheets. At anaesthetic induction, the anaesthetic practitioner must always be ready to **quickly** place the patient in the Trendelenburg position, if aspiration of gastric contents is likely.

Triad of Anaesthesia

Describes the three principle components of anaesthesia:
◊ Analgesia ◊ Hypnosis ◊ Paralysis

Triage

The examination of emergency patients, with the view to assigning degrees of urgency and priorities for treatment.

Tricuspid Valve

The one-way heart valve which allows blood to flow from the right atrium to the right ventricle.

-tripsy

Signifies crushing or breaking. In surgery, describes a procedure where a structure is intentionally crushed.

Triggering

Initiating inspiration in association with the patient's respiratory effort. A ventilator may be triggered by one of several methods:

Pressure: The ventilator delivers a breath when the airway pressure decreases, as the patient makes an inspiratory effort.

Flow: A constant flow is delivered throughout the respiratory cycle, and a change in the constant flow, caused by patient inspiration, is detected by the expiratory limb's flow sensor, which then triggers the ventilator to deliver a breath.

Time: The ventilator cycles at a frequency determined by the set respiratory rate, or by the inspiration to expiration ratio.

Trismus (Lockjaw)

The tight closing of the mouth, due to jaw muscle spasm, caused by an underlying pathology, such as tetanus.

Triturate

Verb: Can mean the reduction of a substance's particle size by crushing and grinding into a powder, or the dilution of a powdered drug with an inert powdered substance, such as lactose.

Troponin

A group of three proteins that take part in regulating heart and skeletal muscle contractions. Following injury, such as myocardial infarction (MI), the heart releases troponin into the bloodstream, and so serves as a marker for MI.

Trousseau's Sign

Spontaneous peripheral venous thrombosis; with carpopedal (hand & wrist) spasm, caused by low levels of calcium or BP cuff pressure higher than systolic pressure.

Tubercolosis (TB)

Bacterial infection caught through inhaling airborne droplets from coughs and sneezes of person with TB infection of the lungs, but is otherwise not infectious. The lungs are the main infection point, but other sites are lymph nodes, bones, joints, bladder, brain, nervous system, digestive and reproductive organs.

Tuberculin Syringe

A 1 ml syringe, for shallow subcutaneous and intradermal use.

Tunnelled Central Venous Catheter

A tube with an entrance in a vein near the right clavicle (collar bone), or in the neck (eg, internal jugular or subclavian), and feeds to the superior vena cava/right atrium, with a distal part tunnelled under the chest, to an exit site, to be anchored by a dacron cuff, under the skin, before leading to two or three venous access lumens. Tunnelling makes the catheter more secure for long term use, and the dacron cuff reduces infection risk. Examples: Hickman, Broviac (paeds), Leonard, and Groshong lines.

Tuohy Needle

A hollow (for stylet and catheter) hypodermic 16g or 18g needle, with a Huber tip and wings to push against - suitable for inserting epidural catheters. The blunted tip reduces the chance of accidentally piercing the *dura mater*, into the subdural space. The stylet prevents a skin plug from blocking the needle. Lengths are 80 to 150 mm, with 1 cm markings. See Appendix A100 (pg 521).

Two Bag Test

Anaesthetic machine/circuit leak test, after breathing system, vapouriser, and ventilator checks. See Appendix A107 (pg 531).

U + Es Test

See Urea and Electrolytes (U+E) Test.

Unintentional Dural Puncture (UDP)

A complication of epidural placement, when the anaesthetist accidentally pierces the dura mater, causing CSF to leak into the epidural space, leading to Post Dural Puncture Headache (PDPH).

Unmeasured Anions

Anions (**albumin**, phosphates, sulphates, ketones, acetate, lactate) that can be the cause of a High Anion Gap Metabolic Acidosis.

Unstable Angina

The least serious form of Acute Coronary Syndrome, where

cardiac blood supply is significantly reduced, but has not progressed to infarction (so no permanent cardiac muscle damage).

Upper Airway Obstruction

Partial or complete obstruction above the level of the larynx.

Complete: Inability to talk, cough, or breathe; tracheal tug. May be cyanosis and see-saw chest/abdomen movement. Few, if any, sounds of breathing. A life-threatening condition, leading to cardiac arrest, requiring immediate management.

Partial: Ability to breathe, with effort, and may include stridor.

Treatment: Remove the obstruction (forceps/suction/Heimlich manoeuvre); Nasal or oral airway adjunct; Head tilt/chin lift; Intubation, Positive End Expiratory Pressure; Oxygen; Tracheostomy - for severe stridor, or large tumour.

Uraemia (Uremia)

Excess urea and creatinine wastes, in the blood, due to kidney failure, is called azotaemia. If azotaemia is severe enough to causes sickness, the condition becomes *uraemia*.

Urea (Carbamide)

The final product of breaking down (catabolising) the amino acids that make up proteins, and sent by the bloodstream to the kidneys for filtration and excretion. A low level is not considered to be problematic, and is normal in pregnancy. A high level of blood urea can indicate dehydration, heart problems, bleeding of the G.I. tract, or kidney dysfunction. Normal range is 2.5 – 7 mmol/litre.

Urea and Electrolytes (U+Es) Test

Test (gold cap) for heart and kidney function, and blood chemistry, through the balance of urea, bicarbonate (HCO_3^-), potassium (K), sodium (Na), creatinine, chloride (Cl-), calcium (Ca), and magnesium (Mg). Also, measures pH, and glucose. Any imbalance can help indicate the cause of a cardiac arrest.

Urticaria (Hives)

An allergic reaction to a drug, pollen, insect bite, or food, causing a raised red itchy rash. **Treatment**: Steroids or 10 mg of Chlorphenamine (antihistamine) as a slow intravenous bolus.

Uvula

The (palatine) uvula is the soft tissue that hangs down the back of the soft palate. The uvula directs food down the oesophagus, and stops it from backing up to the nose. The Uvula is one of the landmarks for intubation.

Vaccine-induced Immune Thrombotic Thrombocytopaenia

VITT: Blood clots and low platelet count caused by some Covid-19 vaccines (Johnson & Johnson, Astra Zeneca). The condition is similar to heparin induced thrombocytopaenia.

Vacuum Insulated Evaporator (VIE)

A large volume pressure vessel that serves as the main storage for a cryogenic liquid gas, such as liquid oxygen, below -150 °C. One litre of liquid oxygen converts to 840 litre at atmospheric pressure.

Vagal Manoeuvre

Stimulation of the Vagus nerve, which can reduce heart electrical impulses, thereby reducing heart rate and blood pressure.

Example vagal manoeuvres:

- Gagging
- Coughing
- Valsalva manouevre
- Immerse face in cold water

Vagus Nerve (Cranial Nerve X)

Vagus, meaning "wanderer", is the tenth and most complex of twelve paired cranial nerves, lying medial and posterior to the internal jugular vein and carotid artery, and extending below the head, to the neck, chest and abdomen, where they contribute to the innervation (nerve supply) of the viscera. The Vagus nerve regulates digest, rest, and repair activity, and provides sensory and **parasympathetic** motor nerve supply to the heart, thorax, and abdomen, plus sensory impulses from the ear, via the auricular branch of the Vagas nerve - the Arnold Nerve. Vagal activity provides a parasympathetic calming effect to the organs, after a typical adrenaline "fight/flight" episode, with effectiveness described as vagal tone. 80-90% of the nerve fibres in the vagus nerve are **sensory** (afferent) nerves, which communicate the state of the secretory glands and viscera (inc throat, heart, lungs, abdomen, and tongue, intestines, and stomach) to the brain. **Motor** function is to the neck muscle, for speech and swallowing, the tissues, and regulation of heart rate, respiration rate, digestion, coughing, vomiting, sneezing, and swallowing.

Vallecula

A crevice or depression in something. In the airway, the Vallecula is a furrow, between the base of the tongue and the epiglottis, which serves to prevent the constant triggering of the swallowing reflex, by acting as a spit trap.

Valsalva Manoeuvre

Taking a deep breath and, keeping the mouth closed and nostrils pinched, attempt exhalation. If there is a surgical need to increase the patient's intra-thoracic pressure, the anaesthetist will conduct a Valsalva Manoeuvre, by using the APL valve and reservoir bag to force an expiration, against a closed Glottis, and hold it for about ten seconds, with a pressure of approximately 4 kPa (40 cmH_2O).

Vancomycin

Glycopeptide antibiotic, for: skin, soft tissue, bone, and joint infections, plus endocarditis and pneumonia. A common allergic reaction is *Vancomycin Flushing Syndrome*.

Vancomycin Flushing Syndrome

Previously known as *Red Man Syndrome*, an anaphylactoidal reaction to vancomycin, with symptoms: angioedema, itchy skin, weakness, back and chest pain, rash on the face/neck/upper torso.

Vapour

The gas phase of a normally liquid or solid substance.

Vapourisation

The reversible process where a change of temperature causes a substance to convert from liquid to its gaseous (vapour) form.

Vapouriser

Delivery system of a vapourised volatile agent, such as Sevoflurane, is made through a hermetically sealed unit, called a *vapouriser*. In modern anaesthetic machines, the delivery mechanism is of the plenum type, where the positive pressure carrier gas passes through the vapouriser to provide the impetus to move the volatile agent towards the patient, with the concentration determined by a manually dialled control unit, to govern how much gas splits (variable by-pass) toward the agent. Different volatile agents have different saturation vapour pressures, so can only be used with vapourisers that have been designed for them which means, in practice, vapourisers function within different temperature ranges. See also *Plenum Vapouriser*.

Varix

A dilated varicose vein – with a meandering course.

Vascath

A specialised (temporary) central venous catheter, with 2 or 3 lumens, used in dialysis. It is usually inserted via the subclavian, jugular, or femoral vessels. The tip should lie in the superior vena cava, just above the right atrium. Duration: 3 months.

Vascularisation

Development of new blood (vascular) vessels within tissue.

Vasoactive

A substance that causes a change in blood vessel diameter, by constriction (vasoconstrictor) or dilation (vasodilator).

Vasoconstrictor (Vasopressor)

A substance that causes blood vessel constriction, causing reduced blood flow and increased blood pressure. Acts on the Somatic Nervous System. Often used in resuscitation, and to treat hypotension in surgical patients. Do not use during haemorrhage.

Example vasoconstrictors...

☺ Adrenaline ☺ Ephedrine ☺ Metaraminol

☺ Methoxamine ☺ Noradrenaline ☺ Phenylephrine

See Appendix A109 (pg 533).

Vasodilators

Drugs to relax smooth muscle of blood vessels, causing dilation and, consequently, a drop in blood pressure. Vasodilators are commonly given to treat hypertension, heart failure, and angina.

Examples: Hydralazine, Minoxidil, Ramipril and Benazepril.

Vasopressor

See Vasoconstrictor.

Vasopressin (Anti Diuretic Hormone)

Increases the amount of water reabsorbed by the kidneys, and constricts arterioles, which tends to raise arterial blood pressure.

Vasovagal (Reflexive) Syncope

Patients can experience syncope (fainting) due to heart valve problems, anaemia, or other physical conditions, or because of emotional stress, such as when the vagus nerve becomes overstimulated, causing slow heart rate, and blood vessels to dilate, especially in the lower legs. As a result, blood pressure drops, and the reduced blood flow to the brain causes fainting. Patients may experience vasovagal syncope because of the sight of needles, blood, or during a local or regional procedure. **Warning signs**: nausea, yawning, vision disturbance, pale skin, dizziness, dilated pupils, seeing black spots, tunnel vision, feeling warm, clammy skin. **Treatment**: In acute vasovagal episodes, lie the patient down for a few minutes, before helping them to rise slowly.

Vecuronium Bromide

Non-depolarising neuromuscular blocking agent, at intubation. Can cause hypotension. Produces less histamine release than atracurium or vecuronium, so might be more suitable for asthmatics. Dose 0.1 mg/kg from a 2 mg/ml supply.

Veins

Veins carry blood towards the heart, and drain de-oxygenated blood towards the right atrium. An exception being the pulmonary vein, which takes oxygenated blood from the lungs to the left atrium. Unlike arteries, veins do not have pressure to prevent any backing up of blood so, instead, they contain one-way valves.

Major Veins:

Jugular:

Drains de-oxygenated blood from the neck and face.

Femoral:

Between External Iliac and Popliteal veins; drains the lower extremities.

Subclavian:

Connects the Axillary and Internal Jugular veins.

Inferior Vena Cava:

Drains lower and middle body into the right atrium of the heart

Superior Vena Cava:

Drains the body above the diaphragm.

Venous Admixture

Shunted (not oxygenated) blood mixed with oxygenated blood, producing lower arterial O_2 partial pressure (paO_2) than normal.

Venous Insufficiency

Blood returns to the heart through veins, which contain 1-way valves to prevent blood flowing backward. If valves in leg veins fail to check the back flow, blood will pool in the lower legs, due to gravity, and cause DVT, ulceration, and varicose veins.

Venous Thromboembolism

A blood clot that develops in a vein, such as in the upper leg (Deep Vein Thrombosis). If the clot detaches and moves through the bloodstream to lodge elsewhere, it is an *embolism*. If the embolism forms in a lung, it is known as a pulmonary embolism

(PE). Venous thromboembolism (VTE) refers to both deep vein thrombosis (DVT) and pulmonary embolism.

Ventilation

Gas flow in and out of the lungs. Pressure gradients make oxygen flow from the atmosphere to the alveoli, and CO_2 from alveoli to the atmosphere. Anticipation of poor ventilation due to: old age, chronic respiratory difficulty, no teeth, Retrognathia, obesity, spinal or jaw deformity, or enlarged thyroid. See also *Minute*, *Alveolar*, and *Dead Space ventilation*.

Ventilation Modes

Pressure controlled: the respiratory rate and maximum airway pressure are pre-set, and the anaesthetic machine delivers gas until the set pressure is reached.

Volume controlled: the respiratory rate and tidal volume are pre-set, and the anaesthetic machine will deliver gas, at whatever pressure is necessary, until the required volume has been reached (risk of barotrauma).

Pressure Support: *Assisted Spontaneous Breathing*: the anaesthetic machine detects the patient's attempts to breathe, and assists with the inspiration effort.

Note: Lung compliance is one of the factors in choosing the optimum ventilation mode.

Ventilation/Perfusion (V/Q) Ratio

A common cause of hypoxaemia, V/Q ratio illustrates the relationship between **V**, the volume of air (gas) that reaches the alveoli, and **Q**, the volume of blood that flows through the lung capillaries. V/Q is used to assess the efficiency of how ventilation and perfusion are matched. Normal ventilation is 4 litre/minute, and normal perfusion is 5 litre/minute, so mean V/Q ratio is 0.8. Any other value is a V/Q mismatch (a feature of COPD). A **low** ratio means ventilation volume is low, compared with the perfusion volume, which may be normal, and might indicate: airway obstruction, pneumonia, pulmonary oedema, asthma, or bronchitis. Low V/Q ratio can cause *hypoxic pulmonary vasoconstriction*. If V/Q=0, there may be a left to right pulmonary shunt. A **high** ratio means ventilation may be normal, but blood flow (perfusion) is poor, such as occurs with emphysema (COPD), pulmonary embolism (most common, and caused by eg DVT), heart disease, and alveolar dead space. See Appendix A110 (pg 534).

Ventilator

A mechanical device that provides a breathing service to a patient, who is unable to breathe for themselves. The two main types are *piston* and *bag in bottle*. A piston system is electronically controlled, electrically driven, and usually hidden within the anaesthetic machine. The bag in bottle ventilator is usually external to the body of the anaesthetic machine, and is easy to see. The Fresh Gas Flow (FGF) is contained within the bellows bag, which is compressed by the driving gas (air or oxygen) in the chamber. Any failure of the bellows or driving gas supply is illustrated by the bellows not reaching its expected height, or collapsing completely if there is a major leak of the driving gas.

Ventilator Settings

Patient ventilation machine settings. See Appendix A111 (pg 535).

Ventilatory Response to Anaesthesia

Volatile anaesthetics tend to increase respiratory rate, decrease tidal volume, and blunt ventilatory responses to hypercapnia and hypoxia. When subject to some volatile agents, such as isoflurane, patients respond with a reduced tidal volume, and an increased rate of breathing. Additionally, both the respiratory and hypoxic drives are obtunded (de-sensitised), which means the natural sensitivity to levels of oxygen and carbon dioxide is diminished.

Ventral

Towards the abdomen, rather than the spine, or the anterior, rather than posterior; as with a *Ventral Hernia* of the abdomen.

Ventricular Fibrillation (VF)

Chaotic heart rhythm, in electrical chaos. No blood is pumped from the heart, and there is no pulse. The ECG trace lacks P-waves, QRS complexes, and T-waves. Action is to follow Life Support protocols. See *AED* + Appendix A112 (pg 536).

Ventricular Tachycardia (VT)

Wide QRS complex, and regular and fast ventricle beating, which is too fast for them to fill with sufficient blood between beats. Pulseless VT can lead to Ventricular Fibrillation. Action for pulseless VT is defibrillation. See *AED* + Appendix A112 (pg 536).

Symptoms

⚐ Palpitations ⚐ Vertigo ⚐ Breathless ⚐ Sweating ⚐ Nausea

Treatment

√ Cardioversion √ Drugs √ Surgery
√ Defibrillation √ Radio frequency ablation

Venturi (air-entrainment) Mask

Colour coded high flow mask devices that deliver inspired air mixed with a known oxygen concentration, 24-50%, for patients, such as those with hypoxic drive, and on controlled oxygen therapy. Mask colour indicates how much (%) oxygen is delivered to the patient, governed by the size of the venturi constriction.

Verapamil

Calcium channel blocker that slows AV node conduction, and lowers blood pressure.

Vesicant

A drug/agent which causes blistering (vesicates) or other tissue damage when extravasation (leaks out of vein) occurs. **Action**: stop infusion, aspirate from the cannula. Example vesicants are calcium chloride, digoxin, gentamicin, potassium chloride, high concentration saline solution, and vancomycin.

Viscera

Refers to the internal organs. Visceral pain occurs in the abdomen (eg, appendicitis), pelvis, intestines, or chest, and is a more vague pain than somatic pain, which is localised, and causes a general discomfort which may be difficult to pinpoint.

Viscus

Pertaining to organs within body cavities, such as the abdomen.

Visual Infusion Phlebitis (VIP) Score

A system to determine the stage (0-5) of phlebitis at a peripheral cannula site, using visual clues and pain levels. A high score suggests treatment for thrombophlebitis (clot in vein), and a need to resite the cannula.

Vital Capacity

The maximum volume of air that can be expelled with a rapid exhalation: The sum of Tidal, Inspiratory, and Expiratory Reserve Volumes. Typically, six litres (adult).

Vital Signs

The physiological signs that indicate life signs, primarily: temperature, pulse rate, respiratory rate, and blood pressure.

Vitamin K

A fat soluble vitamin, which helps promote blood clotting.

VivaSight-DL Endotracheal and Bronchial Tube

Camera guided double lumen endotracheal/bronchial tube, to isolate one lung. See Appendix A113 (pg 537).

VO2max

The maximal rate of oxygen consumption, found during exercise fitness testing, when increased workload does not produce increased oxygen consumption, resulting in the need for anaerobic respiration. A young adult male rate might be 45 ml/kg/min, 40 for a female. Endurance athlete values might reach 90 ml/kg/min.

Vocal Cords (Folds)

Two thin folds of mucus membrane, inside the larynx, which close to form sounds. By laryngoscope, the cords appear like a V shaped grey/white doorway, with the space between (glottis) being the entry point for an ET tube, into the trachea. The *epiglottis* is the landmark above the cords (looks like a curved canopy).

Voice Box

Common name for the Larynx.

Volatile Anaesthetic Agents

Vaporised anaesthetics, packaged as liquids, but evaporate for administration by inhalation. The agents affect all parts of the

CNS, with effectiveness determined by rate of uptake by the circulatory system, concentration in the alveoli, and partial pressure in the CNS. The concentration is determined by ① the *concentration effect*, which produces a higher FA/FI ratio ② an efficient ventilation, so agent diffused to the blood is quickly replaced from the supply ③ a larger lung capacity means less concentration, so slower onset. For a given concentration of volatile agent, partial pressure decreases with altitude, so concentration must be increased (increase flow) as compensation. Volatile agents (except sevoflurane and nitrous oxide) can cause respiratory depression. **Example Agents**: Desflurane, Sevoflurane, and Isoflurane.

Note: In circle systems, the vapouriser dial setting (%) does not exactly match the amount the machine delivers, because the patient also receives some of the agent already in the circuit.

Common **side effects** include: Nausea, respiratory depression, hypotension or hypertension, vertigo, arrhythmias, vomiting, coughing, agitation. A more rare side effect is Malignant hyperthermia. Volatiles are **contraindicated** in pneumothorax and in pulmonary hypertension – because they increase pulmonary vascular resistance. See also *Second Gas Effect*.

Voltarol

Brand name for Diclofenac Sodium.

Volume of Distribution (VD)

The apparent volume of fluid in which the drug dose must be diluted to produce the observed drug concentration in the blood plasma: amount of drug in the body divided by drug concentration in the plasma. If the drug distributes into the tissues easily, it will have a lower concentration in the plasma, and a high VD.

Volutrauma

Lung damage where alveoli become filled with fluid, caused by a high ventilator tidal volume. Possibly due to patient size and lung compliance not being properly considered. A common condition with ARDS and blood transfusion patients.

Von Willebrand Factor

Plasma glycoprotein that helps platelets stick together.

V/Q Mismatch

A condition where parts of a lung receive adequate oxygen but inadequate perfusion (perhaps due to pulmonary embolism), known as *Dead Space* V/Q mismatch, or adequate perfusion and inadequate oxygen (perhaps airway obstruction), known as *Shunt* V/Q mismatch. See *Ventilation/Perfusion Ratio*.

V/Q Ratio

See Ventilation/Perfusion Ratio.

Warfarin

An anticoagulant (and antagonist for Vitamin K). Results from an INR test indicate the effectiveness of Warfarin. Takes 24-48 hours to take effect. If a Warfarin patient has a major haemorrhage, FFP is usually given - for coagulation.

Wash In

The phase describing the exponentially increasing concentration in the alveoli, of an inhaled agent such as Sevoflurane, until it equilibrates with the inspired concentration. The two factors that determine the speed of uptake are cardiac output and an agent's blood solubility. High cardiac output increases equilibration time, as does a higher blood solubility.

Wash Out

The phase describing the exponentially decreasing concentration of an agent, in the alveoli, to elimination (expiration).

Water For Injections (WFI)

Distilled hypotonic and non pyrogenic sterile water, a solvent for powdered drugs, producing a solution with a specific concentration. Also, used to dilute existing solutions to lower concentrations.

Water Vapour

A constituent of alveolar gases, contributing ~47 mmHg (6.2 kPa) to total alveolar pressure. Water vapour is one factor responsible for alveolar oxygen pressure of 104 mmHg (13.8 kPa) being lower than the atmospheric oxygen pressure of 160 mmHg (21 kPa).

Waters Circuit

A Mapleson C circuit with an incorporated soda lime CO_2 absorber. Designed by an American Dr - Ralph Waters. Rarely used, if at all, because the CO_2 absorber was bulky, and the patient was at risk of breathing in soda lime.

Weight/Volume (Mass/Volume) Concentration

The density of a solution, using specific gravity of water as a reference value, 1 g per ml. Pharmacologically, W/V is the method to describe most intravenous drug concentrations, and the ability to produce a particular concentration from two other concentrations is a key skill for anaesthetic assistants.

Wells Score

A number which indicates how likely a patient is at risk of suffering deep vein thrombosis, or pulmonary embolism. Score criteria includes leg swelling, cancer, previous DVT, leg paralysis, tenderness, bedridden, oedema, vein prominence (not varicose).

Wheal

A swelling, just under the skin, which occurs, for example, when a local anaesthetic is administered, before insertion of a cannula.

Wheezing

When an anaesthetised patient is wheezing, the underlying cause must be addressed, with common causes including:

- Δ Partial obstruction of ETT
- Δ ETT abutting the carina
- Δ Endobronchial intubation
- Δ Bronchospasm
- Δ Pulmonary oedema
- Δ Pulmonary embolism
- Δ Gastric aspiration
- Δ Tension pneumothorax
- Δ Foreign body in the bronchus

White Blood Cell (Leukocyte)

See Leukocyte.

Wilson Risk Factor Score

A grading system for predicting difficult intubation, based on dispositions of: **W**eight, **H**eight, **H**ead/neck movement, **P**rominence of teeth, and aspect of the **M**andible.

Winters' Formula

Calculation to predict the arterial CO_2 pressure ($paCO_2$) that should occur if there has been a functional respiratory compensation for a metabolic acidosis: $\mathbf{paCO_2 = (1.5 * HCO_3^-) + 8 \pm 2}$ **mmHg**.

∞ If the blood gas $paCO_2$ corresponds with the calculated value, a *respiratory compensation* is occurring.

∞ If the $paCO_2$ is higher than calculated, there may also be a secondary **respiratory acidosis** (mixed acidosis) present.

∞ If the $paCO_2$ is lower than the calculated value, there may be a secondary **respiratory alkalosis** occurring.

Whole Blood Transfusion

Given when blood products are unavailable (battlefield). The extra volume can cause Transfusion Associated Circulatory Overload.

World Health Organisation "Five Moments"

WHO protocol for hand hygiene: **Before** touching a patient, **before** clean/aseptic procedures, **after** body fluid exposure/risk, **after** touching a patient, **after** touching patient surroundings.

Wound Dressings

Dressing with wound protection. If the dressing does not provide any other function, it is *passive*. If it creates a moist environment for the wound, it promotes healing, so is an *active* dressing. Another type of dressing is *interactive*, because it adds to the function of an *active* dressing, by interacting with the wound with, for example, the removal of some of the wound exudate (drained liquid). *Occlusive* dressings are air and water tight.

W/V

See Weight/Volume.

Xiphoid Process

The cartilage extension of the inferior sternum, which serves as the superior landmark for the sterile field in, for example, laparoscopy.

Xylocaine

Brand name for Lidocaine.

Young's Formula

Paediatric (2-12 years) drug dose formula, when specific dosage instructions are absent: average adult dose * age / (age + 12).

Zithromax

A macrolide sub-class antibiotic, derived from Erythromycin.

Appendices

Please note:

The following protocols, equipment, and setting up descriptions are for illustration purposes only. Refer to local policies and formal guidelines, as appropriate, for relevant equipment, preparations, and protocols.

☆ ☆ ☆ ☆ ☆ ☆ ☆ ☆ ☆

A1: Abdominal Aortic An

Description

A dilation of the abdominal aorta. The aneurysm usually does not cause any symptoms, unless it ruptures, which is more likely if it is more than 2″ (5 cm) in diameter (double normal size). When aneurysms rupture, fatality is very likely. Men, over the age of 65, are at most risk of having an abdominal aortic aneurysm.

Two common methods to repair an Abdominal Aortic Aneurysm:

1. *Grafting*

A surgical excision of the affected aorta, and replacement with a graft. This is a major operation, which leaves significant scarring.

2. *Endovascular Repair*

The section of aorta is repaired, by passing a tube from inside one of the leg arteries, and into the aneurysm. The tube is then passed across the widened aneurysm, and fixed to the good aorta wall with metal clips. This is safer, and less invasive, than above, and there is no scarring, because there is no incision to be made.

A2: Acid Reflux

Risk factors

- Non-fasted patient
- Previous gastric surgery
- Hiatus hernia
- Peptic ulcers
- Pregnancy
- Old age
- Nasogastric tube
- Reduced level of consciousness
- Drugs (Opiates, Volatile agents)
- Bowel obstruction or raised intra-abdominal pressure

Recognition

- Laryngospasm
- Airway obstruction
- Bronchospasm
- Tachycardia
- Hypotension
- Low oxygen saturation
- Severe coughing
- Soiling at the mouth

Management

- Trendelenburg position
- Suction of oropharynx
- 100% oxygen
- Cricoid pressure
- Rapid Sequence Induction
- Tracheal suctioning
- PEEP (5 cmH_2O).

Note: If aspiration risk, recover patient in the left lateral position.

A3: Aintree Intubation Catheter

AIC : Radio opaque, 56 cm long – an adaption of the Cook Airway Exchange Catheter, with internal diameter of 4.8 mm, allowing it to be pre-loaded onto a 4.2 mm fibre-optic intubating bronchoscope, with the directable distal 3 cm left exposed. The external diameter of 6.5 mm allows ET (endotracheal) tubes, with minimum internal diameter of 7 mm, to be loaded onto the catheter. The AIC allows intubation via a Laryngeal Mask Airway (LMA), or Proseal. The AIC can be used to ventilate the patient, by fitting a 15 mm *Rapi-Fit* connector onto the proximal end of the AIC, to which an Ambu bag may be attached (the other connector is for jet ventilation).

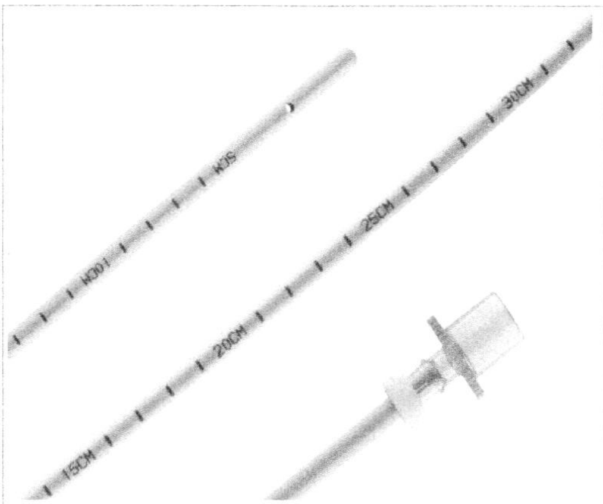

Ventilation with the Aintree Intubation Catheter

- Insert the LMA.
- Railroad the AIC over the lubricated bronchoscope.

☞ Tape the proximal end to the bronchoscope.

☞ Pass the lubricated AIC/bronchoscope through the LMA, into the trachea.

☞ Remove the bronchoscope - leaving the AIC in the trachea.

☞ Remove the LMA - leaving the AIC in place.

Endotracheal intubation with an LMA

☞ Railroad the AIC over the lubricated bronchoscope.

☞ Tape the proximal end of the AIC to the scope.

☞ Pass the lubricated AIC/scope through the LMA.

☞ Advance until the carina is seen.

☞ Remove the tape from the AIC/scope.

☞ Hold the AIC secure - remove the scope.

☞ Deflate the LMA, hold the AIC secure, remove the LMA.

> ☞ If ventilation required...
>
> *Attach Rapifit connector to AIC; attach BVM to ventilate.*

☞ Railroad the ETT over the AIC.

☞ Pass the scope through the AIC (acts as bougie).

☞ Hold the AIC secure - advance the ETT into the trachea.

☞ Inflate the ETT cuff.

☞ Confirm intubation with CO_2 etc.

☞ Remove the AIC/scope.

A4: Anaesthesia Types

Epidural	Injection of a local analgesic into the epidural space, blocking the spinal nerves.
General	Unconsciousness induced by inhalation, IV, or a combination of both techniques. Cough reflex is inhibited (by propofol); aspiration risk; increased intrapulmonary shunt.
Local	Local application of topical or injected analgesic.
Regional	An analgesic blocks sensation to a limb.
Spinal	Injection of local anaesthetic into cerebrospinal fluid of subarachnoid space around the lower spinal nerves.
TIVA	Total Intravenous Anaesthesia (no gases).

A5: Anaesthetic Drug Syringe Preparation

Example Induction phase:

Drug	***Syringe***	***Function***
Propofol 1%	2 * 20 ml	Anaesthesia
Fentanyl	2 ml	Analgesia, quick onset
Ondansetron	2 ml	Antiemetic
Atracurium	5 ml	Muscle relaxant
Diclofenac	5 ml	NSAID
Morphine	10 ml	Analgesia, long duration
Dexamethazone	2 ml	Steroidal anti-inflammatory

Cardiac arrest drugs:

Drug	***Dose***	***Syringe***	***Notes***
Adrenaline	1 mg	10 ml	1 in 10,000 minijet
Adrenaline	3 mg	10 ml	3 in 10,000 minijet
Atropine	1 mg	10 ml	1 in 10,000 minijet
Amiodarone	300 mg	10 ml	3.00%
Calcium chloride	10 ml	10 ml	10% concentration
Naloxone	400 mcg/ml	1 ml	Opioid antagonist
Sodium bicarbonate	50 mmol	50 ml	Antacid

Emergency drugs:

Drug	***Syringe***	***Treats***
Metaraminol	20 ml	Hypotension
Ephedrine	10 ml	Hypotension
Atropine	2 ml	Bradycardia
Glycopyrronium	2 ml	Bradycardia
Suxamethonium	2 ml	Muscle relaxant

Commonly used iv induction agents:

- Propofol, 1.5-3 mg/kg
- Thiopentone, 100-150 mg, over 10 seconds (adult dose)
- Ketamine, 1-4.5 mg/kg

A6: Anaesthetic Induction

Equipment (example)

- IV in situ, drip stand, fluid warmer
- Face mask, catheter mount, filter
- LMAs, ET tubes, lubricating gel
- Syringe to inflate LMA/tube cuff
- Ties/tapes, pads (eyes) for LMA/ET tube
- McGill forceps
- Working laryngoscopes and selection of blades
- Bougies and stylets
- Suction tubing, Yankeur, suction catheters
- Monitoring equipment (ECG, Oximetry, BP, CO_2)
- Nasogastric tube and bile bag
- Clean pillow, canvass, blanket, tilting patient trolley

Patient arrival

- Position patient comfortably
- Check documentation and patient ID
- Verify procedure and marking
- Perform other safety checks (fasting, metalwork, allergies)
- Fit monitoring

- Assist with IV cannulation

Induction

- ☞ Hand Laryngoscope to Anaesthetist (left hand)
- ☞ Place ET tube in Anaesthetist's other hand
- ☞ Apply B.U.R.P. as necessary
- ☞ When ET tube in position, attach circuit
- ☞ Inflate cuff (listen for leak)
- ☞ Tie in ET tube
- ☞ Check ET tube cuff pressure
- ☞ Tape to eyes
- ☞ Ensure correct level of end tidal CO_2
- ☞ Validate intubation (condensation, bilateral chest rising,...)

Mallampati Grading (www.mdCalc.com)

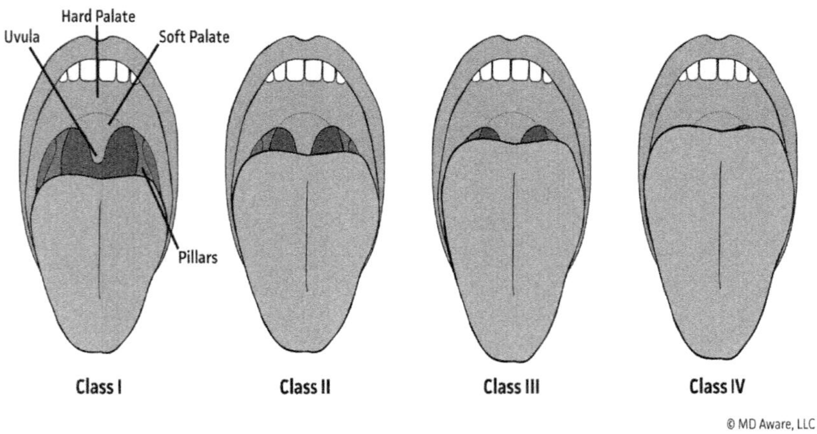

A7: Anaesthetic Machine Checks

The specific checks for a particular type of machine are determined by local policy, which may stipulate compliance with manufacturer's instructions, or other published guidelines. Note: daily checks are much shorter than the following....

Example FULL checking routine (Aestiva)

Initial Setup

- Set system switch to off/standby
- Set ventilation switch to *Bag* mode
- Switch off auxiliary oxygen flow
- Ensure all attachments and lines are clear and undamaged
- Position the machine and apply the brake
- Switch on power (stops battery draining)
- Ensure gas cylinders (Oxygen, N_2O, Air) are closed
- Ensure soda lime is fresh, and the drain valve is closed
- Clean/decontaminate the machine
- Fit the required vaporisers, and top up
- Ensure the vaporisers switch on mutually exclusively

Accessories

- Fit monitoring lines
- Ensure new/undamaged circuit attached
- Fit new suction tubing/Yankeur

Check draw for leads

- Invasive monitoring cables
- Temperature cable
- Nerve Stimulator

Have available: Neostigmine/Glycopyrolate, Metaraminol, Atropine, airways, syringes, needles, tapes.

Negative Pressure Leak Test

- Tug test gas lines for secure fitting
- Turn all flow controls 1½ turns anti-clockwise
- Fit bulb test device into Auxiliary Common Gas Outlet (ACGO)
- Switch on ACGO
- Switch vaporiser on @ 1%
- Deflate bulb (flow control floats should move)
- Bulb should not reinflate within 30 secs
- Repeat steps 4-6 for each vaporiser
- Turn off all gas flow controls (clockwise)
- Turn ACGO (Auxiliary Common Gas Outlet) off
- Remove test device
- Depress drain button for 10 seconds

Vaporiser back-pressure test

① System switch and top monitor on

② Set O_2 (oxygen) flow @ 6 L

③ Ensure O_2 flow is steady, and bobbins move freely

④ Adjust vaporiser to 1% - 1 click at a time

Ensure oxygen flow doesn't drop more than 1 L through range, otherwise either the vaporiser or the machine is faulty. If all is well, switch off the vaporisers.

Gas Cylinder Checks

☞ Set gas flows @ 1 L

☞ Turn on and check level of each gas cylinder

☞ Ensure bobbins move freely

☞ Cylinders off - drain gases until gauges drop to nil

Other Line Checks

☞ Check man LP gas pressures (4 bar)

☞ Check suction

☞ Ensure active scavenging flow tube shows green

☞ Ensure auxiliary oxygen flows

Oxygen Calibration

⊶ Unplug O_2 sensor

⊶ Do a 21% calibration test

⊶ If successful (30-40 secs), refit the sensor

⊶ If unsuccessful, do a 100% calibration test.

⊶ If still unsuccessful, replace the sensor.

Hypoxic Guard

☞ Switch N_2O and O_2 flows to minimum (clockwise)

☞ Increase N_2O; check O_2 maintains 21% partial pressure

☞ Switch off O_2, N_2O should drop first

☞ Set O_2, N_2O, Air @ 1 L

☞ Disconnect main O_2 supply; wait for alarm

☞ Ensure N_2O drops before O_2 - Air still flows

☞ Reconnect O_2 supply; check O_2 flow returns to 1 L

☞ Switch off N_2O and Air

☞ Allow O_2 flow for 1 minute (to flush volatile agents)

PAW (airway pressure) Alarm Checks

Ensure pressures are maintained by an effective APL valve.

☞ Set oxygen flow @ 0.5 L*

☞ Occlude patient end of circuit (reservoir bag)

☞ Set APL valve @ 30 cmH_2O **

☞ Flush to 30 cmH_2O; force "Sustained PAW" alarm

☞ Set APL valve @ 70 cmH_2O

☞ Flush to 40 cmH_2O

☞ Force "High PAW" alarm

☞ Turn APL valve off

* *Compensates for sampling line "leak".*

** *Normal lung pressure is 20-30 cmH_2O.*

Ventilator Settings

Ύ Set: Vt = 400 ml

Ύ Breath rate = 12

- I:E = 1:2
- Set Volume mode

Ventilator Operation

- Set the ventilation switch to *Vent* mode
- Set oxygen flow to minimum
- Flush with oxygen to fill bellows
- Ensure VTE level reaches 90% VT (360 ml) within 6 cycles
- Ensure one-way inspiratory valve rises on inspiration
- Ensure one-way expiratory valve rises on expiration
- Disconnect reservoir bag to force "bellows" alarm
- Reconnect reservoir bag
- Flush bellows
- With bellows at highest point, set switch to *Bag* mode

If bellows fall more than 100 ml/min, there is a ventilator leak.

Standby Mode

- Set system switch to *standby*
- Open APL valve fully
- Switch gas flows off
- Refit sampling line (if removed during testing)

A8: Anaphylaxis

Common Causes

- Dairy products
- Bee stings
- Aspirin
- Nuts
- Shellfish
- Blood products
- Latex
- Eggs
- Contrast media
- ACE inhibitors
- Antibiotics

Anaesthesia

Anaphylaxis may be caused by: chlorhexidine, NM blocking agents (Atracurium etc), induction agents, opioids, local anaesthetics, inhalational agents, antibiotics, contrast media.

Note: The anaesthetised patient, suffering anaphylaxis, may appear to have airway obstruction or cardiovascular collapse.

Key indicators

- Sudden onset and progression of symptoms
- Shortness of breath
- Rash or swelling of lips or eyelids
- Angioedema (swelling of tissues)

Symptoms

- Collapse
- Skin flushing
- Inspiratory stridor
- Urticaria
- Sense of doom
- Hypotension
- Vasodilation
- Cardiovascular shock

- Laryngeal oedema
- Expiratory wheeze
- Abdominal pain
- Difficulty in swallowing
- Throat and mouth swelling
- Nausea

Note: In food allergies, swelling usually starts in the mouth and tongue, progressing to upper airway obstruction.

Assessment

- Airway: examine for oedema, stridor, wheezing
- Breathing: measure respiratory rate
- Circulation: pulse, BP, and capillary refill
- Disability: response level (Alert, Voice, Pain, Unresponsive)
- Exposure: assess body for urticaria and angioedema

Treatment

- Patient flat & raise legs - if breathing unimpaired
- Adrenaline* (Epinephrine)
- High flow oxygen
- IV crystalloids (adult:500 ml, child:20 ml/kg)
- IV Chlorphenamine**
- IV Hydrocortisone***

** Intravenous Adrenaline (Epinephrine)*

Adult = 50 microgram;   Child = 10 microgram/kg

(If IV access not available, use the IM route.)

Intramuscular Adrenaline

Age group	***Dosage 1:1000***
Adults	500 microgram (0.5 ml)
Child, over 12 years	500 microgram (0.5 ml)
Child, 6-12 years	300 microgram (0.3 ml)
Child, under 6 years	150 microgram (0.15 ml)

** ***Chlorphenamine*** *and* *** ***Hydrocortisone*** (IM or slow IV)

Age group	***Chlorphenamine***	***Hydrocortisone***
Adult or child over 12	**10** mg	**200** mg
Child, over 6 - 12 years	**5** mg	**100** mg
Child 0.5 - 6 years	**2.5** mg	**50** mg
Child, under 6 months	**250** mcg/kg	**25** mg

A9: Anion Gap (AG)

Metabolic Acidosis Types...

Normal Anion Gap (NAGMA)

An AG of 4-12 mmol/litre suggests metabolic acidosis might be due to **increased chloride** (perhaps from saline administration), **decreased acid excretion**, or **loss of HCO_3^-**, resulting from (RAGED) **R**enal tubular acidosis, **A**ddison's Disease, **GI** issue (*diarrhoea, pancreatic fistula), **E**xcessive chlorine, **D**iuretics. {*diarrhoea is the most common cause of **NAGMA**}

High Anion Gap (HAGMA)

An AG > 12 mmol/L suggests accumulation of unmeasured anions (organic acids): ketones, lactate, from kidney failure, hypovolaemic shock, toxins, aspirin (a salicylate), methanol, paracetamol, iron, or carbon monoxide. High AG symptoms: fatigue, deep breaths, vomiting, shock, hypotension, ventricular arrhythmias. Note: In complex cases, there may be a HAGMA without high Anion Gap.

A10: Antiemetic Classes

Class	*Indications*	*Examples*
Antihistamine	Motion and morning sickness in pregnancy, and opioid nausea.	**Cyclizine**, Diphenhydramine, Meclozine, Promethazine.
Benzodiazepine	Sedation, anxiety, muscle relaxation, anti-convulsion.	Midazolam, Lorazepam
Steroid	Low dose given at the onset of G. A.	**Dexamethasone**
5-HT3 receptor antagonists	Block serotonin receptors in CNS and GI tract. To treat post-op and cytotoxic drug nausea & vomiting.	Dolasetron, Mirtazapine, **Ondansetron**

A11: APGAR Score

Note: A score above 6 is normal.

	0	***1***	***2***
Appearance	Blue or pale all over	Blue at extremities ; pink body	No cyanosis; body and extremities pink
Pulse rate	Absent	< 100	≥ 100
Grimace	No response to stimu-lation	Feeble cry when stimulated	Cry or pull away when stimulated
Activity	None	Some flexion	Flexed arms/legs, resist extension
Respiration	Absent	Irregular, gasping	Strong, lusty cry

A12: Arterial Blood Gases

Example Normal Ranges

Parameter	***Description***	***Range***
pH	Acid status	**7.35 – 7.45**
paCO2	CO2 pressure	**4.7 – 6 kPa** (35-45 mmHg)
HCO3-	Bicarbonate	**22–26 mmol/L**
Base excess	Bicarbonate +/-	-2 - +2 mmol/L
paO2	Oxygen pressure	10 – 13 kPa (75-100 mmHg)
SaO2	Oxygen saturation	> 94%
Lactate	Product of glycolysis	0.5 – 1.5 mmol/L
Hb	Haemoglobin	120 – 172 g/L

Acid-Base Status

<u>Note</u>: When $paCO_2$ and HCO_3^- are both low, or both high, but pH has returned to the normal range, compensation has taken place.

pH	$paCO_2$	HCO_3^-	Acid Status
↓	✓	↓	Metabolic acidosis (CO_2 normal)
↓	↓	↓	Metabolic acidosis + respiratory compensation occurring
↓	↑	✓	Acute respiratory acidosis (HCO_3^- normal)
↓	↑	↑	Chronic respiratory acidosis + metabolic compensation occurring
↓	↑	↓	Combined respiratory & metabolic acidosis
↑	✓	↑	Metabolic alkalosis (CO_2 normal)
↑	↑	↑	Metabolic alkalosis + respiratory compensation occurring
↑	↓	✓	Acute respiratory alkalosis (HCO_3^- normal)
↑	↓	↓	Respiratory alkalosis + metabolic compensation occurring
↑	↓	↑	Combined respiratory & metabolic alkalosis

A13: Arterial Line

Arterial Line Functions

Real-time measurement of arterial blood pressure; Frequent drawing of blood samples for lab testing; Blood sampling for measurement of blood gases, with slow saline flush of 2 ml/hour.

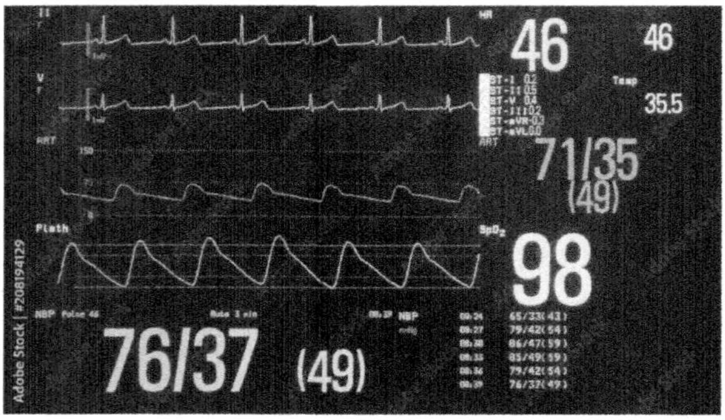

The arterial waveform reflects cardiac output and systemic vascular resistance, with the upstroke reflecting systole, the dicrotic notch representing closure of the aortic valve, and the downstroke reflecting diastole. Once in-situ, a continuous Heparin infusion may be used to maintain the patency of the arterial cannula. Note: the image shows bradycardia (46) and hypotension (71/35).

Equipment

- Drip stand and transducer clamp
- Pressure bag and 500 ml bag of saline (may be Heparinised)
- Transducer set, monitor cable, 20 ml syringe
- BD Flow Switch, Insyte, Abbocath (20g), or arterial catheter
- "Arterial" stickers

- Chlorhexadine (2%) spray
- Tegaderm dressings: 1 big, 1 small (place first)
- 1% Lidocaine
- 1, 3, 10 ml syringes, and drawing up needle

Setup

- Fit saline bag into pressure bag
- Close arterial line clamps/valves and tighten connections
- Remove end tube section + valve from arterial line
- Fit 20 ml syringe to end section (saline label)
- Fit bung to end of arterial line
- Close drip roller clamp, then spike the saline bag
- Pressure to 300 mmHg
- Open drip roller clamp
- Flush air bubbles (tubing and ports)
- Close end-most valve
- Fix "Arterial" labels
- Fit transducer to clamp on drip stand
- Prime separate end section with saline
- Replace port caps with bungs

Connecting

- Dorsiflex patient's wrist over padding and inco-pad
- Spray 2% chlorhexadine to insertion site
- Create wheal at insertion site with 1% Lidocaine
- Palpate pulse with two fingers - track course of vessel
- Insert arterial needle (Abbocath etc) at 30° - 60° angle
- Advance needle until pulsatile arterial blood appears
- Withdraw needle through catheter, or use Seldinger Technique

Seldinger technique

- Advance guide-wire through needle
- Remove needle
- Advance plastic catheter over guide-wire
- Remove guide-wire

Complete the connections

- Connect the end section
- Turn valve to "on" position
- Aspirate arterial blood, and flush with saline
- Turn valve off (until arterial line connected to main tubing)
- Remove syringe, and connect main arterial tubing
- Secure catheter (suture, dressings)
- Fit first dressing from hand towards elbow
- Fit second dressing in opposite direction

Transducing an arterial line

- Switch 3-way tap in tubing open to air, and off to patient.
- Press zero button on monitor to observe zeroing complete.
- Switch 3-way tap off to air, and open to patient.
- Ensure transducer point of reference, and observe trace.
- Waveform should be pulsatile, with dicrotic notch.

Cautions

- Transducer should be level with zero point (mid Axilla).
- Limit use of 3-way taps.
- Remove air bubbles from system.
- Calibrate transducer to atmospheric pressure regularly.

Removing the line

- Prepare a dressing pack at the bedside
- Place patient's arm on the bed, with dressing facing up
- Remove the dressing
- Check puncture, suture integrity, catheter position
- Clean the area around the site
- Remove sutures whilst holding the arterial line in place
- Place sterile gauze over the insertion site
- Apply pressure (5 min) whilst withdrawing the line
- Apply clear dressing over the site
- Check that the line has been removed

Note 1: The arterial line measures arterial blood pressure relative to ambient pressure. By zeroing the arterial line with the transducer at the same level as the right atrium, the transducer establishes ambient pressure as the nil (zero) reference value, from which the arterial pressure is measured. By zeroing with the transducer at the "zero" level, there is no hydrostatic pressure in the line tubing to cause any artefact pressure values. If, after zeroing, the height of the transducer changes, relative to the height of the patient's right atrium, then the measurement will be made against a different hydrostatic (head) of fluid pressure. Therefore, maintaining the transducer at the same vertical level as the right atrium assures accuracy.

Note 2:

(i) An occasional flush will disperse any debris which might otherwise cause an obstruction.

(ii) With air in the line, the air bubbles will absorb some of the line pressure, causing damping of the waveform, and an incorrect pressure reading.

(iii) If the patient is lower than the transducer, the monitor will show an incorrect lower value.

(iv) For every 10 cm (4 inch) below the right atrium, the arterial transducer will read an extra 7.6 mmHg of pressure, due to the extra column of saline.

(v) A normal arterial waveform shows a dicrotic notch, when the aortic valve closes.

(vi) Square wave test: Fast flushing should produce a square wave. If not, there may be air in the line.

Dicrotic Notch (Courtesy The Free Dictionary)

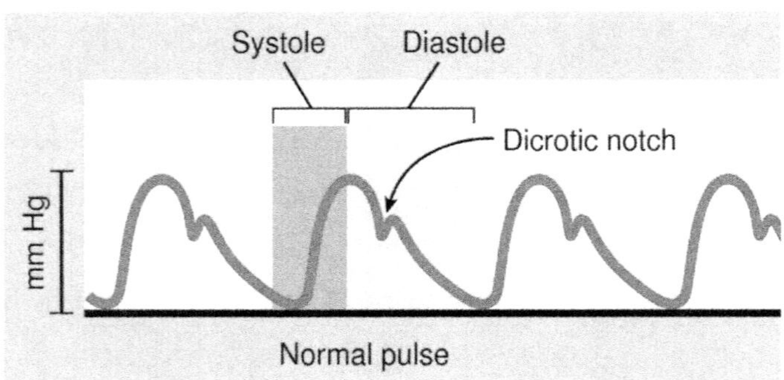

A13b: Arterial Square Wave Test

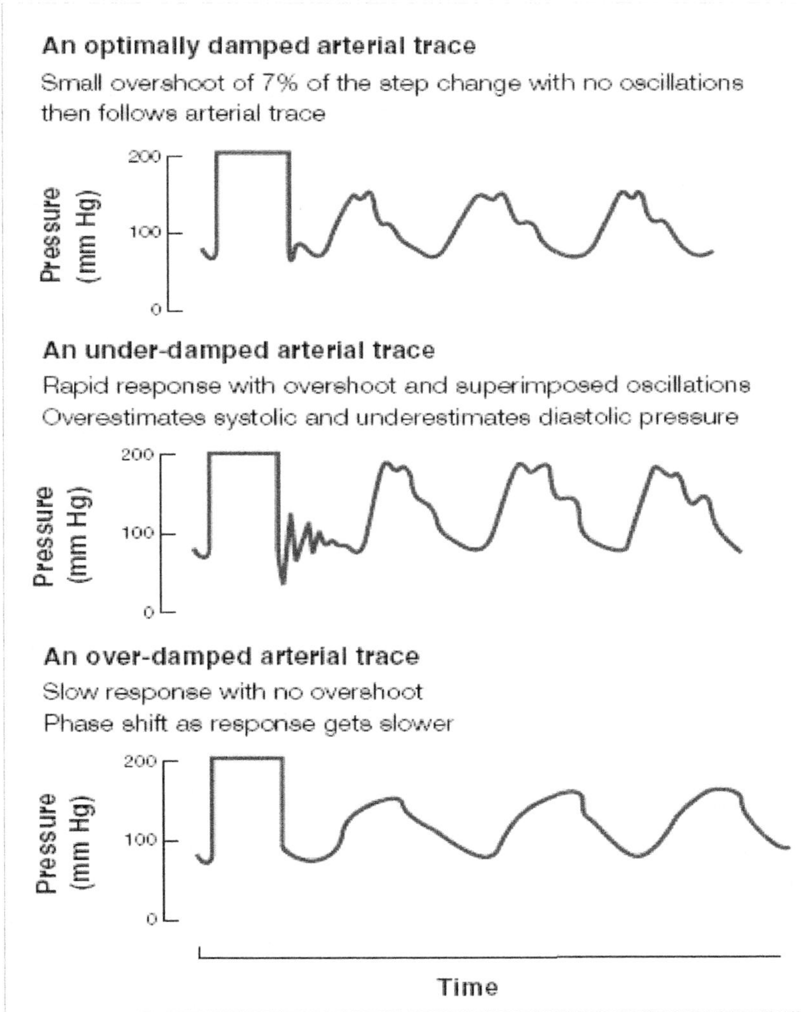

Image courtesy of Anaesthesia UK.

A14: Aspiration of Gastric Contents

Risk factors

- ☠ Pregnancy
- ☠ Peptic ulcers
- ☠ Old age
- ☠ Difficult intubation
- ☠ Hiatus hernia
- ☠ Non-fasted
- ☠ Inadequate anaesthesia
- ☠ Gas insufflation
- ☠ Bowel obstruction
- ☠ Previous gastric surgery
- ☠ Nasogastric tube in situ
- ☠ Reduced consciousness
- ☠ Drugs & Volatiles
- ☠ Raised intra-abdominal pressure

Recognition

- Laryngospasm
- Bronchospasm
- Coughing
- Tachycardia
- Hypotension
- Airway obstruction
- Low oxygen saturation

Management

- Head down
- Suction
- O2
- Anaesthesia
- RSI

Precaution: If there is a risk of aspiration, the patient should be recovered in the left lateral position.

A15: Asystole

Treatment Cycle

- Start CPR (30:2)
- Give Adrenaline 1 mg, intravenous, asap
- Continue CPR 30:2 until airway secured, then continuously
- Treat reversible causes
- After 2 minutes, check status
- If VF/VT, change to shockable algorithm
- Otherwise, give 1 mg Adrenaline, intravenous

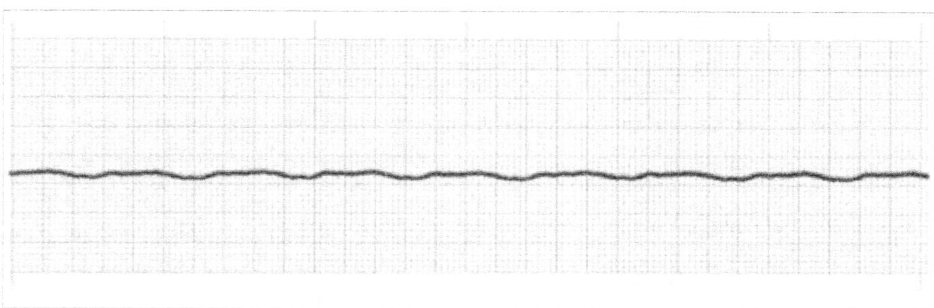

A16: Atelectasis Types

Obstructive (Resorptive)

Airway blockage (tumour, inflammation, foreign object, blood clot) prevents gases reaching the alveoli. Gases already in the alveoli diffuse into the bloodstream, but the obstruction prevents new gas from replenishing the alveoli, causing them to collapse.

Adhesive

Impaired or lack of surfactant makes alveoli walls stick together.

Compressive

External pressure (eg, pleural effusion, pneumothorax) forces gas out of the alveoli, and prevents expansion.

Absorption

When the patient is receiving 100% O_2 (oxygen), nitrogen washes out of the lungs and is replaced by new O_2. In absorption atelectasis, the O_2 diffuses from alveoli to the blood quicker than the alveoli can be replenished by the supply, so less gas enters the alveoli than what diffuses to the blood, causing a negative pressure (wrt atmosphere), causing some alveoli to collapse.

A17: Atrial Fibrillation

Causes

- Heart valve disease
- Old age
- Hypoxia
- Pulmonary embolism
- Ischaemic heart disease
- Excess alcohol
- Acute myocardial infarction

Symptoms and signs

- Feeling feint
- Dizziness
- Shortness of breath
- Palpitation
- Tiredness
- No ECG P-wave

Management options

- Anticoagulation with low molecular weight Heparin or
- Above plus rate control with Digoxin or
- Immediate anticoagulation with low molecular weight Heparin plus cardioversion.

ECG trace - note absence of P-waves:

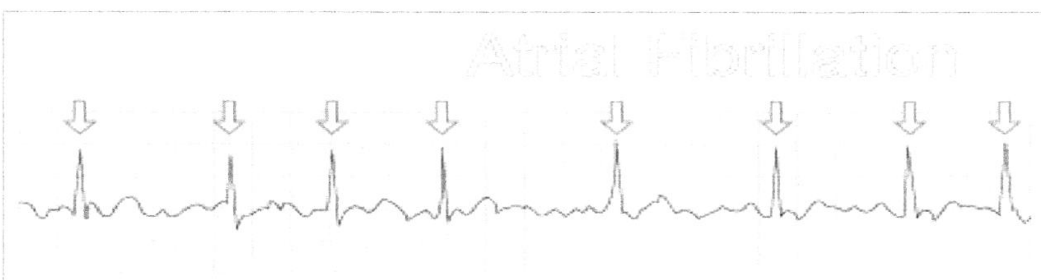

Image, courtesy of Nottingham University

A18: Awake Intubation

Equipment

- Fibreoptic stack and flexible intubating endoscope
- Suction tubing: cut to fit scope
- Uno-flush cleaning solution
- Oxygen source, oxygen line (Hudson mask set)
- Epidural pack
- Nasal ventilating sponge (yellow tip)
- MAD nasal cone and MADgic LMA
- Phenylephrine/Lidocaine spray (blue box)
- Anti-fogging agent (scrub team)
- K-Y gel and Instillagel (have available)
- Syringe driver
- Electro-cath (curly wurly) and syringes: 1, 2, 5, 20 ml
- Remifentanil
- 1% Lidocaine (max 4 mg/kg)
- Lidocaine & phenylephrine (blue pencil case)
- Xylocaine – nasal spray
- Atropine 500 microgram or Glycopyrrolate 200 microgram (dries mucus membrane)
- Diazepam 2 mg

- ⚒ Cocaine - for nasal intubation
- ⚒ Bowls and paper towels for vomit

Setting up

- Put camera stack in anaesthetic room; plug in
- Don sterile gloves
- Retrieve bronchoscope from sterile store
- Thread line through top port - leaves 4"-5" to yellow tag
- Tape Epidural line to scope
- Remove piston from 5 ml syringe
- Put CVC sticker on syringe
- Fit bung to syringe
- Tape syringe, bung down, to top shelf of stack
- Fill syringe with anti-fogging liquid

A19: Beta Blockers

Beta-adrenergic antagonists: Inotropic drugs that block effects of Adrenaline on the heart and blood vessels, weaken effects of the Sympathetic Nervous System on heart conductivity, and reduce blood pressure and heart rate. Used in the management of cardiac arrhythmias, myocardial infarctions, and hypertension.

Example conditions/agents

Condition	*Agents*
Cardiac arrhythmia	Esmolol, Sotalol
Congestive heart failure	Bisoprolol, Carteolol
Hypertension	Atenolol, Esmolol, Labetalol
Migraine	Timolol
Myocardial infarction	Atenolol, Metoprolol

Note 1: Esmolol has short duration of action, and can be useful in preventing hypertension and tachycardia following intubation.

Note 2: Beta-blockers can cause bronchospasm in asthmatics.

A20: Blood

Functions of Blood

① Transports gases, nutrients, waste products

② Regulates hormonal balance, body temperature

③ Protection: clotting, circulates leukocytes against infection

Blood Constituents

Blood is a suspension of cells in plasma. Cells are 45% of total blood volume, with the remaining 55% being plasma.

- Plasma
- Red blood cells (erythrocytes, RBCs)
- White blood cells (leukocytes, WBCs)
- Platelets (thrombocytes)

Adult (70 kg) blood volume

- 5 litre circulating blood (men:70 ml/kg, females:65 ml/kg)
- 1 litre in the heart, artery and capillary circulations
- 1 litre in the pulmonary circulation
- 3 litres in the venous circulation

Plasma

Plasma constitutes 55% of total blood fluid, and is 90% water. The other 10% of dissolved substances are mostly proteins. These dissolved substances are circulated throughout the body, and diffuse from areas of higher to lower concentration, into tissues and cells. Waste materials flow in the opposite direction, where they go on to be removed by the kidneys or lungs. There are approximately 2.7 – 3 litres of plasma in an average adult.

Plasma functions

- ☞ Transports platelets and blood cells
- ☞ Contains a few hours of reserve protein
- ☞ Carries drugs to site of action
- ☞ Resists blood flow – it is viscous
- ☞ Draws fluid into blood vessels, preventing oedema

Red Blood Cells (Erythrocytes)

Red blood cells contain haemoglobin, an iron-containing protein, which facilitates transportation of oxygen by reversibly binding to this respiratory gas, and greatly increasing its solubility in blood. In contrast, carbon dioxide is almost entirely transported extracellularly, dissolved in plasma as bicarbonate ions. Red cells live for 120 days, and have a density of 5 million/mm^3.

White Blood Cells (Leukocytes)

Made in bone marrow, WBCs exist in blood and lymph, to fight infection. Types are granulocytes, monocytes, and lymphocytes. White cell density is 5,000 – 10,000/mm^3.

Platelets

Platelets are the first substance to arrive at a wound site, where they cover the breach by "adhesion", and release chemical messengers, into the blood, to attract more platelets – a process of "aggregation". Platelets are transfused when a patient:

- Has a low platelet count (thrombocytopenia)
- Has significant bleeding
- Has platelets which function abnormally
- Has bone marrow failure
- Following a transplant or chemotherapy treatments
- To treat leukaemia

There are 150,000-450,000 platelets per micro-litre of blood, or 150–450 billion per litre. Each unit (240 billion) of platelets raises the count by approximately 5,000 platelets per microlitre. A low platelet count can result in uncontrolled bleeding, and a high count might result in heart attack or stroke. (Platelets must be stored at 22° C, and must not be put through a rapid infuser)

A21: Blood Groups

Blood grouping is determined by the antigens (surface markers) found on RBCs (Red Blood Cells). *See also Appendix A21b.*

Antibody

A protein in plasma, type A or B, that alerts the immune system to attack foreign substances (antigens).

Antigen (Agglutinogen)

A foreign substance that is attacked by antibodies. Antigens attached to the plasma membrane on the surface of an RBC (red blood cell) are markers which prevent the body from producing antibodies for that type (A or B). The body makes antibodies for the antigen types that are NOT on the cell membrane.

RhD Antigen

If red blood cells have the RhD antigen on their surface, the blood type is known as Rhesus Positive, otherwise Rhesus Negative.

Blood Groups

Type A RBCs have type A antigens on their surfaces, and their immune system makes antibodies only for type B antigens. These antibodies do not recognise (key doesn't fit lock) type A antigens, so they ignore them.

Type B RBCs have type B antigens on their surfaces; the immune system makes antibodies only for type A antigens. These antibodies do not recognise type B antigens, so they ignore them.

Type AB RBCs have types A and B antigens on their surfaces, so blood does not make antibodies for either type A or B antigens.

Type O RBCs have no antigens on their surfaces, so make antibodies for both type A and type B antigens. O Positive types can receive blood from O Positive or O Negative donors. Type O Negative are universal donors, whereas O Positive blood can be donated to any (A, B, AB, O) Rhesus **Positive** blood type only.

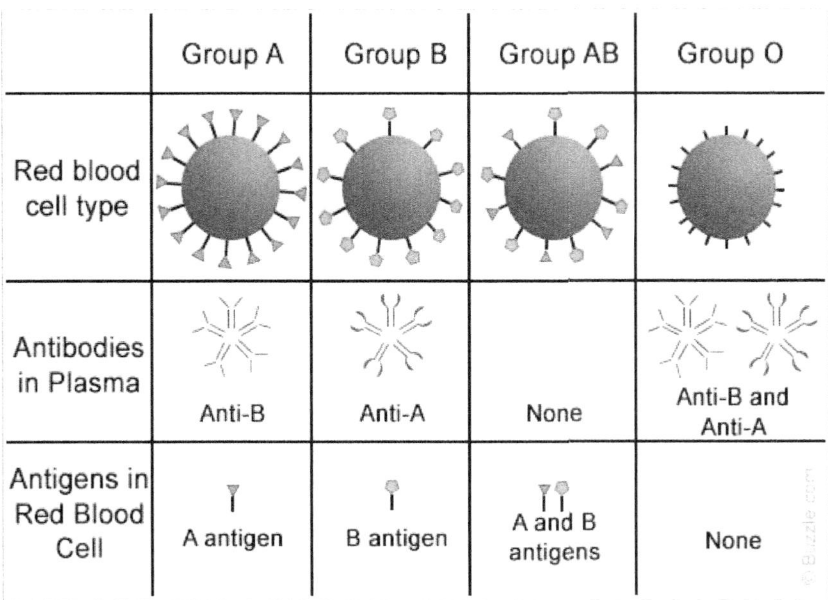

A21b: Blood Group Compatibility

Donor	Recipient							
	O-	O+	A-	A+	B-	B+	AB-	AB+
O-	√	√	√	√	√	√	√	√
O+		√		√		√		√
A-			√	√			√	√
A+				√				√
B-					√	√	√	√
B+						√		√
AB-							√	√
AB+								√

A24: Blood Test Bottle Cap Colours

Colour	***Common Tests***
Gold	Biochemistry, Thyroid, U&Es, Thyroid
Grey	Glucose, Lactate (blood , CSF)
Light blue	Clotting/Factors, Prothrombin, Thrombophilia, Lupus, INR
Lavender	Full Blood Count, Viscosity, Sickle cell, HIV
Pink	Group & Save, Cross Match
Red	Immunology
White	Immunology
Yellow	Transplant immunology

A25: Blood Transfusion - Preparation

Equipment

- Drip stand and giving set.
- Infusion pump - if required.
- Fluid warmer.
- Patient notes & prescription chart.
- Blood compatibility form.
- Unit of blood/blood product.
- Gloves.
- Saline and alcohol wipes.
- Syringe and needle.

Administration

Meet the patient

- 10 minutes (max) before transfusion, record observations: pulse, temperature, blood pressure, respiration rate.
- Discuss and explain transfusion procedure with the patient.
- Establish venous access (before fetching the blood).
- Fetch the blood product from the blood bank.

Identity checks

- Ask the patient to state their name and date of birth. Confirm identity against notes and wristband - do not transfuse unless the patient has a valid wristband.
- Verify the label (Name, DOB, NHS number) on the blood product against the patient's notes and wristband.
- Verify the blood group/expiry date/unit number against the compatibility form and patient notes.
- If the supplied blood group is different from the patient's group, ensure this fact is mentioned on the compatibility from.
- Check prescription/compatibility forms for special instructions.

Infusion process

- Assess the patient's condition for the transfusion process.
- Determine whether the patient has had adverse reactions to previous transfusions.
- Ensure patency and security of the cannula, and check for swelling, inflammation, or pain.
- If the cannula has been used to administer anything but 0.9% saline, flush with 10 ml 0.9% saline, prior to transfusion.
- Ensure the blood has a separate line from any other infusion.
- Feed the transfusion line through the warming device.
- Using aseptic technique, prime the giving set.
- Attach the infusion line to the cannula.
- Give a slow infusion in the first 15 minutes, because this is

when reactions (agitated, rash, hypotension, tachycardia, pyrexia, ...) are usually seen, then set the prescribed rate.

Management

- Assess the patient at regular intervals, during infusion.
- Prevent circulatory overload - maintain a fluid balance chart.
- When the transfusion has finished, flush the cannula (saline) and cap off - or remove the cannula, if it is no longer required.
- Dispose of sharps.
- Log transfusion to Blood Safety and Quality Regulations:
    1. Number of each unit given.
    2. Start date and time of each unit.
    3. Finish date and time of each unit given.

A26: Bronchospasm

Bronchospasm is an abnormal, reversible, and rapid spasm of the smooth muscle of the bronchioles, resulting in narrowing and obstruction. Signs: low sats, cough, may be expiratory wheeze. Bronchospasm is a major characteristic of asthma and bronchitis, and can present on its own, or as part of anaphylaxis, or some other underlying pathology.

Process

The bronchial smooth muscle goes into a state of contraction (bronchospasm), which narrows the bronchiole. The mucosa become swollen and inflamed, which further reduces the bronchial diameter. Additionally, bronchial glands produce excessive amounts of sticky mucus, which is difficult to cough out, and which may form plugs in the bronchus, further obstructing the flow of air.

When bronchi become obstructed, greater pressures are needed to push air through them, in order to meet the body's requirement for oxygen. Breathing, during bronchospasm, requires more effort than normal. The excessive amounts of mucus, caught in the bronchi, are irritating, and often trigger coughing.

Causes

- Asthma (most common)
- Chronic obstructive airway disease
- Pulmonary oedema
- Anaphylaxis
- Pneumothorax
- Aspiration
- Laryngospasm
- Reversal from anaesthesia
- Bronchitis
- Isoflurane/Desflurane introduced too quickly
- Recent upper respiratory infection
- Thiopentone, Atracurium, Mivacurium, Morphine, NSAIDs; Antibiotics
- Airway manipulation/irritation: when patient only lightly anaesthetised
- Histamine release, or noxious stimuli

Signs

- Prolonged expiration
- Expiratory wheezing (unless complete obstruction)
- Increased peak inspiratory airway pressure during IPPV
- Reduced exhaled tidal volume
- Shark-fin capnograph – increasing wave size, slope up L to R

Note:

► When intubated, ventilation may become difficult, and there may be a rise in airway pressure. In severe cases, silent chest may occur i.e., so little gas flow in or out that no sound is heard during auscultation.

► Absolute bronchospasm may be difficult to distinguish from oesophageal intubation.

► Airway obstruction can produce a "shark fin" capnograph (prolonged expiration and narrow airway).

► A blocked circuit, or blocked or misplaced ETT can mimic bronchospasm.

Bronchospasm occurs equally during intubation and maintenance phases of GA. During induction, bronchospasm usually occurs due to airway irritation (e.g., laryngoscopy). During the maintenance phase, bronchospasm usually occurs due to allergic reaction.

Risk Factors

- Asthma or COPD
- Smoking
- Upper respiratory tract infection

Treatment (intra-operative)

- Stop stimulation.
- Ventilate manually with 100% oxygen.
- Call for help.
- Consider allergic reactions.
- Deepen anaesthesia (volatile agents are bronchodilators).

- Ketamine (the only bronchodilating anaesthetic agent).
- Ensure high airway pressure not caused by endobronchial intubation or kinked tube.
- Slightly withdraw ET Tube/LMA.
- IV or intratracheal lidocaine, 1-2 mg/kg.
- Give salbutamol ($\beta 2$ agonist) through circuit inspiratory limb, by inhaler or nebulizer.
- Have Hydrocortisone, Magnesium, Ketamine on standby.
- In extreme cases, give Adrenaline infusion.
- Intravenous steroids.

Bronchospasm Capnogram – Shark Fin

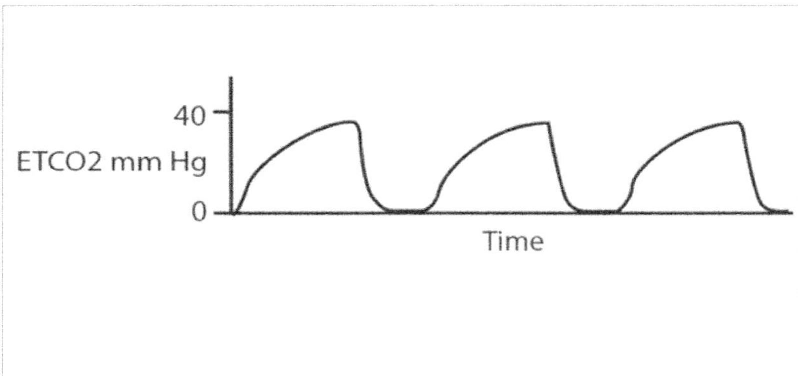

Note: A shark fin trace can also mean COPD or obstructed ET tube.

A27: Bronchial Tree

The trachea divides into left and right main (primary) bronchi, at the tracheal bifurcation. The right main bronchus divides into three lobar (secondary) bronchi, serving the three right lung lobes. The left main bronchus divides into two lobar bronchi of the left lung, serving the two left lung lobes. *Note*: The extra lobar bronchus of the right lung is known as the Eparterial Bronchus, and supplies the superior lobe of the right lung - the most superior secondary bronchi; it arises above the pulmonary artery level, giving its name, "eparterial". (Distributions inferior to the pulmonary artery are termed "hyparterial.").

A **lobar** (secondary) **bronchus** divides into segmental (tertiary) bronchi (9-10); each serving a bronchopulmonary segment.

A **segmental bronchus** branches into progressively smaller sub-segmental bronchi.

Sub-segmental bronchi branch into terminal bronchioles.

Terminal bronchioles branch into respiratory bronchioles, marking the start of the respiratory zone.

Respiratory bronchioles branch into alveolar ducts, then to alveolar sacs, in which are the alveoli.

Structures

Bronchi have cartilaginous support, which prevents them

collapsing due to, for example, allergens.

Bronchioles, alternatively, are not supported by cartilage; their diameter is governed by smooth muscle contraction/dilation.

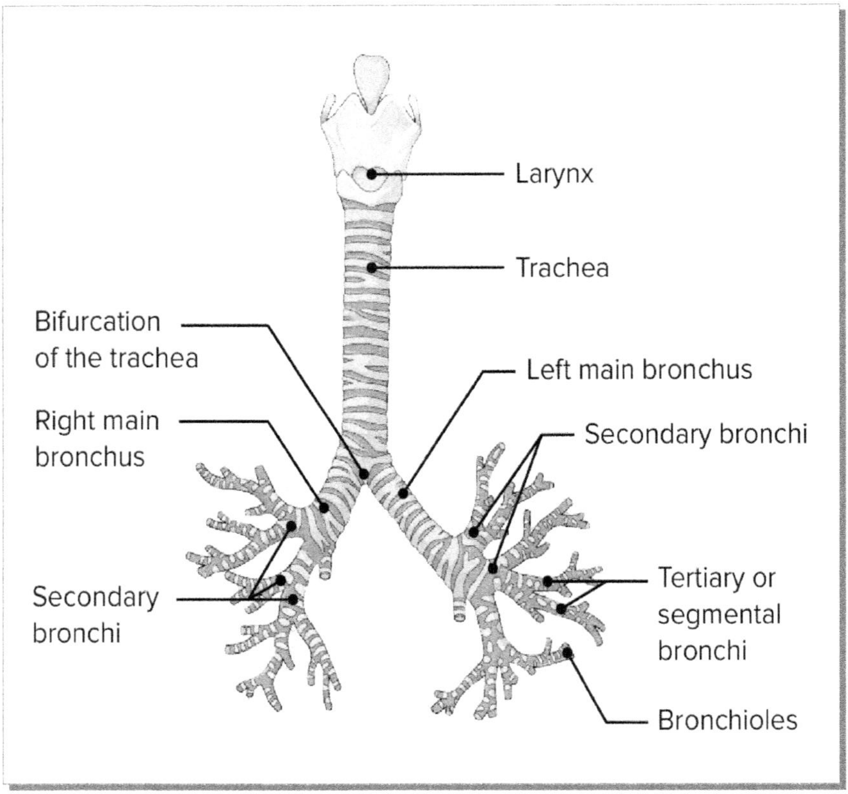

A28: Caesarian Section

Level of urgency is identified by four categories

Category	*Description*
1	Requires immediate (within 15 mins) delivery; a threat to mother or baby.
2	Requires urgent (within 30 mins) delivery; compromised mother or baby, but not immediately life-threatening.
3	Requires early delivery; neither mother not baby compromised.
4	Elective delivery at a time suited to the mother and staff.

Examples of Category 1 Cases

- Major haemorrhage
- Profound and persistent foetal bradycardia
- Prolapsed cord
- Shoulder dystocia
- Uterine rupture

Complications of Epidural

- Dural tap
- Total spinal
- Local anaesthetic overdose
- Bloody tap
- Adhesive Arachnoiditis
- Hypotension

Contraindications to Spinal/Epidural

- Septicaemia
- Amide allergy
- Hypovolaemia
- Coagulopathy
- Insertion site infection
- CV instability
- Raised intra-cranial pressure

Massive Obstetric Haemorrhage

A major cause of maternal death and morbidity. Defined as:

- Blood loss > 1500 ml, or
- A decrease in haemoglobin > 4 g/dl, or
- Acute transfusion requirements > 4 units

The gravid uterus receives up to 12% of cardiac output, thus obstetric haemorrhage can be unexpected and life threatening.

See also Appendix A73.

A29: Caesarian Section, G.A.

Acid Aspiration Prophylaxis

Emergency Case

- If Ranitidine (if allowed?) has not been administered during the labour, give 50 mg (in 20 ml saline) I.V.
- 10 mg metoclopramide I.V.

Elective Case

- Ranitidine (if allowed?) 150 mg, oral, the night before.
- Ranitidine 150 mg and metoclopramide 10 mg, oral, 2-4 hours before the procedure.

Intubation

- Have a second anaesthetist present.
- Confirm choice of rescue device (LMA/Proseal/ILMA).
- Prepare a difficult intubation device, such as Glidescope.
- Establish I.V. Access: 16 gauge.
- Put mother in left lateral tilt (until delivery), to prevent aortocaval compression, maternal hypotension, foetal problems.
- Give 30 ml 0.3 M sodium citrate antacid prophylaxis.

- Optimise head/neck position, and place suction under pillow.
- Pre-oxygenate for 3+ minutes.
- Administer Thiopentone; apply cricoid pressure.
- Administer 1.5 – 2 mg/kg Suxamethonium,
- Intubate.
- Ventilate with 2% Isoflurane in 50:50 O_2:N_2O (1st minute).
- Reduce to 1% Isoflurane.

Delivery

- After (immediately) deliveries: 5 IU Syntocinon (Oxytocin) IV.
- Start syntocinon infusion, 40 IU/500 ml saline at 10 IU/hour.
- Oxygen concentration can be reduced to 30%.
- Ask the surgeon if the left tilt can be removed.
- Morphine/Paracetamol/PR Diclofenac.

Note: 2 ml of i.v. 1:1,000 Salbutamol acts as an antagonist (relaxes uterus) of Syntocinon when e.g., doing a manual removal of the placenta (gives more space for surgeon).

After all deliveries

- Consider a nasogastric tube to drain the stomach.
- Have suction catheters ready.
- Have oxygen cylinder/hudson mask available.

A30: Cannulation

Procedure

☞ Wash hands, don gloves.

☞ Open the cannula wings.

☞ Slightly withdraw and replace the needle – this will make it glide easier when cannulating.

☞ Unscrew cannula cap (back), and place upright in the tray.

☞ Remove the cannula sheath.

☞ Secure the vein with your non-dominant hand from below, by gently pulling on the skin, distal to the insertion site.

☞ Warn the patient of a sharp scratch.

☞ Insert the cannula directly above the vein, through the skin (10-30°) – ensuring the bevel is facing upwards.

☞ Observe for flashback in the cannula chamber.

☞ Decrease angle twixt needle and skin, then advance needle another 2 mm, after flashback, to ensure in the vein lumen.

☞ Withdraw the introducer needle slightly, so that its point is inside of the plastic tubing.

☞ Advance the cannula fully into the vein.

☞ Release the tourniquet.

☞ Place sterile gauze directly underneath cannula hub.

☞ Apply pressure to the proximal vein, close to the tip of the cannula, to reduce bleeding.

☞ Gently pull the introducer needle backwards, whilst holding the cannula in position.

☞ Connect luer lock-cap, or extension set, to the cannula hub.

☞ Dispose of the introducer needle, into a sharps container.

Common Volume (B is preferred)

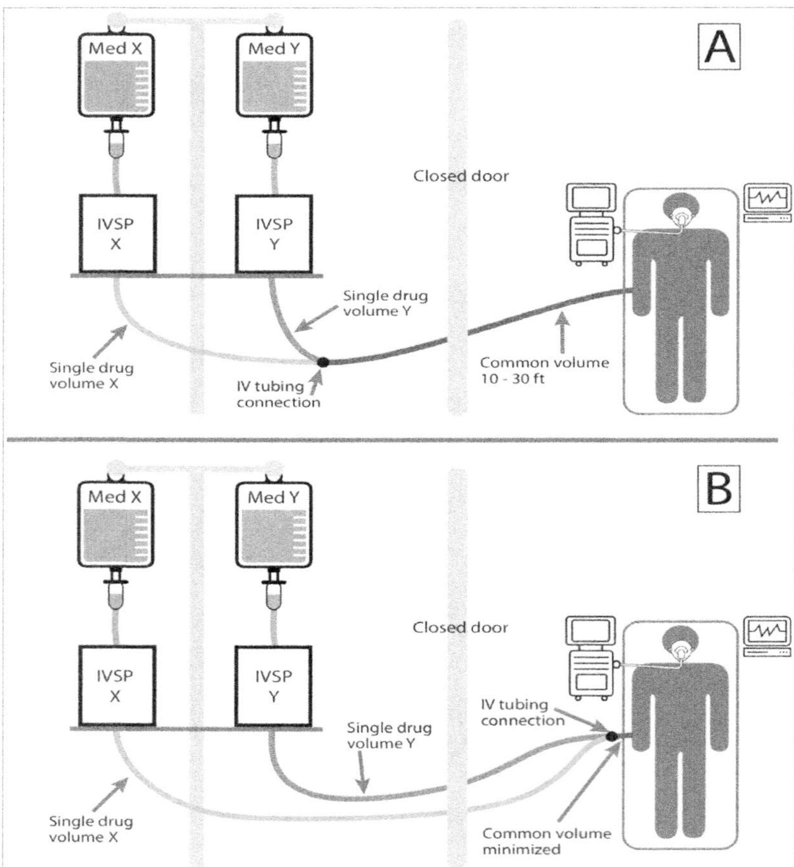

A31: Capnogram

Capnogram Format:

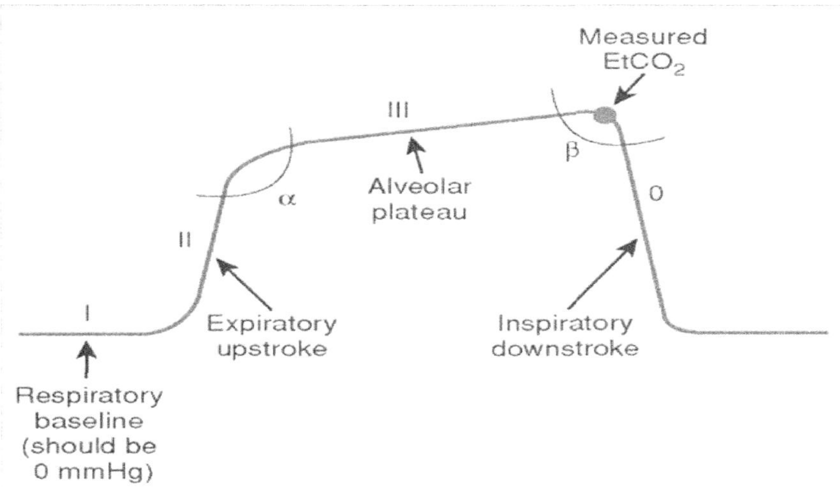

<u>Note 1</u>: The **α** angle is the transition from mixed alveolar and dead space CO_2 to only alveolar CO_2. If α angle > 90°, there may be ventilation/perfusion (V/Q) mismatch.

<u>Note 2</u>: The **β** angle is the transition from expiration (end tidal CO_2) to inspiration. If rebreathing, the β angle might be > 90°.

A31b: Capnogram Examples

Hyperventilation (Decrease in $ETCO_2$)

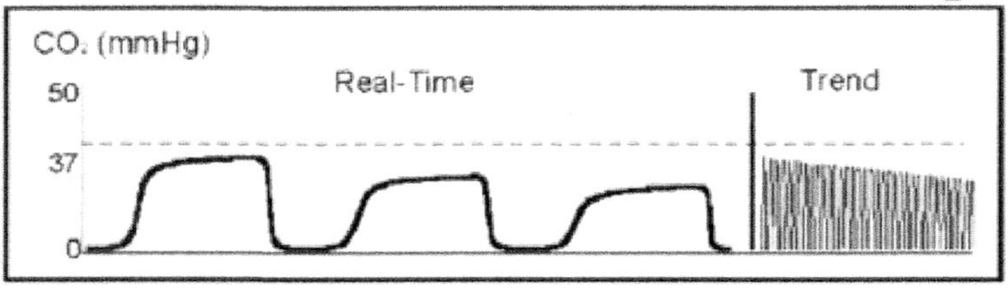

Possible Causes:

- Increase in respiratory rate
- Increase in tidal volume
- Decrease in metabolic rate
- Fall in body temperature

Inadequate Seal Around ET Tube

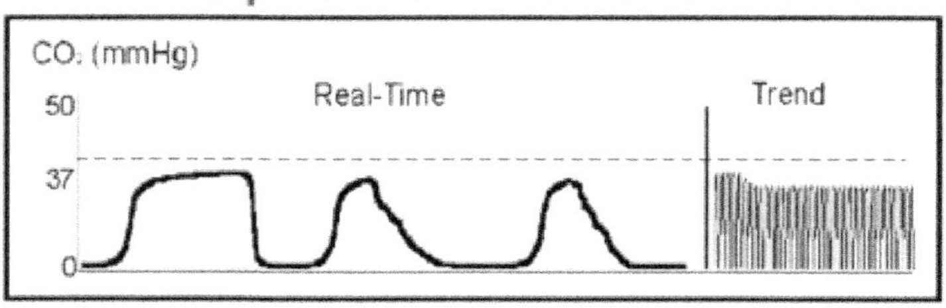

Possible Causes:

- Leaky or deflated endotracheal or tracheostomy cuff
- Artificial airway is too small for the patient

Muscle Relaxants (curare cleft)

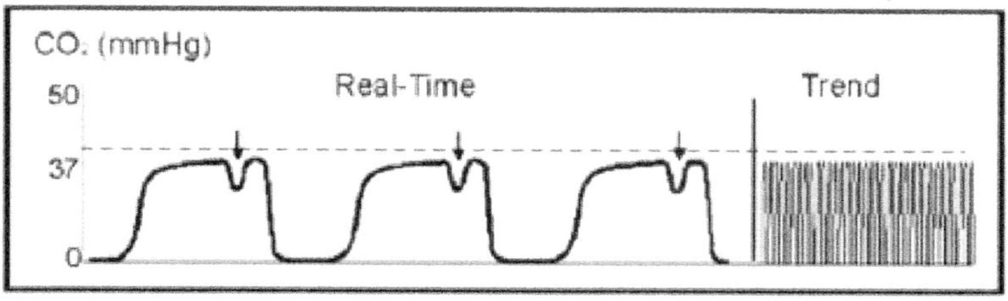

- Appear when muscle relaxants begin to subside
- Depth of cleft is inversely proportional to degree of drug activity

Obstruction in Airway or Breathing Circuit

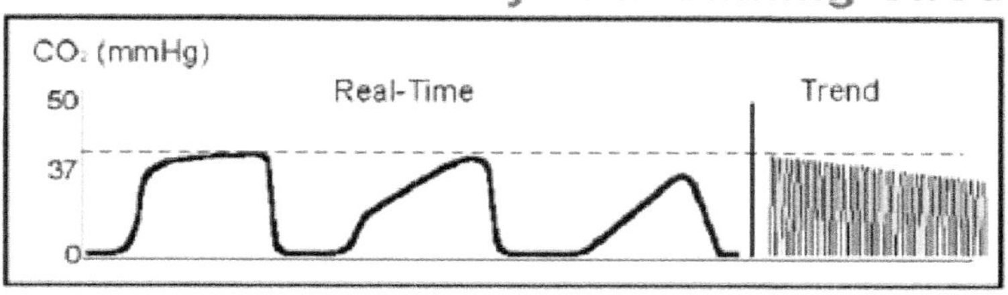

Possible Causes:

- Partially kinked or occluded artificial airway
- Presence of foreign body in the airway
- Obstruction in expiratory limb of breathing circuit
- Bronchospasm

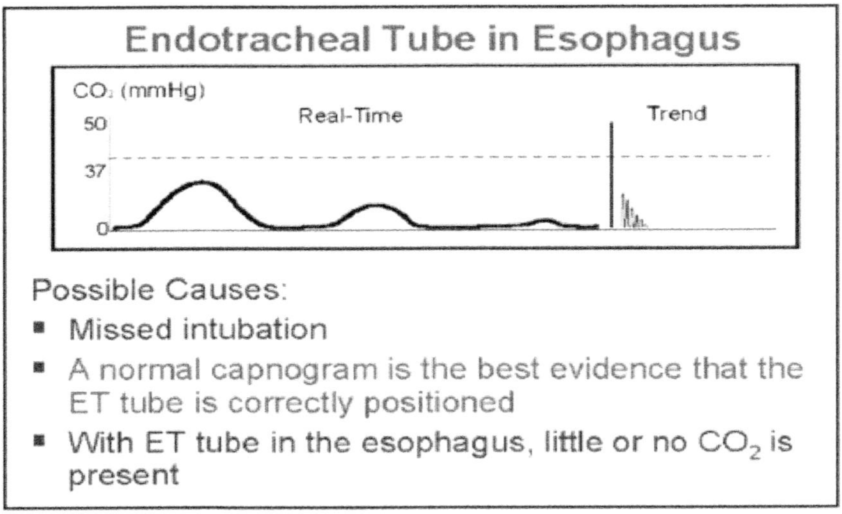

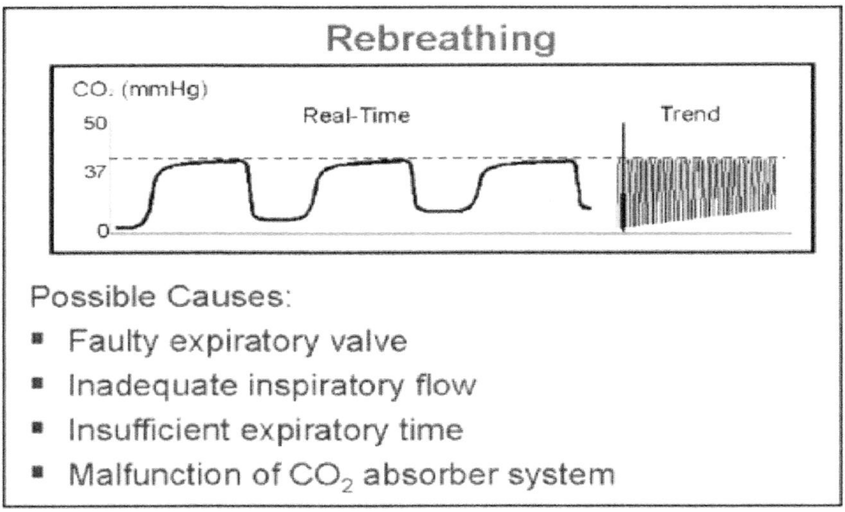

Images courtesy of CapnoAcademy.

A32: Cardioversion

Conversion of an arrhythmia to a sinus rhythm. In synchronised electrical cardioversion, the patient is anaesthetised, ventilated, has a bite block fitted, defibrillator pads attached, and a shock delivered to the myocardium - synchronously with an R-wave.

Defibrillator energy levels

Condition	***Biphasic***	***Monophasic***
Atrial fibrillation	120-150 joules	200-360 joules
Atrial flutter	70-120 joules	100-150 joules
Ventricular tachycardia	120-150 joules	200-360 joules

Pharmacological cardioversion

IV Amiodarone – 300 mg over 1 hour.

A33: Cell Salvage

Overview

Step 1: Suction

As the surgeon makes the incision, blood oozes from the dissected tissues and begins to pool. The blood is sucked away via a dual lumen tube, which mixes the blood immediately with an anticoagulant. Both are then sucked into a reservoir connected to a vacuum pump. The anticoagulant is either Heparin or Citrate.

Step 2: Collection and filtration

The blood and anticoagulant collect in the reservoir, and filtered to remove large clots and debris.

Step 3: Preparation

Blood and anticoagulant are drawn from the reservoir, into a centrifuge, to be processed.

Step 4: Separation

Sterile isotonic (0.9%) saline solution is pumped into the centrifuge bowl. The force supplied by the centrifuge holds the dense red blood cells against the outer wall of the bowl. The less dense white blood cells, platelets, plasma, clotting factors and anticoagulant, move toward the centre of the bowl, where they spill over into a waste bag.

Step 5: Waste disposal

Waste, including white blood cells, platelets, plasma, anticoagulant, fat, clotting factors, and free plasma haemoglobin, are collected, and disposed of as clinical waste.

Step 6: Red cell salvage

Packed red blood cells, separated from waste products, are collected in a separate bag. The quality of the collected red cells depends upon the volume of wash solution used, degree of concentration achieved, quality of the blood prior to washing, type of surgery, and the presence of various substances that remain in the red cell pack.

Step 7: Re-infusion

Red blood cells can then be re-infused immediately, or post-surgery, with a limit of six hours for re-infusion.

Note: Swabs and sponges are weighed before placing them into a bowl of anticoagulant. The blood from the bowl is then taken to the reservoir, and processed the same as the other surgical field. (Step 3), to ensure that all blood is salvaged.

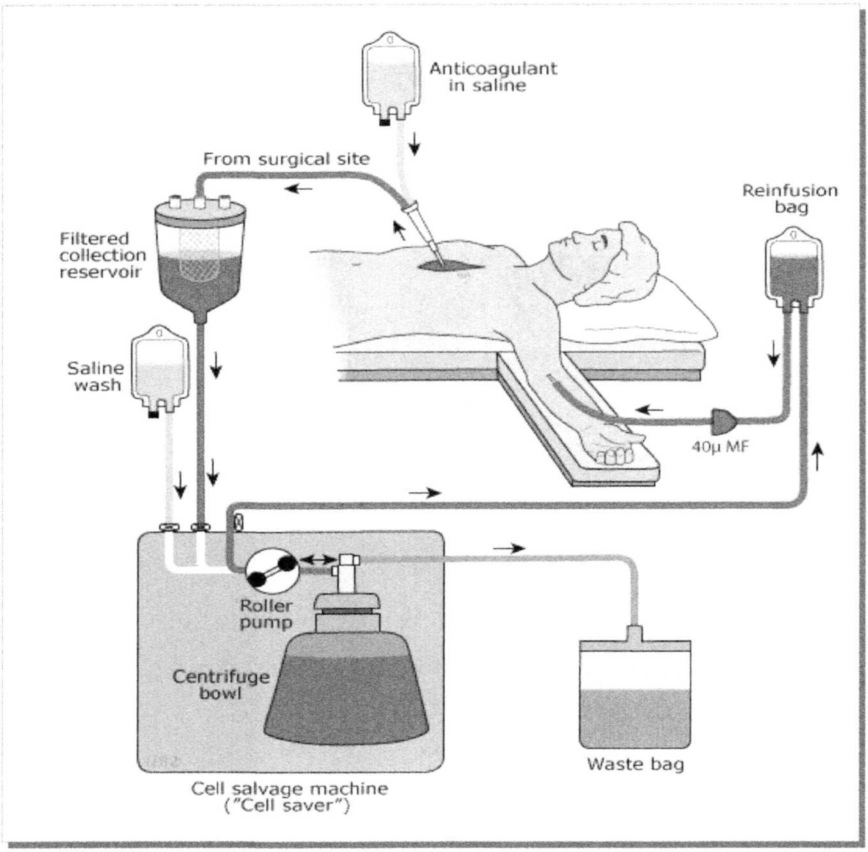

Cell Salvage Operation

Equipment:

- Cell Saver machine
- Power source, and 2 power cables.
- 3 litre reservoir cannister
- Vacuum tube (suction: -80 to -120 mmHg)
- Aspiration & Anticoagulant (A&A) set
- Centrifuge pack (R,Y,B lines, re-infusion bag, waste bag)

⚒ 2 * 1 litre bags of Normal Saline (wash).

⚒ 1 litre Heparinised (30 k IU) saline (or 15 k IU in ½ litre).

Setup:

Ƴ Fit reservoir - inline with W caps.

Ƴ Occlude drain on reservoir.

Ƴ Fit Vacuum tube to reservoir and bottom vacuum source: Y-Y.

Ƴ Hang Heparinised anticoagulant saline.

Ƴ Plug in both power leads.

Collection:

◇ Pass A&A tubing set to sterile field.

◇ Receive back spiked line for Hep/saline, and suction tube.

* Spike Hep/saline .

* Fit suction tube to reservoir.

◇ Switch suction on.

◇ Prime reservoir filter with 100-200 Hep/saline, then clamp off.

◇ When blood enters reservoir, switch Hep/saline back on @ 1 drop/sec.

◇ When 600-800 ml collected in reservoir, setup wash system.

Wash system:

☞ Hang Normal Saline bags.

☞ Fit Centrifuge.

☞ Hang re-infusion bag from top pig-tail on IV pole.

☞ Close the 2 side clamps (R) on re-infusion bag.

- ☞ Hang waste bag on front pins; check drain port is closed.
- ☞ Close clamps on spiked Y Normal Saline lines.
- ☞ Open front panels; thread tubing (RYB) through line sensor.
- ☞ Thread tubing (RYB) around pump...
- ☞ Y spiked lines to clamped Normal Saline bags.
- ☞ B (unclamped) to re-infusion bag.
- ☞ R to reservoir drain (R).
- ☞ Load pump and air detector.
- ☞ Close pump lever and manifold door.
- ☞ Open side clamp.
- ☞ Unclamp line (Y) from 1 Normal Saline bag.
- ☞ Open clamp (R) from reservoir
- ☞ Switch wash system on.
- ☞ When system loaded, press **Start** (enters *Standby* mode).

Troubleshooting

Message	***Actions***
Bowl type choice	If using white bowl adaptor, press "Yes" Otherwise, press "No"
Saline bag empty	Open clamp to bag, and spike in bag. Check tubing in air detector. Close clamp to unused spike. Check tubing placement in valves.
Centrifuge cover	Check inlet and outlet tubing placement.

not closed	
Waste bag full	Empty or change waste bag, ensuring bowl is empty.
Air detected in fill cycle	If reservoir empty, wash partial bowl or wait for more blood. If reservoir not empty: ♦ Check tubing in air detector. ♦ Check suction < 200 mmHg. ♦ Open clamp on stepdown connector to red line. ♦ Check placement of tubing in valves placement.
Long empty cycle	Check tubing placement. Verify bowl size. Check for occlusions in effluent, red, and blue lines. Check bowl displacement. Air in waste bag.
Clamped line detected	Check for kinks or occlusions in tubing. Ensure clamps on reinfusion bag and reservoir are open.

A34: Central Venous Catheter

Gives continuous measurement of...

- Blood Pressure
- Vascular tone
- Patient's response to treatment

Provides long term access for...

- Repeated toxic drugs
- Hydration
- Blood administration
- Repeated specimen collection
- Parenteral nutrition

Benefits...

- Drugs, irritant to peripheral veins, can be given centrally.
- Multi-lumens reduce need for peripheral cannulation.
- Rapid fluid infusion (short length, large bore cannulae only)

Catheter types

- Tunnelled
- Non-tunnelled (typical in theatres, ICU)
- Peripherally inserted

⚐ (Totally) Implanted Vascular Access Devices

Equipment – Central Line (non-tunnelled)

- 500 ml bag of saline, pressure bag, drip stand
- Ultrasound machine
- Transducer set & monitor cable
- Pink Chlorhexidine spray, 2%
- CVP pack + trolley, swabs, blades, sutures, and 3-way taps
- Sonosite ultrasound set
- Nasogastric tube, (Ryles) bag
- McGill forceps
- Luer lock syringes

Insertion sites

- Internal Jugular vein.
- External Jugular vein.
- Subclavian (higher risk of pneumothorax).
- Brachial/anti-cubital fossa.
- Femoral (greater risk of sepsis).

Note:

- Internal Jugular vein is preferred insertion point.
- Supine/Trendelenburg: vein engorgement, avoids embolus.
- If the guidewire gets stuck, the introducer and guidewire should be removed as a single unit.

Placement method

- Anaesthetist scrubs
- Patient placed 20º head down *
- Open sterile CVP pack
- Squirt saline into sterile tray
- Syringe of saline - flushes lines
- Pink spray to insertion site (e.g., jugular)
- Ultrasound gel couplant to insertion site
- Transparent sterile drape over patient face and chest
- Gel on ultrasound probe & in plastic sheath
- Probe in sheath, roll back sheath over cable
- Cannulate vein with a needle (Seldinger technique)
- Push guide wire through the needle
- Remove needle
- Feed cannula over guide wire and into the vein **
- Withdraw guide wire
- Suture in place

* Prevents air entering cannula during insertion - air embolus.
** If cannula goes too far into right atrium, ECG becomes irregular.

Line patency

The line could become blocked: by blood clot, precipitate (inadequate flushing between medications), or fat embolism (due to parenteral nutrition). Patency is maintained by continuous infusion (keeps vein open) and intermittent flushing, using pulsatile (push-pause) method, to create turbulent flow. Heparinised saline used for flushing - to disperse blood clots. Flush and cap all lumens.

Air Embolism

To reduce risk of embolism, use Luer lock syringes, and put patient in Trendelenburg position (at insertion). Unused connections should be clamped. If an embolism occurs, the patient should be placed head down and on left side.

CVP measurement

- Ensure patency of catheter.
- Position patient (retain position for readings).
- Ensure transducer level with patient's mid Axilla.
- Calibrate monitor: off to patient, open to air.
- Press 'BP zero' button.

The CVP waveform should fluctuate in response to atrial pressure changes in the cardiac cycle. An irregular ECG wave occurs when the catheter is too far into the atrium.

Complications

- Air embolus (if infusion or monitoring lines disconnected).
- Dysrhythmia from over insertion of catheter into right Atrium.
- Catheter displacement, causing cardiac arrhythmia.
- Catheter occlusion - regularly flush line.
- Haemorrhage - especially in thrombolytic therapy.
- Heart puncture causes cardiac tamponade.

- Lung puncture causes pneumothorax.

Normal parameters for a healthy patient...

5-10 cmH_2O at mid Axilla. A low reading suggests either fluid loss from haemorrhage (trauma or surgery), poor return due to shock, or excessive diuresis due to *diabetes mellitus* or diuretics.

A high reading could be due to...

- Hypervolaemia
- Congestive heart failure
- Increased intra-thoracic pressure
- Lumen occlusion (cannula against vein wall, thrombus)
- High blood viscosity
- Artefact (viscous drugs or fluid remaining in line)
- User error

Five lumen central line

Proximal	Orange	Parenteral nutrition
Medial	Blue	Inotropes
Medial	Yellow	Drugs
Medial	Purple	Drugs
Distal	Green	CVP monitoring

Contraindications...

☠ Infected insertion site

☠ Coagulopathy

☠ Vein injury

Removing the Central line...

- Place patient supine – to avoid air embolism.
- Prepare dressing pack at patient's side.
- Turn off infusions.
- Place patient in Trendelenburg - 10 minutes before removal.
- Explain Valsalva manoeuvre to patient.
- Remove dressing around line, and clean site.
- Remove sutures whilst holding central line in place.
- Place sterile gauze over puncture site.
- Ask patient to perform Valsalva manoeuvre.
- Remove line at 90 degree angle, apply pressure.
- Tell patient to breathe normally.
- Cover gauze site with occlusive dressing.

A35: Combitube

Note: The white pilot balloon is for the distal cuff, and is inflated (10-15 ml) first. The blue pilot balloon (50-80 ml) is for the proximal cuff.

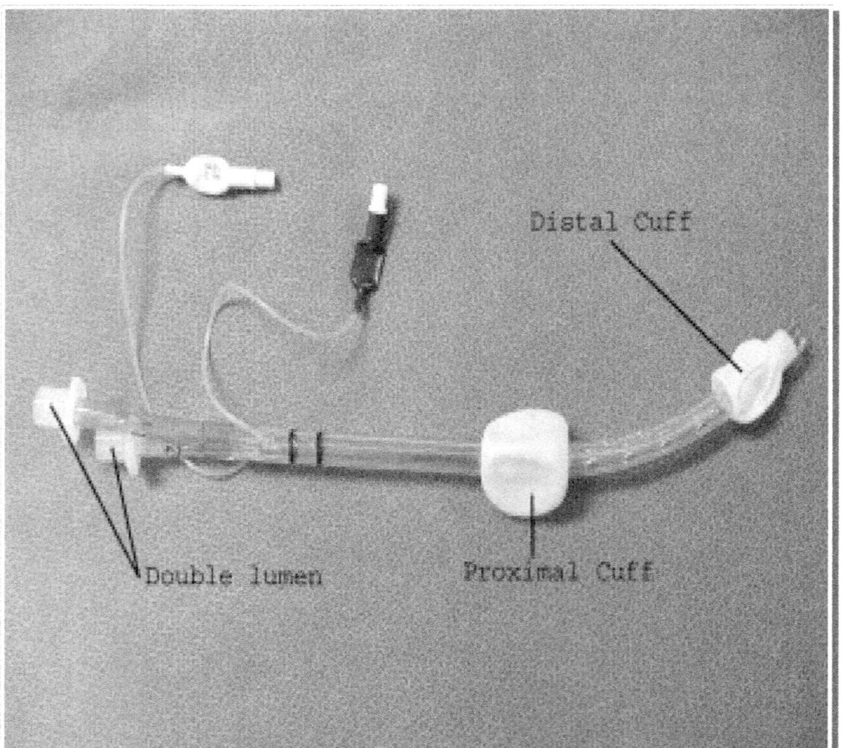

A36: Cricothyrotomy

An emergency airway access procedure, where an opening is made into the cricothyroid membrane (CTM), to allow access (intubation) to the airway inferior to the glottis. Care should be made to avoid the vocal cords, which lie approximately 1 cm superior to the cricothyroid membrane.

There are three distinct cricothyrotomy techniques:

Technique	***Description***
Needle catheter	A needle catheter is placed directly into the cricothyroid space.
Percutaneous dilational	*Seldinger technique:* A guide wire is inserted through a needle or catheter. An airway catheter is then introduced over a dilator, which is threaded over the guide wire.
Scalpel	An incision is made into the cricothyroid space, then a tracheostomy or endotracheal tube is introduced.

In anaesthetic settings, the scalpel technique is most commonly used, and is referred to as an *emergency surgical airway*.

Emergency Surgical Airway

Equipment:

- 🛠 Clear chlorhexadine and gallipot
- 🛠 Fenestrated drape
- 🛠 Sterile gauze
- 🛠 Sterile gel (for ET tube)
- 🛠 Surgical marking pen (if needed)
- 🛠 No 10 blade/scalpel
- 🛠 Blunt dilating forceps (in case blunt dissection needed)
- 🛠 Tracheal hook
- 🛠 Trousseau dilator
- 🛠 Size 6 (I.D.) cuffed ETT (ET tube) & 10 ml syringe

Steps:

- ☞ Use neck extension, to better expose the CTM.
- ☞ Clean (clear chlorhexadine) the front of neck (time permitting).
- ☞ Drape (fenestrated) the area (time permitting).
- ☞ Locate the membrane – between thyroid/cricoid cartilages.
- ☞ Stabilise the thyroid and cricoid cartilages (free hand).
- ☞ Horizontally incise CTM by 3-4 cm.
- ☞ Turn the blade 90° - blunt edge toward the head.
- ☞ Slide a bougie along the blade, into the trachea.
- ☞ Withdraw the blade.

☞ Railroad lubricated ETT over the bougie, into trachea.

☞ Remove bougie.

☞ Connect oxygen supply.

☞ Inflate ET tube cuff.

☞ Confirm correct ET tube placement (CO_2, misting, etc).

☞ Secure the ET tube.

***Note 1**:* Maintain aseptic principles throughout.

***Note 2**:* Use a head ring, to steady the head, and place a bolster or pillows between the shoulders.

***Note 3**:* When oxygenating via cricothyroid cannula, inspiration should take 1 second, and expiration should take 3-4 seconds.

A37: Decompression Sickness

Description

The generic term to describe a number of physiological assaults on a diver's body, caused by "ascending" from a higher ambient pressure (deep), to a lower one (shallow), without allowing enough time for dissolved gases to come out of solution from the blood and tissues. For shallow water dives, where air is the breathing medium, the dissolved gas is nitrogen; for commercial divers, who dive to much greater depths, helium will be the dissolved gas. As the diver nears the surface, the previously dissolved gas comes out of solution, and expands in line with the reduction in pressure, and the bubbles so formed create obstructions in the bloodstream and joints, or impinge on nervous tissue.

The "Bends"

Commonly, decompression sickness is described as "the bends", but this is a corruption of terminology; one of the most significant symptoms of decompression sickness is lower back pain and the tendency for the diver to adopt a bent over posture. Commercial divers came to label this condition as being "bent up" or having a "bend". To describe this condition as *the bends* is akin to describing someone as suffering from *the heart attacks*. In both cases, the plural is incorrect and inappropriate.

Symptoms

- ♿ Headache
- ♿ Joint pain
- ♿ Death
- ♿ Paralysis
- ♿ Loss of balance
- ♿ Vision disturbance

Treatment

Immediately place the patient in a decompression (hyperbaric) chamber, and pressurise to a depth of at least 33 feet (10 metres), then comply with an appropriate decompression table, such as US Navy table 6, or Royal Navy table 62, for example.

A38: Delta Ratio (Δ)

Delta ratio = (AG-12) / (24-HCO_3^-)

Delta Ratio	*Meaning*
< 0.4	A normal-AG metabolic acidosis (hyperchloraemic).
0.4 - 0.9	Mixed NAGMA and HAGMA, with normal kidney function, and acidic anions excreted in urine, as in ketoacidosis or lactic acid (OR kidney failure). {Small diff between diff HCO_3^- and diff AG}
1 to 2	Pure high-AG metabolic acidosis. {Diff AG > diff HCO_3^-}
> 2	HAGMA + either metabolic akalosis or a compensated respiratory acidosis. {Diff AG much > diff HCO_3^-}

A39: Diabetes Mellitus

Causes

Diabetes Mellitus is the condition where the body's ability to regulate blood sugar is impaired, and occurs when the pancreas does not produce enough insulin to help glucose enter the cells, or the insulin which is produced does not work properly (insulin resistance). An insulin deficiency causes the body to metabolise amino acids and triglycerides, instead of glucose.

Glucose

Glucose comes from digested carbohydrates, and is produced by the liver. Typical carbohydrate sources are bread, vegetables, and fruit. Because the diabetic cannot make proper use of glucose, it builds up in the blood, but is not used as fuel.

Insulin

Insulin is the hormone, produced by the pancreas, which allows glucose to enter cells, where it is used as fuel for energy. When blood sugar is high, insulin is released into the circulation, causing cells to convert glucose into glycogen (glycogenesis), and store it in the liver and muscle tissue.

Glucagon

A hormone, produced in the pancreas, which is released into the bloodstream in response to low blood glucose levels. Glucagon triggers the body into breaking down its stores of glycogen into glucose, which is then released back into the bloodstream. Together with insulin, glucagon maintains optimal blood sugar levels.

Type 1 Diabetes (insulin dependent)

Type 1 develops when the insulin producing cells in the body have been destroyed, so the body has an absence of insulin, resulting in too much sugar (hyperglycaemia) in the bloodstream. Onset is usually before the age of 40, and accounts for between 5 and 15 per cent of all instances of diabetes. Treatment is by daily insulin injections, a healthy diet, and regular physical activity.

Type 2 Diabetes (non-insulin dependent)

Type 2 is when the body does not make enough insulin, or the insulin produced does not work properly (insulin resistance); onset is usually after the age of 40, or 25 in Africans and South Asians. Type 2 diabetes accounts for 85-95 per cent of all cases, and is treated with a healthy diet and increased physical activity. Medication and supplemental insulin may also be required.

Blood sugar levels (mmol/litre)

Subject type	***Before meals***	***2 hours after meals***
Non diabetic	3.6 - 5.4	< 7.7
Type 2 diabetic	4 - 7	< 8.5
Type 1 diabetic (adult)	4 - 7	5 - 9
Type 1 diabetic (child)	4 - 8	< 10

A40: Difficult Intubation

Unanticipated difficult/failed intubation, four main stages:

- **Plan A:** Attempt facemask ventilation & ET intubation.
  If unsuccessful, try plan B.

- **Plan B:** Oxygenate and insert a supraglottic (LMA) device.
  If unsuccessful, try plan C.

- **Plan C:** Attempt face mack ventilation.
  If unsuccessful, perform plan D.

- **Plan D:** Conduct Front Of Neck Access (FONA).

Priority, throughout, is ventilation – NOT intubation.

Indications for a potentially difficult airway include:

- Less than 3″ (7 cm) between mandible and hyoid bone
- Less than 5″ (12.5 cm) sternomental distance
- Less than 35° neck extension
- Poorly visualized uvula
- Short, thick neck
- Receding mandible (e.g. Pierre Robin Syndrome)
- Protruding teeth

A41: Double Lumen Endobronchial/Endotracheal Tube

Left Robertshaw double-lumen tube

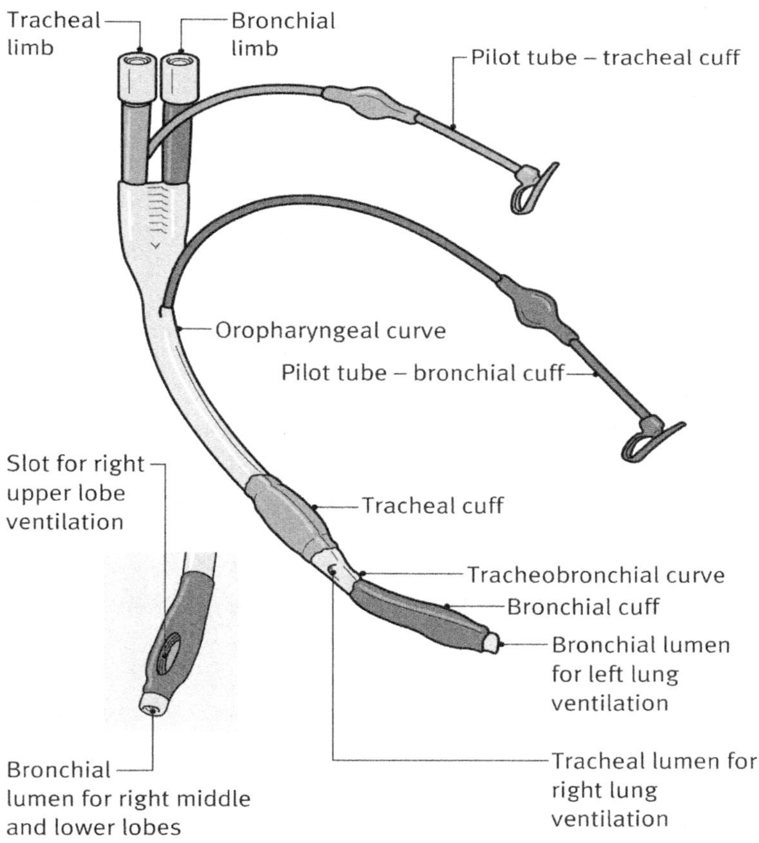

Inset, tip of right-sided Robertshaw. Reproduced, with permission, from the Department of Medical Illustration, Wythenshawe Hospital, Manchester, UK.

A42: Drug Administration

Prescription Checks

- Validate the prescription against the patient.
- A second qualified person confirms above.
- Check drug, dose, strength, route, date, signature (Dr).
- Record the Controlled Drug in the drawings book.
- Sign the prescription chart.
- Aseptic precautions: wash hands, wear gloves.
- Adopt a new syringe and drawing up needle.
- If using a powdered agent mix water with the agent.
- For liquid agents, draw up the solvent, then the drug.
- Ensure the administration site is not contaminated.
- Inform an awake patient what is happening.
- Monitor base readings before injecting.
- Monitor for reactions e.g., heart rate, allergy.

A43: Early Warning Score (NEWS2)

	3	2	1	0	1	2	3
RR	< 9		9 - 11	12 - 20		21 - 24	> 24
SpO2 1	< 92	92-93	94-95	> 95			
SpO2 2 (HRF)	< 84	84-85	86-87	**Target 88-92**, > 92 on air	93-94 on O2	95-96 on O2	> 96 on O2
Air or O2		O2		Air			
SBP	<= 90	91-100	101-110	111-219			> 219
Pulse, minute	<= 40		41-50	51-90	91-110	111-130	> 130
ACVPU				Alert			CVPU
Temp °C	<= 35		35.1 - 36	36.1 - 38	38.1 - 39	>= 40	

SpO2 2: This row, if patient has Hypercapnic Respiratory Failure.

CVPU: Where **C**=new onset **C**onfusion/agitation, and responds to **V**oice, **P**ain, or is **U**nresponsive.

A44: Electroconvulsive Therapy

Equipment

- 🛠 Tilting trolley with padded sides
- 🛠 Monitoring
- 🛠 Small gauge cannula/tourniquet/skin wipe/dressing/flush
- 🛠 Face mask, filter, oxygen supply
- 🛠 Oral airway (Guedel pattern)
- 🛠 Mouth guard
- 🛠 Propofol, suxamethonium, ondansetron (available)

Procedure

- Conduct pre-anaesthetic checks, and confirm consent.
- Remove dentures, hearing aids, jewellery, contact lenses/glasses.
- Attach monitoring.
- Establish venous access.
- Pre-oxygenate.
- Anaesthetic induction (propofol).
- Muscle relaxant (suxamethonium).

- Insert airway.
- Continue oxygenation.
- Replace airway with mouth guard.
- Psychiatrist chooses dose and bilateral or unilateral method.
- Psychiatrist places paddles and administers energy.
- Patient has a seizure for 10 – 60 seconds:

  If seizure is short, repeat (?) propofol, suxamethonium, treatment.

  If seizure is too long, intravenous Diazepam may be given.
- When seizure stops, replace mouth guard with airway.
- When ECG normalised, ventilate with facemask.
- Wait for spontaneous breathing.

A45: Electrolytes

An electrolyte is an ionic mineral found in intracellular (ICF) and extracellular (ECF) fluids and tissues. An electrolyte is formed when a substance (solute) is dissolved in water, and it disassociates into its component ions, each of which carries either a positive or negative charge, with the result that the solution becomes electrically conductive – essential for muscle and nerve activity.

If an electrolyte has more protons (positive) than electrons (negative), it is a positive ion, or cation, and is indicated by a plus sign(s). So, for example, the magnesium electrolyte, which has two more protons than electrons, is indicated by labelling it with a double plus (++). Conversely, if an ion has one more electron that protons, it will be indicated with a single minus sign.

Collectively, electrolytes:

- Allow nutrients to enter and waste products to leave cells
- Maintain homoeostasis, especially fluid balance
- Maintaining proper pH
- Aid in nerve excitability
- Enable muscle contraction
- Endocrine secretion

- Create osmotic pressure to keep fluids in compartments.
- Membrane permeability, buffering body fluids, and controlling the movement of fluids between compartments.

The seven most important body electrolytes are Sodium (Na^+), Potassium (K^+), Calcium (Ca^{++}), Chloride (Cl^-), Bicarbonate (HCO_3^-), Magnesium (Mg^{++}), and Phosphate (HPO_4^-).

Sodium is the prime cation in ECF, and plays an important role in cellular osmosis; chloride is the prime anion in ECF. Within cells, potassium is the prime cation.

Electrolytes are essential for human life, with good sources being fruits and vegetables.

Main Electrolyte Serum Values

Bicarbonate	HCO_3^-	22-26 mmol/L
Calcium	Ca^+	2.2-2.6 mmol/L
Chloride	Cl^-	98-108 mmol/L
Magnesium	Mg^+	0.7-1.1 mmol/L
Phosphate	PO_4^-	0.8-1.5 mmol/L
Potassium	K^+	3.5-5.2 mmol/L
Sodium	Na^+	135-145 mmol/L

A46: Emergency Anaesthesia: Basics

Setting up

- Establish IV access
- Provide a tilting trolley or table
- Ready monitoring and temperature probes
- Central Venous Pressure monitoring equipment
- Arterial line equipment
- Intubation equipment plus bougies and suction
- "Difficult" intubation trolley
- Induction and emergency drugs
- Ventilator
- Fluids and fluid warming device
- Forced air warming device
- Syringe pumps

Note: Suxamethonium is contra-indicated in burns patients.

Blood loss

A loss of greater than 15% circulating volume causes tachycardia and vasoconstriction. Although systolic pressure may be maintained, the vasoconstriction may cause a rise in diastolic pressure, with a consequent fall in pulse pressure (difference between diastolic and systolic pressures). The ability to compensate for blood loss is reduced in frail and elderly patients. If haemorrhage continues, BP and urine output will fall. Oxygen saturation may also fall.

Transfusion

The priority is to restore circulating blood volume. Initially, give 0.9% saline, then blood.

Manual In Line Stabilisation (MILS)

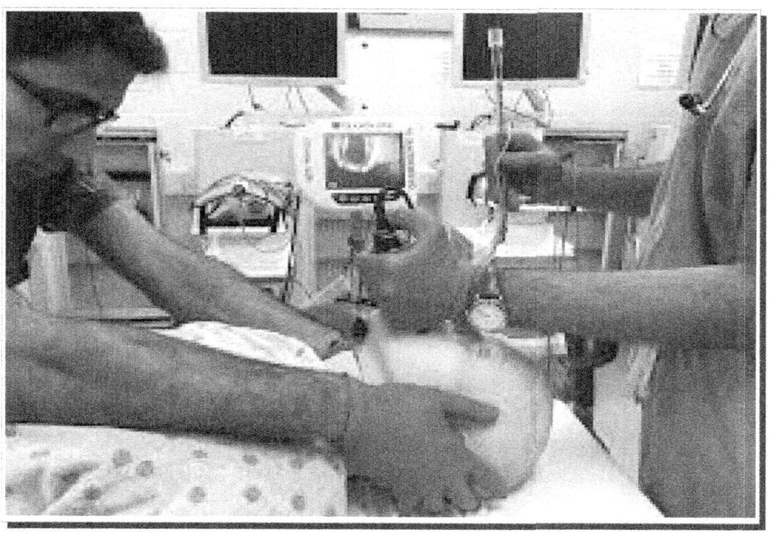

A47: Epidural Block

Usage

The advantage of *epidural* over *spinal* anaesthesia is its ability to maintain continuous anaesthesia after placement of the epidural catheter, making it suitable for lengthy procedures. Epidural blocks can also be used postoperatively, using smaller amounts of local anaesthetic drugs, or in combination with other agents. With an Epidural block, a patient may still be able to walk - unlike with a Spinal block. Drugs used include Marcaine and opioids.

Description

A Tuohy needle. 16-17g, is positioned outside of the dural mater membrane, in the fat filled epidural space, through which nerves pass, after leaving the spinal cord.

The epidural space is identified by loss of resistance to a syringe, filled with saline or air, when the needle passes through the *ligamentum flavum*. Either a bolus dose of local anaesthetic is injected, or a plastic catheter is fed through the Tuohy needle, in order to permit a continuous or occasional infusion technique.

A Lumbar block is performed more commonly than a Thoracic block, and the epidural space is widest (0.5 cm) at this level. If the Tuohy needle is inserted too deeply, and a tear made in the dura, the CSF leakage can give the patient a headache (PDPH) or, even cause permanent damage, vis a vis **adhesive arachnoiditis**.

Indications	Post-op, intra-op, and palliative pain; trauma; Obstetrics.
Contra-indications	Raised intra-cranial pressure; spinal deformity; infection; obesity; allergic to opiates; neurologically diseased.
Advantages	Stable analgesia without peaks/troughs; increased patient mobility; fewer G.I. problems; better respiratory function; more patient satisfaction.
Disadvantages	Motor sensory weakness; catheter may dislodge; careful monitoring required.
Analgesics	1. Fentanyl (fast action and absorption into epidural fat). 2. Bupivacaine (15-20 minutes before action; 6-12 hours duration).
Emergency drugs	Atropine, Ephedrine, Naloxone.
Prohibitions	Avoid Trendelenburg position.

Complications:

Adhesive Arachnoiditis	Puncture and injection into the dural space, giving life long severe pain.
CSF leakage	Headache, nausea
Infection	Backache, spasm, pyrexia, paralysis.
Spinal haematoma	Back/leg pain, urinary retention
Motor weakness	Leg tingling or numbness. Treat with

	positioning and decreasing infusion rate
Hypotension	Stop infusion and give oxygen. Have Naloxone available
Breathing difficulty	Stop infusion, sit patient up, give oxygen, check catheter patency
Bradycardia	Stop epidural, give oxygen. Have available: Atropine, Naloxone, and Ephedrine
Urinary retention	Catheterise, give fluids
Itching	Cool flannel, Ondansetron

Venous access

- Large bore cannula
- 1% Lidocaine
- Dressing
- 5 ml syringe, orange needle
- Saline flush

Equipment

- Gallipot
- Pink Chlorhexidine spray
- Sterile Epidural pack
- Tuohy needle (16g)
- 20 ml saline
- Marcaine 0.5% + 2% Lidocaine
- Flexigrid and Tegaderm dressing

Method

- Sit the patient up, with feet on a stool.
- Spray the patient's back with pink chlorhexidine.
- Open the Epidural pack for the anaesthetist.
- Squirt saline onto the sterile tray.
- Show Lidocaine/date to anaesthetist; drop onto tray.
- Anaesthetist drapes the back of the patient.
- Anaesthetist injects the Lidocaine.
- Anaesthetist inserts the trocar into the Epidural space.
- Anaesthetist injects into the trocar.
- Anaesthetist inserts the catheter through the trocar.
- Anaesthetist removes the trocar.
- Tape (mefix) the Epidural catheter to the skin.
- Fix Flexigrid over the insertion site.

Contraindications

- Coagulopathy - bleeding into the epidural space
- Skin infection at injection site
- Raised intracranial pressure
- Hypovolaemia
- Neurological disorder (e.g., multiple sclerosis)
- Fixed cardiac output state (e.g., heart block)
- Abnormality of vertebral column
- Uncooperative patient

- Prophylactic low dose heparin

How an Epidural differs from a Spinal

An Epidural may be given at a Cervical, Thoracic, or Lumbar site; a Spinal must be given below L2, to avoid piercing the spinal cord.

Onset of analgesia is 25-30 minutes for an Epidural, but 5 minutes for a Spinal. The indwelling catheter of an Epidural allows topping-up of analgesia; a Spinal is a one shot injection.

The larger space with the Epidural requires a larger dose (10-20 ml); a Spinal dose is 1.5 - 3.5 ml.

A49: Epileptic Fit

Tonic-clonic seizure (aka grand mal)

The classic type of epileptic seizure, consisting of two phases to a tonic-clonic seizure: the tonic phase and the clonic phase. In the tonic phase, the body becomes rigid; in the clonic phase, there is uncontrolled jerking. Tonic-clonic seizures may or may not be preceded by an aura (changed behaviour, senses), and are often followed by headache, confusion, and sleep. They may last just a few mere seconds, or continue for several minutes.

If a tonic-clonic seizure does not resolve, or if such seizures follow each other in rapid succession, seek emergency help. The person could be in a life-threatening state known as *Status Epilepticus*.

Signs

- Stiffness
- Fall to the floor
- Loss of consciousness
- Jerking/convulsions
- Irregular breathing
- Blueness around the mouth

Tonic-clonic seizure first aid

- Protect patient from injury - nearby objects etc.
- Cushion their head
- Look for an epilepsy identity card/jewellery
- After seizure, place in recovery position

- Calmly reassure patient
- Stroke hand/hair
- Call ambulance if first/prolonged/repeated seizures

Don't...

- Restrain patient's movements
- Put anything in patient's mouth
- Move them (unless in danger)
- Give food or drink
- Attempt to wake them up

Focal (partial) seizure

When patient is unaware of surroundings. They may pluck at clothes, smack their lips, swallow repeatedly, or wander around. In this case, protect from danger, and reassure them.

A50: Failed Intubation

Difficult Airway Society Protocol ...

- Call for help
- Make 3-4 intubation attempts, with different manouevres
- Maintain cricoid pressure, if appropriate
- Trendelenburg and airway suction, as required
- Insert oral airway
- Ventilate with 100% oxygen
- Wake patient up

If ventilation proves difficult, try an LMA. If ineffective, and laryngospasm has been excluded, perform a cricothyroid puncture (14 g cannula?). See also Appendix A40 (pg 424).

A51: Febrile Convulsion

Description

Seizures which occurs in children (6 months – 3 years) with a fever over 39°C (102.2°F). These most typically occur during the early stages of a viral infection, while the temperature is rapidly rising. The convulsions occur because the electrical systems in the brain have not yet matured sufficiently to cope with the stress of a high temperature, and usually last up to 5 minutes. Immediate treatment is to place the child in the recovery position.

Symptoms

- Loss of consciousness
- Stiffness
- Cessation of breathing for up to 30 seconds
- Loss of control of the bladder or bowel
- Spasms of both limbs or the face muscles
- Eyes roll upwards

A52: Fibreoptic Intubation Equipment

Scope Equipment

- Camera stack
- Light source
- Flexible intubating bronchoscope
- Scope cleaner
- Bronchoscope cleaning sponge
- Anti-fogging agent

Airway Equipment

- Mepore tape
- Laryngoscopes
- McGill forceps
- LMAs on standby
- Endotracheal or nasal tube
- Suction tubing: cut to fit scope
- Nasal breathing sponge
- Oxygen eg, Euro mask

Miscellaneous

- Head wrap & sponges
- Eye tapes & pads
- Swabs
- Lubricating gel (Instillagel)
- Cuff inflation syringe
- 5 ml syringe, green needle

A53: Glasgow Coma Scale

Response	Score
Eye opening (E)	
Spontaneous	E4
To verbal command	E3
To pain	E2
No response	E1
Best motor response (M)	
Obeys commands	M6
Localises pain	M5
Withdraws to pain	M4
Abnormal flexion to pain	M3
Extension to pain	M2
No response	M1

Best verbal response (V)	
Oriented and converses	V5
Disoriented and converses	V4
Inappropriate words	V3
Incomprehensible sounds	V2
No response	V1

The total score describes the neurological (disability) state:

Mild	13-15
Moderate	9-12
Severe	3-8 (Coma)

A54: Haemorrhage (Adult)

Haemorrhage Classifications

Class I: Less than 15% blood loss may go undetected, and may not require management.

Class II: 15-30% loss can produce tachycardia, anxiety, and lower pulse pressure. Fluid/blood administration may be required.

Class III: 30-40% loss is an emergency, requiring oxygen treatment, and immediate fluid and blood administration. Symptoms include tachycardia, hypotension, reduced peripheral perfusion (cool extremities), and reduced urine output.

Class IV: Above 40% blood loss is life threatening, and has similar signs to class III, but with greater tachycardia, and minimal urine output. Treatment is similar to that of Class III.

Major Haemorrhage

At least 20% loss of blood volume inside one hour, or at least 50% loss in three hours (infants,: 90 ml/kg body weight, and other children: 80 ml/kg). Also, bleeding that leads to systolic BP < 90 mHg, or heart rate > 100 beats/minute.

Major Haemorrhage – Immediate Actions

{Partial example algorithm is courtesy of St Thomas's Hospital}

√ Control bleeding through compression, elevation, or by surgical means, such as packing.

√ Give 15 L/min oxygen using non-rebreather mask.

√ Obtain a blood Cross Match (**pink** bottle cap), Full Blood Count (**purple** cap), and Clotting factors (**blue** cap) assays.

√ Obtain large bore (14g, 16g) venous access.

√ Set up fluid warmer for intravenous products.

√ Apply body warming blanket to maintain temp > 36°.

√ Until blood products are ready, give 500 ml crystalloids, as necessary to maintain palpable pulse.

√ Catheterise.

√ Give 1-2 g tranexamic acid over 10 minutes.

√ Monitor Calcium and Hb.

√ Repeat fibrinogen, FBC, and clotting factors each hour.

Blood Product Administration

- Until blood group is known, give 1-2 units of O neg blood.
- As soon as there are 2 Group/Save samples recorded, order 6 units of group specific blood (no cross matching), plus 3 units FFP.
- Administer 1-2 units group specific blood.
- Administer FFP, when thawed/ready.
- If more blood administered, give blood:FFP in 2:1 ratio.
- Consider other blood products with Haematology Consultant.

Blood Product Summary

Red Blood Cells	Issue 6 group specific units	Immediately blood group known
Fresh Frozen Plasma	Thaw and issue 3 units when blood group known. Then thaw 1 unit FFP for every 2 units RBCs.	45 minutes to thaw
Cryoprecipitate	Thaw and issue 2-4 pools cryo as required, for every 15 units RBCs.	45 minutes to thaw
Platelets	Issue 2 pools as required for every 15 units RBCs.	1-2 hours for delivery
Other	Beriplex 25 iu/kg for emergency reversal of Warfarin. Novoseven 3 * 2 mg	Immediately available once Consultant Haematologist authorised

Target Parameters

- Haemoglobin (Hb) > 90 g/litre
- Platelets > 75 * 10^9/litre
- INR < 1.5
- APTT (Activated Partial Thromboplastin clot Time) < 45

- Fibrinogen > 150 mg/deciLitre
- Ratio RBCs:FFP < 2:1
- Peripheral pulse palpable
- Heart rate < 100 bpm
- Urine output > 30 ml/hour
- Temperature > 36° C
- pH > 7.3 (arterial blood gas)

Controlling Bleeding

If possible, **direct pressure** should be used. If ineffective or impractical, apply a haemostatic agent (Tranexamic Acid [1 g over 10 min], Floseal, NovoSeven etc) to e.g., junctional (armpit, neck, groin, abdomen) wounds; ensure the agent is delivered in a gauze that supports tight wound packing. Apply as much pressure as possible to the bleeding vessel, for at least three minutes. In massive haemorrhage, the therapeutic aim is to maintain tissue oxygenation, and to restore circulating volume and haemoglobin levels.

A55: The Heart

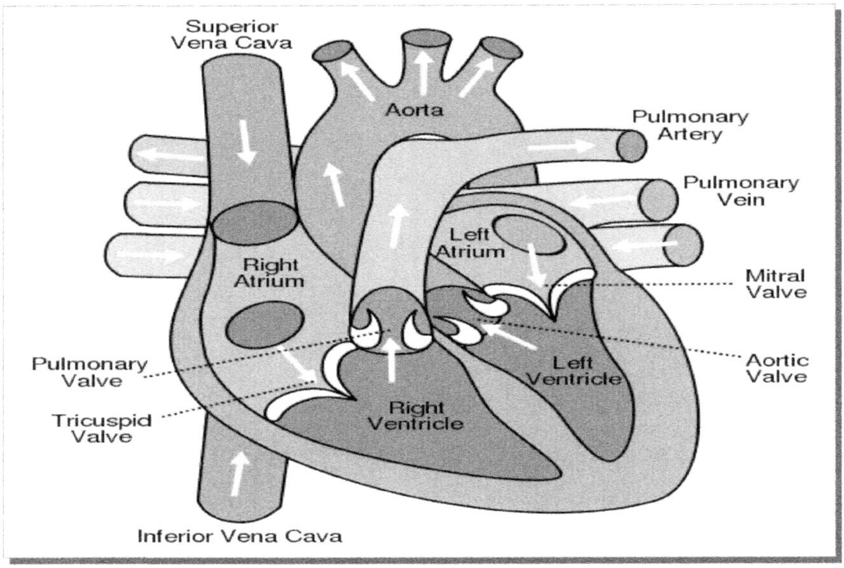

Heart Chambers

Each side of the heart comprises an upper (atria) and lower chamber (ventricle). Left and right chambers are separated by a wall of muscle, called a septum.

The right atrium receives de-oxygenated blood from the vena cava, and ejects it into the right ventricle, which sends it to the lungs, via the pulmonary arteries, for re-oxygenation and removal of waste products (CO_2,...). The left atrium receives oxygenated blood from the lungs (pulmonary veins), to eject into the left ventricle, for delivery to the aorta (systemic circulation).

Heart Linings

Endocardium: Protective membrane lining the inside of the atria and ventricles, and the outer surface of valves.

Pericardium: Double inner serous membrane and outer fibrous tissue, which encloses the heart.

Epicardium: Protective layer of serous membrane, connecting the inner pericardium to the outer myocardium (heart muscle).

Heart Valves

Valve	***Function***
Tricuspid	Regulates blood flow between R atrium/ventricle.
Pulmonary	Controls blood flow from R ventricle into the pulmonary arteries.
Bicuspid (Mitral)	Lets oxygenated blood from the lungs pass from the L atrium into the L ventricle.
Aortic	Oxygenated blood passes from the L ventricle into the aorta, then is distributed to the whole body.

Jugular Venous Distention

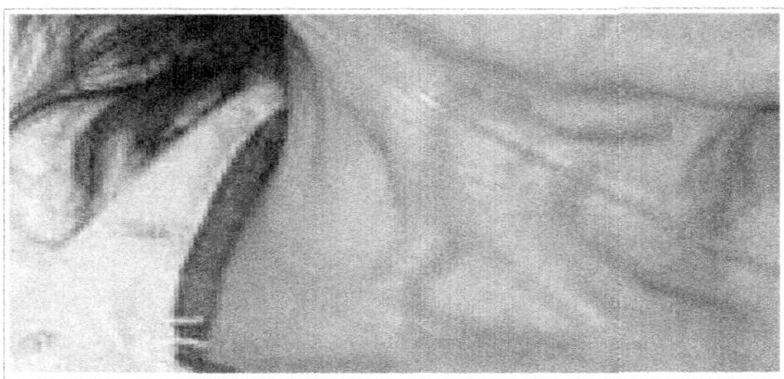

A56: High Spinal Block

Symptoms

Tingling in hands, breathing difficulty, bradycardia, hypotension.

Management

Stop the Epidural (if present), tilt the mother to the left, give high flow oxygen, intubate – if necessary.

Circulation

Treat hypotension with fluids and 3 mg bolus of Ephedrine. Bradycardia may be treated with 0.6 mg i.v. Atropine.

Risk factors increased by...

- High dose of anaesthetic
- High BMI
- High lumbar insertion
- Needle gauge too fine

A57: Human Factors

The scientific discipline concerned with the understanding of interactions between humans and other elements of a system, and the profession which applies theory, principles, data and methods, to produce system designs in order to optimise human well-being and overall system performance. *The Institute of Ergonomics and Human Factors, 2017.*

Human Factors refers to: "Environmental, organisational and job factors, and human and individual characteristics, which influence behaviour, at work, in a way which can affect health and safety".

In 1991, Continental Airlines began the first human factors training programme, labelled *Crew Coordination Concept* workshops, as a consequence of the realisation that blaming individuals, such as Pilots and Maintenance crew, for error, failed to recognise the workplace and situational factors which contribute to failure events.

Following the Continental Airlines experience, the central theme of understanding Human Factors, and associated implications for safety, has come to be based on the model, known as *The Dirty Dozen*, which was developed for Transport Canada (1993), by Gordon Dupont, and universally adopted.

Dirty Dozen Human Factors

Lack of knowledge: Shortage of training and information.

Norms: Expected rules of behaviour become “normal”. Existing norms do not make procedures right.

Distractions: The primary cause of forgetfulness.

Lack of Communication: Only 30% or verbal communication is received and understood. Use written checklists.

Lack of resources: People and equipment.

Lack of awareness: Failure to recognise a situation.

Pressure: Ask for extra help. Communicate concerns.

Fatigue: Physical and mental.

Lack of Assertiveness: Failure to raise concerns.

Complacency: Overconfidence from repeatedly performing a task.

Lack of teamwork: Discuss how a task should be executed.

Stress: Any factor which causes tension.

A58: Hyperventilation

Caused by

- Anxiety/pain
- Stimulants
- Excessive intake of aspirin (a salicylate)
- Asthma
- Chronic obstructive pulmonary disease
- Pulmonary embolism
- Infection such as pneumonia or sepsis
- Congestive heart failure
- Heart attack
- Diabetic ketoacidosis

Biochemistry

Hyperventilation has little effect on arterial oxygen partial pressure (pO_2), and almost no effect on oxygen saturation. Its main effect is to lower partial pressure of carbon dioxide (pCO_2), producing respiratory alkalosis. Secondary hypocalcaemia also occurs.

Symptoms

- Wheezing and shortness of breath during attack

- Pain/discomfort in the chest
- Feeling of choking or suffocation
- Palpitations
- Tingling in the fingers, toes, and around mouth
- Muscle spasms in the hands and feet
- Dizziness
- Weakness
- Tinnitus
- Sweating
- Loss of consciousness
- Trousseau's sign
- Chvostek's sign

Note: The process of breathing in and out of a paper bag, in order to increase the level of carbon dioxide in the blood, is no longer recommended, because the carbon dioxide level can rise too high.

A59: Hypothermia

Symptoms include...

- ◆ Acidosis
- ◆ Bradycardia
- ◆ Coma
- ◆ Confusion
- ◆ Hypotension
- ◆ Vasoconstriction
- ◆ Muscle rigidity
- ◆ Shivering
- ◆ Decreased E_TCO_2

Swiss Staging System

I	35-32° C	Conscious and shivering
II	32-28° C	Impaired consciousness, not shivering
III	28-24° C	Unconscious, not shivering, has vital signs
IV	< 24° C	Not breathing, no vital signs
V		Irreversible hypothermia, death

Hypothermia can lead to...

- Cardiac arrest
- Delayed wound healing
- Prolonged recovery
- Surgical site infection
- Venous Thrombo-embolism

A60: Hypoventilation

Hypoventilation causes an increased concentration of CO_2 (carbon dioxide) in the blood and cerebrospinal fluid. The increase in H^+ ion concentration means a lower pH (more acidic), which is detected by the central chemoreceptors, and passed on to the medulla, which then triggers an increase in the respiratory drive (minute volume), until a normal CO_2 level is restored.

Caused by

- Hypopnoea: the breathing is too shallow
- Bradypnoea: the breathing is too slow
- Diminished lung function

Carbon dioxide

Whilst either slow or shallow breathing may occur with hypoventilation, the rate or depth of breathing is not diagnostic, since hypoventilation, by definition, occurs if there is an increase in blood carbon dioxide levels. If the body retains too much CO_2, due to impaired respiratory function, the body's pH drops and become more acidic, creating respiratory acidosis.

Alveolar hypoventilation is when the arterial carbon dioxide partial pressure ($paCO_2$) exceeds the more normal 45 mmHg.

Symptoms

- Cyanosis secondary to hypoxaemia
- Impairment of sleep due to nocturnal hypercapnia
- Morning fatigue and lethargy
- Mental confusion and headaches
- Chronic hypercapnia

Triggers

- Excessive opiate analgesics
- Insufficient analgesia
- Inadequate reversal of muscle relaxants

If left untreated, cyanosis, polycythemia, pulmonary hypertension, and congestive heart failure may occur.

A61: Hypoxia

Four Types of Hypoxia

Anaemic: Deficient number of red blood cells or Hb molecules to carry available O_2 (eg, carboxyhaemoglobin).

Circulatory: Aka *Stagnant/Ischaemic*; The circulation is unable to deliver enough perfusion to oxygenate the tissues.

Histotoxic: Inability of mitochondria to produce ATP, due to toxins, especially cyanide poisoning.

Hypoxic: Insufficient O_2 supplied from the lungs to the blood.

Hypoxia Causes

- Airway obstruction
- O_2 supply problem
- Deflated ETT cuff
- Hypovolaemia
- Volatiles
- Bronchospasm
- Atelectasis (causes shunt)
- Displaced/blocked ETT/LMA
- Circuit blockage
- Drugs
- High spinal
- Pneumothorax

When O_2 saturation falls, quickly isolate the cause, which might be ① Sats probe position ② Poor peripheral perfusion (try an ear Sats probe) ③ Sats probe failure (test your own finger)

Symptoms

- Cyanosis
- Tachycardia
- Hypertension
- Agitation
- Restlessness
- Tachypnoea
- Nostril flaring
- Discoloured skin
- Noisy breathing
- Falling partial pressure of arterial oxygen (paO_2)
- Need accessory muscles to breathe

Effects

Reduction in oxygen partial pressure causes increased CO_2 partial pressure, with resultant increased respiratory effort.

If hypoxia untreated, results in ...

- Bradycardia
- Cardiac arrest
- Convulsions
- Hypotension
- Unconsciousness

.

Treatment

- Sit the patient up
- Administer oxygen
- Intubate
- Treat the cause
- BVM (no catheter mount, angle piece, filter) with jaw thrust

> Note: Systemic arteries dilate in response to hypoxia, but pulmonary arteries constrict.

Caution: When O_2 saturation falls, quickly isolate the cause, which might be ① Sats probe position ② Poor peripheral perfusion (try an ear probe) ③ Probe failure (test your own finger) ④ Failed oxygen supply ⑤ Circuit/ETT blockage ⑥ ETT displaced ⑦ ETT cuff deflated.

A62: Infection Risk

Risk Factors

- ASA rating > 2
- Blood transfusion
- Corticosteroid use
- Diabetes Mellitus
- Electrocautery
- Obesity
- Hypothermia
- Malnutrition
- Adrenaline injection
- Hair removal with razor
- Previous irradiation of site
- Extremes of age or systemic factors
- Multiple preoperative comorbidity diagnoses
- Foreign body, recent surgery, wound drains

Reducing Infection Risk

1. Patients should bathe on the day of their surgery.
2. Hair should be cut with clippers – not razors.
3. Skin should be disinfected immediately prior to incision.
4. Give prophylactic antibiotics 1 hour before surgery.
5. Patient should not be cooler than 34° C, before anaesthesia.
6. Surgery should comply with aseptic protocols.
7. Minimum number of people should be present during surgery.
8. Wounds should be dressed with interactive dressings.

A63: Inotropes

Definition

Inotropic: affecting the force of muscular contractions, especially of the heart. β-blocking drugs have negative inotropic effects, whereas positive inotropic drugs increase the strength of cardiac contractions, thereby increasing cardiac output. The short half life of inotropes means that they must be given by continuous infusion.

Positive Inotropic Drugs

Positive inotropes strengthen the heart's contractions, so it can pump more blood with fewer heartbeats. These agents are usually given to patients with cardiomyopathy, or congestive heart failure. Additionally, they may be given to patients who have experienced recent myocardial infarction. In some cases, inotropes are given to patients with cardiogenic shock, such as after cardiac surgery, where their hearts have been weakened.

Digoxin, for example, strengthens the force of the heartbeat by increasing the amount of calcium in the heart's cells, thus stimulating the heart to contract. When the Digoxin reaches the heart muscle, it binds to sodium and potassium receptors, which control the amount of calcium in the heart muscle, by stopping the calcium from leaving the cells. As calcium builds up in the cells, it causes a stronger force of contraction.

Example Positive Inotropes

Adrenaline	Amiodarone	Calcium
Digoxin	Dopamine	Dobutamine
Insulin	Isoprenaline	Milrinone
Noradrenaline	Vasopressin	

Negative Inotropic Drugs

Weaken heart contractions, slow heart rate, and treat hypertension, chronic congestive heart failure, arrhythmias, and angina; sometimes used to reduce stress on the heart, and prevent future heart attacks. Negative inotrope types include beta-blockers, calcium channel blockers, and anti-arrhythmic agents.

Beta-blockers

Block the effects of adrenaline on beta receptors, thus slowing the nerve impulses which travel through the heart. As a result, the heart does not have to work as hard, because it needs less blood and oxygen. Beta-blockers also block the impulses which can cause an arrhythmia. Examples: *Atenolol, Metoprolol, Esmolol.*

Calcium Channel Blockers

Slow the rate at which calcium passes into the heart muscle, and into the vessel walls, which relaxes the vessels. These relaxed vessels let blood flow more easily through them, thereby lowering blood pressure. Examples: *Diltiazem, Nifedipine, Verapamil.*

A64: Jet Ventilator Setup

Jet Ventilator

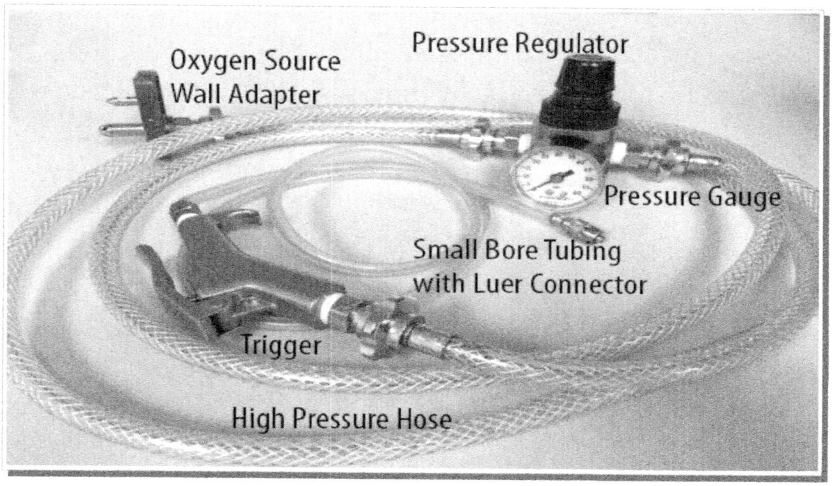

Equipment

- Luer lock connector tube & wide bore extension
- Sampling line filter
- 2 syringe drivers (or tiva)
- Octopus connector or 2 curly wurlies
- Propofol, 50 ml jars and spikes
- Remifentanil (2 * 1 mg)
- Saline bag - spiked
- LMA (or micro laryngeal ET tube)

A65: Laryngospasm

Caused (during light anaesthesia) by:

- Irritation to vocal cords by trauma or obstruction (blood etc)
- Sensitivity to a drug
- Stimulation from the laryngoscope
- Reaction to endotracheal tube insertion/removal
- Aspiration

Symptoms

Partial laryngospasm

- Chest movement with stridor, but little movement of air.
- In spontaneous ventilation, little bag movement.

Complete laryngospasm

- Chest movement without airway noise.
- No bag movement
- Not possible to provide ventilation.

Typical symptoms of airway obstruction:

- See-saw chest/abdomen movement on inspiration
- Tracheal tug
- Stridor (if only partial obstruction)

- Rib retraction

Effects:
Resultant hypoxia and hypercapnia (high CO_2) produces an increased respiratory effort, with noisier breathing.

Violent coughing or breath holding indicates airway obstruction, so requires suction. At induction: laryngospasm breaks up with deeper anaesthesia. Forceful coughs may dislodge foreign material.

Terminating the laryngospasm

Take patient out of Stage II of anaesthesia:

- Deepen anaesthetic with gas or I.V. agent (e.g. Propofol).
- Allow patient to wake up.

Breaking the laryngospasm

- Stop the stimulation e.g., laryngoscope.
- Suction the airway.
- 100% oxygen via Mapleson C circuit - valve partially closed.
- Apply positive pressure ventilation.
- Ensure good mask seal and jaw thrust.
- Call for help.
- If laryngospasm persists, sedate with Propofol.
- Give Suxamethonium (succinylcholine), and intubate.
- Alternatively, apply pressure to the laryngospasm notch.

Avoiding laryngospasm

☞ Do not stimulate the vocal cords in a semi-conscious patient.

☞ Do not extubate in Stage II of anaesthesia.

☞ Extubate awake, or in a deep plane of anaesthesia.

☞ Clear the pharynx of secretions (suction).

Laryngeal Structures

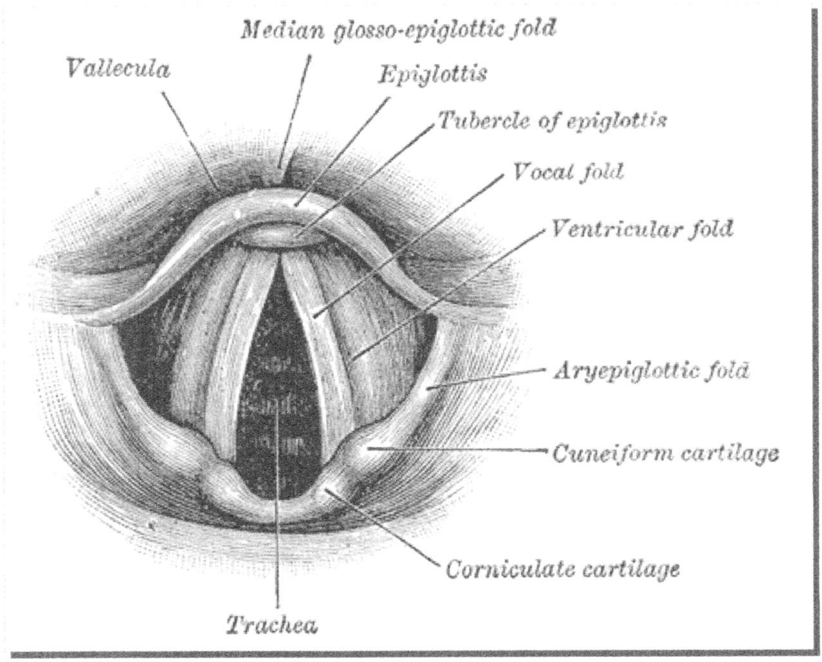

A66: Local Anaesthetic Toxicity

Symptoms

- Dizziness
- Numb mouth
- Numb tongue
- Blurred vision
- Metallic taste
- Hypertension
- Unconsciousness
- Muscular spasms
- Sinus bradycardia
- Cardiovascular collapse

Management

- Stop injecting the local anaesthetic.
- Call for help.
- Maintain the airway, and give 100% oxygen.
- Intubate, if necessary.
- Ensure intravenous access.
- Control seizures (benzodiazepines, thiopentone, or propofol).
- Manage respiratory arrest.
- Follow local guidelines
- Ensure lipid emulsion is available.

A67: Malignant Hyperthermia

Initial signs are tachycardia, increased CO_2, and mixed metabolic/respiratory acidosis; spontaneously breathing patients will deal with the CO_2 by breathing more rapidly; IPPV patients will have higher end tidal CO_2. Arterial Blood Gas shows hypercapnia, respiratory and metabolic acidosis.

Symptoms

- Tachycardia
- Increased end-tidal CO_2
- Tachypnoea - if breathing spontaneously
- Hypotension and arrhythmia
- Increased oxygen consumption
- Metabolic and respiratory acidosis
- Temperature rise several degrees per hour
- Flushed skin and sweating
- Hyperkalaemia and cyanosis
- Dark urine
- Increased muscle rigidity (late sign)

- Inability to relax after Suxamethonium (succinylcholine)
- Rise in serum Potassium

Treatment

- Turn off volatile agents.
- Hyperventilate the patient with high flows of oxygen.
- Use a new anaesthetic machine - flushed for 30 minutes.
- Use a new non-rebreathing circuit.
- Give cool infusion of saline - not Hartmann's.
- Draw up Dantrolene, using filter needles.
- Give Dantrolene: 2-3 mg/kg, then 1 mg/kg.
- Topically cool patient with ice, fluids, cooling blanket.

To collect

- M.H. box, Dantrolene
- Sterile water (without bacteriostatic agent)
- Syringes (50 ml), syringe drivers and connecting lines
- Arterial and Central line kits
- Blood gas and sample bottles

A68: Minimum Alveolar Concentration

For a specific anaesthetic vapour, and a specific class (age etc) of patient, MAC indicates the concentration of the agent, in the alveoli, which would prevent response to a standard surgical stimulus, in 50% of that class of patient. A MAC value is valid when the vapour is given in oxygen, equilibrium (alveolar-brain) has been reached, and no other agents are administered.

The definition of MAC, as a percentage of one atmosphere, is an indirect way of specifying the partial pressure of the agent in the alveoli; for example, if an agent has a MAC of 1, then MAC will be reached, at equilibrium, when the alveoli partial pressure is 1 kPa. Similarly, if the agent has a MAC of 2.5, then the MAC level is reached when the partial pressure is 2.5 kPa. The ambient pressure is not a factor in the MAC concentration, because the above partial pressure is an absolute value.

Statistics

The plot of the distribution of the patients, not responding to the above stimulus, creates a partial pressure to response curve. MAC is the point on this curve, corresponding to the 50% (median) point of the distribution (bell) curve. The sd (standard deviation) of an agent's MAC equates to approximately 10% of that MAC; for example, 1.2 MAC (MAC + 2 sd) should not produce a response to stimulation in ~ 97.7% of patients. Similarly, 1.3 MAC (MAC + 3 sd) should not elicit a response in ~ 99.86% of patients.

Example:

For a 40 year old patient, the MAC value for Sevoflurane is 2.1, which means that the 50% level is reached when the partial pressure of Sevoflurane, in the alveolus, is 2.1% of 1 atm (16 mmHg).

Factors which increase MAC:

- Hypercapnia
- Cocaine
- Decreasing age
- Hyperthermia
- Hypernatraemia
- Thyrotoxicosis
- Sympathoadrenal stimulation
- Increases in ambient pressure

Factors which decrease MAC:

- Nitrous oxide
- Hypocapnia
- Hypothermia
- Hyponatraemia
- Increasing age
- Hypothyroidism
- Hypoxia
- Hypotension
- Anaemia
- Pregnancy
- Sedatives
- Opioids
- Tranquillizers
- Lidocaine
- Magnesium
- Clonidine
- Benzodiazepines
- Acute alcohol abuse

Note: Sex, height, weight & anaesthetic duration do not alter MAC.

A69: Mixed Acid-Base Conditions

Respiratory ($paCO_2$) and metabolic (bicarbonate) changes

	Metabolic Acidosis	Metabolic Alkalosis
Respiratory Acidosis	**CO_2 high, bicarbonate (HCO_3^-) low**. Typical causes: cardiac arrest, multi-organ failure.	**CO_2 high, bicarbonate high**. Seen in COPD patient taking diuretics.
Respiratory Alkalosis	**CO_2 low, bicarbonate low**. Typical patient has renal failure and hyperventilates.	**CO_2 low, bicarbonate high**. Caused by diuretics, liver cirrhosis, high minute volume in COPD.

A70: Nasal Cannula Flow Rates

Flow (L/min)	*O2 delivered (%)*
1	24
2	28
3	32
4	36
5	40
6	44

Oxygen fraction calculation: 20% + (4 * litres of flow).

A71: Nitrous Oxide

Description

During induction, the volume of N_2O, entering the pulmonary capillaries, is greater than the nitrogen moving from the blood, to the alveolus. As a result, the effective volume of the alveoli decreases, thereby increasing the fractional concentration of the remaining gases. This process augments ventilation, as bronchial and tracheal gas is drawn into the alveolus, to make good the diminished alveolar volume. Conversely, at the end of the anaesthetic, N_2O rapidly diffuses from the blood, to the alveoli, reducing the concentration of available oxygen in the alveoli (diffusion hypoxia). Additional oxygen must then be administered to a patient recovering from N_2O anaesthesia, to counteract the potential hypoxia. For prolonged intubations, N_2O has a tendency to diffuse into the endotracheal tube cuff, and the subsequent increase in pressure might cut off the blood supply to surrounding tissues, so the cuff pressure should be regularly checked. Note: N_2O has been the cause of pneumothorax.

Note: N_2O ia stored in liquid form, with a small amount of gas at the top of the cylinder. As the gas is delivered, it is replaced by some of the liquid N_2O, which changes to gaseous form. As a result, the pressure gauge only starts to drop after the liquid portion is depleted, which is when the cylinder is nearly empty.

A72: Non Steroidal Anti Inflammatory Drugs

Action...

NSAIDs suppress the action of COX (cyclo-oxygenase) 1 and 2 inhibitors, which would otherwise produce the prostaglandins which cause pain and inflammation.

Side-effects...

◇ Gastric ulceration
◇ Interactions with other drugs
◇ Asthma (triggers)
◇ Bleeding (affects platelets)
◇ Renal impairment

High risk groups...

◇ Heart problems
◇ Aged 75+
◇ Diabetics (mellitus)
◇ Hypertension
◇ Smokers

Not recommended for...

◇ Kidney disease
◇ Pregnancy
◇ Stomach ulcers
◇ Breastfeeding
◇ Liver disease

Example NSAIDs: Diclofenac, Ibuprofen, Celecoxib, Aspirin.

A73: Obstetric Haemorrhage Classes

Class	*Description*	*Causes*
Antepartum (APH)	Bleeding after 24 weeks gestation and before delivery.	Placental abruption, Placenta praevia, Trauma, Uterine rupture
Primary post-partum (PPH)	Blood loss within 24 hours of delivery: > 500 ml, following a vaginal delivery, and > 1000 ml following a Caesarean section.	Uterine atony, Retained products of conception, Genital tract trauma, Clotting defects, Inverted uterus
Secondary post-partum	Blood loss more than 24 hours after delivery.	Retained products of conception, Puerperal sepsis

A74: Optiflow System

♦ Increases alveolar ventilation and reduces rebreathing by flushing expired gases from the upper airway.

♦ Additional benefits of Optiflow include less thicker secretions, lower irritation to the airways, and reduced nasal bleeding.

♦ Airway pressure dynamically changes depending on the patient's breathing pattern and the flow of gas delivered to the patient.

♦ Optiflow Nasal High Flow reduces inspiratory resistance making inspiration easier, and increases expiratory resistance prolonging expiration. This promotes slow, deep breathing which increases alveolar ventilation.

Setting up

Use aseptic (non touch) technique.

- Connect the AC electrical supply.
- Connect air and oxygen supplies.
- Connect tubing from flow meter to top of pressure manifold.
- Insert humidifier; connect inspiratory tubing to humidifier.
- Store unheated blue extension in ring shape to reduce risk of contamination.
- Fit nasal cannula and connector to blue tubing.
- Attach bag of sterile water for inhalation.

- Set the gas flow rate.
- Ensure the humidifier is set to invasive mode.

The pressure manifold for Optiflow is blue and has a maximum pressure limit of 45 cm/H2O. Ensure that you do not use the pressure manifold for the bubble CPAP system, which is white and has a maximum pressure limit of 17cm/H2O.

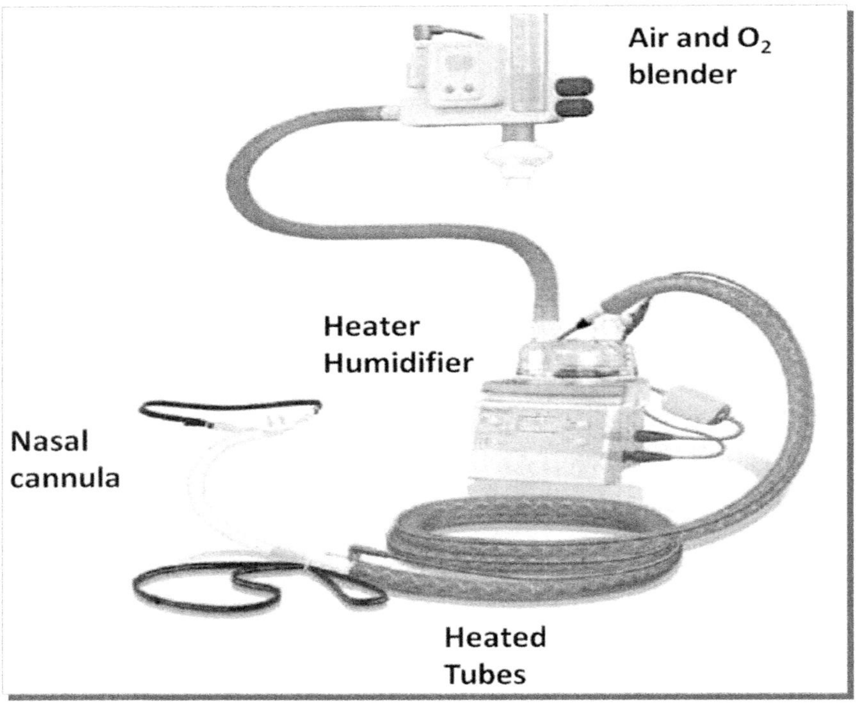

A75: Paediatric Setup

Anaesthetic Room

- Paediatric intubation trolley
- Paediatric circuit & paediatric Ambu bag (BVM)
- Paediatric/adult Yankeurs
- Ayre's T-piece (on ACGO) - small filter, no catheter mount
- 1 litre (or 0.5?) reservoir bag
- Sevoflurane
- Small ECG dots, BP cuffs, Elastoplast sats probe
- 0.5 litre Hartmann's on a burette
- Bare Hugger (under body?)
- Padded cot sides; stool

Intubation Trolley

- LMAs and selection of cuffed and un-cuffed ET tubes
- Selection of laryngoscope blades & bougies & stylets
- Pink tape (trouser legs)
- Size 6,8,10 (lime, blue, black) suction catheters

Kidney Dish

- Swabs & stirette wipes
- 24g (yellow) and 22g (blue) Venflon Catheters
- Tegaderm dressing & dental rolls
- NS primed 5/10 ml syringe and 4 inch 3-way tap extension
- 1 ml syringes: Atropine, Suxamethonium

Theatre (OR)

- Paediatric Ambu bag (BVM)
- Sevoflurane
- Paediatric/adult Yankeurs & small suction catheters
- Ayre's T-piece (on ACGO) & Paediatric circuit
- 1 litre (or 0.5) reservoir bag
- K-Band bandage to hold I.V. cannula in place

Note: If Fentanyl is to be given, make up a 10 microgram/ml solution by combining 1 ml (50 microgram) Fentanyl with 4 ml normal saline, then draw into a 1 ml syringe.

A76: Patient Positions

Supine

When supine, lung and functional residual capacity are reduced, especially in obese patients. A change from erect to supine position increases venous return and stroke volume.

Trendelenburg

Flat and head-down, with the feet angled up by 15-30 degrees.

Lateral

Ensure padding between the knees, and below the lateral aspect of the dependent leg - to prevent damage to the perineal nerve.

Injuries to avoid...

Ulnar Nerve

The most common injury in anaesthetised patients, often due to being compressed between the posterior aspect of the Medial Epicondyle of the elbow, and the bed or arm board.

Brachial Plexus Nerve

Occurs when the plexus is stretched or compressed.

Common Peroneal Nerve

The lateral aspect of the knee is compressed against a stirrup.

Saphenous Nerve

When the Medial Tibial Condyle is compressed by leg supports.

A77: Patient Transfer to Operating Table

Main Goals

- Manage the airway.
- Monitor oxygen saturation.
- Prevent nerve and pressure point damage.

Transferring

- Ensure the airway is disconnected (temporarily).
- Apply the brakes on the trolley and operating table.
- Catheter - hold clear.
- Drains - hold clear.
- Monitoring lines - hold clear.
- Intravenous lines - hold clear.
- Ensure tourniquet won't snag.
- Transfer patient to operating table.
- Ensure suction will reach the patient's airway.

Immediate life support

- Attach the pulse oximetry probe
- Place arm supports

- ☞ Position patient for surgery
- ☞ Protect pressure points
- ☞ Fit tourniquet - if applicable

Physiology

- ☞ Connect the IV line - ensure correct flow rate
- ☞ Attach mono-polar diathermy plate (unless bipolar)
- ☞ Place ankle supports
- ☞ Fit flowtrons
- ☞ Fit Bare Hugger

Field setup

- ☞ Switch on and position table lights
- ☞ After draping and skin prep, switch on Bare Hugger
- ☞ Attach and position suction carousel

A78: Peripheral Nerve Block

Benefits

√ Reduced need for opiates

√ May avoid need for general anaesthesia

√ Better targeted analgesia

√ Shorter recovery and discharge times

√ Less traumatic (no G.A,), especially for elderly

√ Reaction to local anaesthetics more obvious

Suitability

√ Cooperative patients

√ Susceptibility to malignant hyperthermia

√ Susceptibility to airway compromise

Risks

- Nerve damage
- Infection
- Injection into an artery
- Cardiac arrest

Contra-indications

- Existing nerve damage
- History of allergic or local anaesthetic reaction
- Infection at the injection site

A79: pH Calculation

A pH value, between 1 and 14, describes the molarity (M) of [H+] (hydrogen ion concentration) per litre of an aqueous solution, where a value of 7 is neutral - neither acidic or alkaline. The pH is found by the negative logarithm (base 10) of [H+].

The formal definition is given by: **pH = - log10 [H+]**

Example 1

Find the pH of a solution with a [H+] of 0.01 M (0.01 mol per litre).

Solution: The logarithm of 0.01 is -2. The negative of -2 is 2.

Answer: pH is 2.

Example 2

Find the pH of a solution with a [H+] of 0.000,0001

Solution: The log of 0.000,0001 is -7. The negative of -7 is 7.

Answer: pH is 7.

A80: PICC & Hickman Central Lines

Hickman Line Placement

With the patient 30° head down, incisions are made at vein (jugular) entrance and tunnel exit (right chest wall) sites. A needle punctures the vein, and a guide-wire passed through the needle, and the needle is withdrawn. Artery forceps then feed the hickman line between tunnel entry and exit sites, and the distal end of the line is cut to fit the vein length. A sheath is then railroaded over

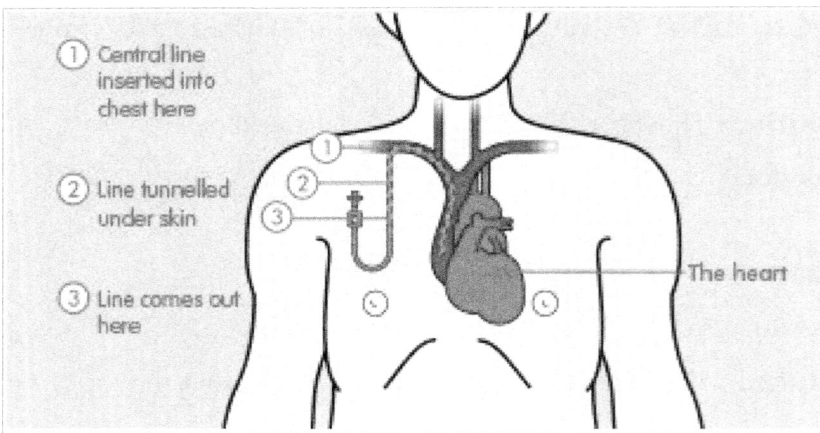

the guide-wire, into the vein, then the guide-wire is withdrawn. The Hickman line is then threaded through the sheath, until it rests at the heart "entrance". Once placement is confirmed, and the lumens flushed for clots, the line is clamped, and lumens sealed with bungs. The wounds are then stitched and dressed, and the outer line is taped to the chest. Lumens have to be regularly flushed, with saline, to prevent blockages. A small Dacron cuff prevents the line from coming out. There is a remote risk of pneumothorax, so x-ray is needed to confirm proper placement.

Peripherally Inserted Central Catheter (PICC)

Inserted into a vein of the upper arm (basilic, brachial, cephalic, medial cubital), and advanced until the catheter tip rests in the distal superior vena cava or cavoatrial junction, leaving the lumens sticking out from the skin.

Risks

Venous thromboembolism (needs frequent flush, and lines capped), infection, peripheral vein damage or phlebitis. PICC lines block more easily than Hickman lines.

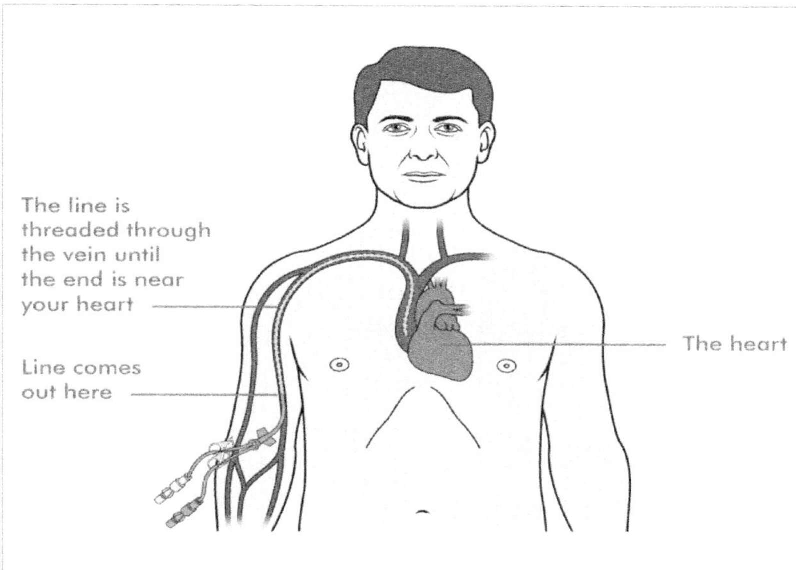

A81: Pneumothorax

A pneumothorax can be open or closed. "Open" is when the chest wall is open to the environment. If pleural cavity pressure is lower than ambient pressure, air is drawn into the cavity, from the environment, and is known as a "sucking wound". A "closed" pneumothorax is when the chest wall is intact. Often, the pneumothorax will cause deviation of the trachea towards the opposite side, where the pressure os lower.

Four main types of pneumothorax:

1 Primary spontaneous pneumothorax:

Unexpected pneumothorax in mostly healthy young adults, particularly males and smokers, caused by a tear in the lung, allowing air to escape into the pleural space, and which usually repairs itself - in 2-3 days.

2 Secondary spontaneous pneumothorax:

A side effect of an underlying lung pathology, such as COPD.

3 Tension pneumothorax:

Occurs when air leaks into the pleural cavity, but is unable to return. The resultant increasing pressure, outside of the lung, can lead to collapse of that lung. Gives a monitor rhythm, but no pulse.

4 Crushing pneumothorax:

Crushing or penetrating chest trauma.

Symptoms

Sudden sharp chest pain	Tachycardia	Chest tightness
Asymmetrical chest rise	Tachypnoea	Fatigue
Shortness of breath	Coughing	

Aspiration

The common method of removing the air is by aspiration through a tube, which has a three-way tap and syringe attached.

Aspiration management

- Local anaesthetic is injected into the drain site.
- Insert the tube through the chest wall.
- Aspirate some air through the syringe.
- Turn off the three-way tap.
- Expel the air in the syringe to the atmosphere.
- Keep aspirating until most of the air is removed.

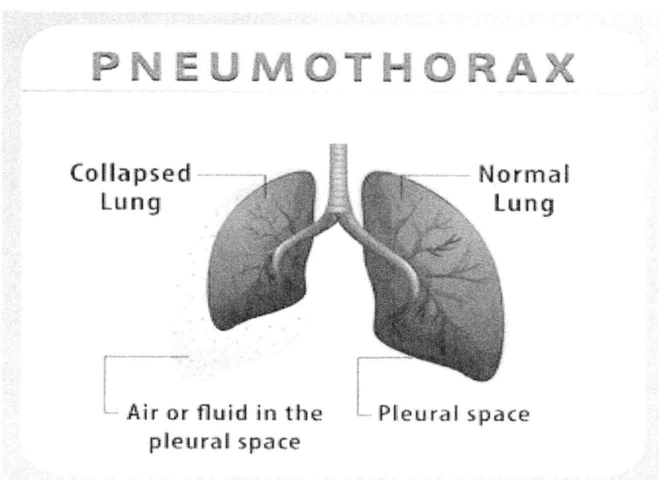

A82: Post Operative Nausea and Vomiting

Factors which increase the likelihood of PONV

- Female
- History or PONV
- Non-smoker
- postoperative opioids

Apfel's rating system for risk of PONV

Number of factors	0	1	2	3	4
Risk rating	10%	20%	40%	60%	80%

Actions to reduce the risk of PONV

- ☞ Use TIVA - avoid general anaesthetics and nitrous oxide
- ☞ Use non-opioid analgesia
- ☞ Give IV fluids and use high flow oxygen

A83: Potassium

Hyperkalaemia

Causes include:

Metabolic acidosis ♣ Endocrine problem ♣ NSAIDs ♣ Renal failure ♣ ACE inhibitors ♣ Beta blockers ♣ Addison's disease

An acidosis causes potassium to move from cells into the plasma, and H+ ions in the other direction.

ECG characteristics of hyperkalemia:

- Tall tented T waves
- QRS widening
- Fusion of QRS-T
- Loss of the ST segment
- P-waves widened and low amplitude, due to slow conduction

Signs include:

- Weakness
- Confusion
- Palpitations
- Nausea
- Tingling

In Cardiac Arrest, immediate IV treatments:

- Calcium gluconate 10 ml of 10% may be given, over 2 minutes, to stabilise the heart muscle from toxic effects. Note: calcium gluconate does not irritate the veins as much as calcium chloride.

- Insulin (10-20 units) to push potassium into the cells, and dextrose to (25 g in 25 ml) to counter hypoglycaemia.
- Salbutamol helps shift K (potassium) into the cells - might be needed when insulin/glucose infusions fail to do so.
- Nebulised salbutamol, 10 mg.
- Sodium bicarbonate 1 mmol/kg of 8.4%, followed by half the dose every 10 minutes. **OR** 500 ml of 1.4%, over two hours – negates acidosis and moves K from extracellular fluid into cells.
- Furosemide and saline infusion can cause the nephrons to excrete K, in patients with normal kidney function.

Hypokalaemia

Causes: Dehydration or...

- Laxatives
- Kidney problems
- Metabolic alkalosis
- Steroids
- GI problems
- Low magnesium
- Diuretics
- Drugs
- Diet deficiency
- Burns
- Vomiting
- Hypothermia

ECG indications:

- Flattened T waves
- Negative T waves
- ST depression
- Prominent U waves

Treatment: Potassium.

A84: Preoperative Assessment

Example Checks

- Patient Identification
- BMI
- Medical History
- Comorbidities
- Current Conditions
- Medications
- Drug Use & History
- Mental State
- Allergies
- Fasting Status
- Dental/mouth Condition
- Previous Anaesthetic Experiences
- Diabetes Mellitus?
- ASA Score
- L.E.M.O.N. Score
- Wilson Score
- Blood Pressure, O_2 saturation, Heart rate, Respiratory rate
- As necessary: Bloods, Sickle Cell, CPET, Pregnancy, ...

A86: Pulmonary Embolism (PE)

Pulmonary Embolism Types

Peripheral

Travels to the lung, producing breathlessness and Pleurisy. This condition can occur due to placement of central (sometimes peripheral) venous lines, chest or abdomen insufflation, or head and neck surgery.

Massive Central

Lodges in a pulmonary artery, and prevents blood from leaving the right side of the heart. As a consequence, there is a significant reduction in cardiac output, resulting in hypotensive collapse and death. CPR may break up the embolus, and thrombolytic drugs, such as Streptokinase or rt-PA, help to dissolve it. To prevent a recurrence, Heparin and Warfarin might be given.

Saddle

The embolism lodges in the pulmonary trunk, and so blocks circulation to both left and right pulmonary arteries.

Pulmonary Embolism Symptoms

- Chest pain
- Coughing (blood?)
- Breathing problems
- Dysrhythmias
- Hypotension
- Cyanosis
- Cardiac arrest
- Sweating
- Fever
- Tachycardia
- Dizziness
- Drop in ETCO2
- Increased Central Venous Pressure

Management

- Give 100% oxygen
- Stop the source of the air/gas
- Discontinue nitrous oxide
- Compress the veins in the open surgical field
- Flood the open veins with saline
- Ensure the surgical field is lower than the heart
- Place the patient head and right side down
- Aspirate the right atrium or ventricle via a central line
- Anticoagulants

Note: hypoxia and hypocapnia are often signs of acute pulmonary embolism.

A87: Pulseless Electrical Activity

Cardiac arrest where the patient has a pulse, but with cardiac electrical activity, that fails to produce cardiac output. PEA usually has an underlying treatable cause which, in emergency situations, is most often hypovolaemia. Performing a pulse check after a rhythm/monitor check will ensure that PEA is identified.

Treatment (NOT shockable)...

- Start CPR (30:2)
- Give Adrenaline 1mg, iv
- Continue CPR 30:2 until airway secured, then continuously
- Treat reversible causes. See Appendix A92.

After 2 minutes, recheck the patient's condition...

- If a pulse is present, start post-resuscitation care.
- If rhythm is VF/VT, change to the shockable algorithm.
- If still in PEA, and no change in ECG appearance: continue CPR and give further adrenaline 1 mg every 3-5 min.

A88: Rapid Sequence Induction

Setting up:

- Tilting trolley or operating table.
- Suction - switched on and placed under the patient's pillow.
- Breathing circuit and oxygen.
- Selection of laryngoscope sizes, e.t. tubes, and blades.
- Bougie, cuff syringe, filter.
- Monitoring equipment.
- Range of oral airways.
- Anaesthetic drugs - induction agent (Thiopentone), Atropine, and Suxamethonium (succinylcholine).
- Have available a nasogastric tube and Magill forceps.

Preparation:

- A tube tie should be placed under the patient's neck.
- Suction turned on and placed under the pillow.
- Bougies/suction catheters at hand.
- Have various sized airways at hand.
- Attach a primed syringe to the inflation port of the e.t. tube.
- Ensure laryngoscope blades are at hand.

Method:

- Pre-oxygenate for 3 minutes (6-8 litres/min), or 8 vital capacity breaths with a non-rebreathing mask.
- Find cricoid cartilage (inform patient).
- Give Thiopentone, or Etomidate if CV problems.
- When patient closes eyes, apply cricoid pressure, with a force of 30 newtons - release if patient tries to vomit.
- When blinking stops, give Suxamethonium (succinylcholine).
- Intubate.
- Inflate the endotracheal tube cuff.
- Ensure a proper placement with end-tidal CO_2 reading.
- Release cricoid pressure when the anaesthetist says so.

Note: Preoxygenation may be supplemented with nasal prongs (15 L/min), to increase the FiO_2. Also, elevating the patient's head (reverse Trendelenburg) by 30° can improve gas exchange.

A89: Recovery

Upon arrival in Recovery

- Quickly assess airway, breathing, circulation
- Give 40% oxygen (6 litre flow)
- Assess skin colour - no cyanosis
- Fit monitors
- Note the time
- Observe the patient

Initial Assessment

- Consciousness level: swallowing, reflexes...
- Oxygen saturation
- Peripheral pulse (rate/force/rhythm)
- Respiratory rate (including depth & nature)
- Blood Pressure
- Temperature
- Perfusion
- Signs of haemorrhage (wound/drain/catheter)

Ongoing Assessment

- ♿ Consciousness level
- ♿ Oxygen saturation
- ♿ Blood pressure & peripheral pulse (rate/force/rhythm)
- ♿ Respiratory rate (including depth & nature)
- ♿ Blood Pressure
- ♿ Temperature
- ♿ Blood glucose (if appropriate)
- ♿ Skin colour
- ♿ Pain control
- ♿ postoperative nausea and vomiting
- ♿ Sensory level from regional blocks
- ♿ Pressure areas
- ♿ Outputs: Urine/wound/drains/stoma/NasoGastric Tube
- ♿ IV flow
- ♿ Dressing patency

A90: Regional Block

Example Block Types

Central (neuraxial)

- Epidural (below knee amputation)
- Spinal (hip, knee)

Peripheral plexus

- Brachial or interscalene (arm/shoulder surgery)
- Supraclavicular (elbow)

Single nerve

- Femoral and sciatic (knee replacement)
- Popliteal (ankle)

Setup

- Block trolley
- Ultrasound set and probe cover
- Inco pads
- 0.5% Chlorhexadine Gluconate OR 2% pink spray
- Sterile gel
- 22g probe needle (50/80/100 mm)

- Nerve stimulator + ECG dots
- 1% Lidocaine
- 5 ml syringe and orange needle
- Gauze swabs
- 1% and 2% Lidocaine/Adrenaline (fridge)
- 20 ml 0.5% Marcaine
- 2 * 20 ml syringes
- Capno Mask

A91: Respiratory Failure (RF) Types

Type I, *Hypoxic*

Hypoxaemia where arterial oxygen partial pressure (paO_2) < 8 kPa (60 mmHg), but without hypercapnia. *Caused by*: Asthma, lung damage, pneumonia, pulmonary embolus, pulmonary oedema.

Type II, *Hypercapnic*

Hypoxaemia with hypercapnia ($paCO_2$ > 6 kPa) and respiratory acidosis. Suggests lung problems. Aim for sats of 88-92%. If too much O_2 is given, hypercapnia can worsen.

Causes: Hypoventilation (due to COPD, drug respiratory depression, poor lung compliance), V/Q mismatch, morbid obesity, shunt, inability to perform proper gas exchange and diffusion.

RF Symptoms

Confusion, seizures, anxiety, cyanosis, coma, coughing up mucous, fatigue, tachycardia, hypertension, increased respiratory effort (tachypnoea, accessory breathing muscle activity, nasal flare).

RF Treatment

Treat the underlying cause, including airway clearance, oxygen, intubation, PEEP, pressure control ventilation, antibiotics (if lung infection), ECMO, tracheotomy, and bronchodilators.

A92: Reversible Causes of Cardiac Arrest

Cause	*Description*
Hypoxia	Causes: Airway obstruction, atelectasis, O_2 failure, misplaced ETT, bronchospasm, pneumothorax, drugs, volatiles, high spinal?
Hypovolaemia	**Absolute**: reduced blood volume from haemorrhage, AAA. **Relative**: vessel dilation.
Hyper/hypo disorders	Abnormal level of: eg, potassium, calcium, glucose, pH (acidosis, alkalosis). *Hypokalaemia is most common.*
Hypothermia	Core body temperature < 35° C.
Thrombosis	Blood clot in a **coronary** or **pulmonary** blood vessel.
Tension pneumothorax	Build up of air in the pleural space.
Cardiac Tamponade	Build up of fluid in the pericardial sac.
Toxins	Anaesthetics, drugs, alcohol?

See also guidelines at: http://www.resus.org.uk

A93: Second Gas Effect

Overview

At gas induction of anaesthesia, the rapid uptake from alveoli to pulmonary capillary blood of high concentrations of nitrous oxide (1st gas), means the nitrous oxide (N_2O) enters capillaries faster than the other gases, causing a void in the lung. The resultant reduced effective lung volume produces increased alveolar concentration of a second gas, such as sevoflurane, making a greater concentration effect (F_A/F_I ratio) that produces a higher (quicker) uptake of that second gas. In simple terms, to reduce gas induction time, add high flow nitrous oxide to the induction scheme.

Mechanism

N_2O (nitrous oxide) has a low *blood:gas partition coefficient*, which means that it is not easily soluble in blood. Once in the bloodstream, the low blood solubility of N_2O means very little becomes "part" of the blood (binding to plasma proteins). Instead, most of it remains unchanged, and quickly travels to the brain, where it exerts its anaesthetic effect.

Second Gas Effect

The rapid uptake (diffusion from alveolar to blood) of high concentrations of N_2O, at induction of inhalational anaesthesia, produces an increase in alveolar concentrations (partial pressures) of second gases, such as a volatile anaesthetic agent and O_2 (oxygen). This is the **Second Gas Effect**, which is a specific type of *Concentration Effect*.

Emergence

During emergence from an anaesthetic that included large amounts of N_2O, elimination of the N_2O from the bloodstream to the alveoli is rapid – because of its low solubility in blood. This rapid elimination dilutes other alveolar gases, such as O_2 which, in turn, may produce alveolar "diffusion hypoxia", also known as the *Fink Effect*. This, essentially, is the second gas effect, but in the opposite direction.

A94: Secondary Survey

Head:

- Skull
- Ears (blood or CSF)
- Eyes for pupil size and reaction (PEARL)
- Lips for colour (cyanosis)
- Jaw for displacement, mouth, teeth
- Skin colour/texture/temperature

Thorax:

- Clavicles
- Sternum
- Ribs

Abdomen:

- Rigidity and guarding
- Pulsating masses
- Bruising
- Pelvis

- Groin (dampness)

Limbs:

- Irregularity, deformity and fractures (compare limbs)
- Flexion and extension without aggravating any injury
- Signs of drug abuse (Needle marks)
- Identity bracelets
- Capillary refill and distal pulses

Back:

- Scapulae for fractures
- Spine for irregularities

History:

- Allergies
- Medication, documents, and previous medical history
- Last meal
- Event - what happened?

A95: Sepsis Signs

Sepsis definition (Sepsis-3): **infection** + 2 or more **SOFA** points (Appendix A97) but, for a preliminary and quick assessment, the following symptoms may help to indicate sepsis.

Early signs (all ages)

- Chills
- Temperature < 36° or > 37.5° C
- Tachycardia (90+)
- Tachypnoea (20+)

Later signs and septic shock

Rash: non-blanching	Tongue/lips: pale/blue/blotchy
Dizziness	Confusion
Muscle pain	Slurred speech
Unconsciousness	Clammy/cold skin
New or changed cough	Fatigue
Sore throat	Vomiting/nausea
Muscle/head aches	Diarrhoea
Low or painful urination	Abdominal pain

Young children (< 12) **sepsis** symptoms, any combination

Non blanching rash (as with meningitis)	Fast/difficult breathing
Blotchy/bluish skin, lips or tongue	Feels cold
Convulsions, vomiting	Inconsolable, sleepy
Jaundice	Bulging soft spots
Doesn't make eye contact	Decreased urination
Temperature < 36° or > 38° C	Infrequent urination

Sepsis Risk Factors

- ☠ Diabetes Mellitis
- ☠ Sickle Cell Disease
- ☠ Splenectomy
- ☠ Long term steroid use
- ☠ Invasive monitors
- ☠ Chemotherapy
- ☠ Age under 1, or over 65 years
- ☠ Difficult childbirth
- ☠ Recent surgery or skin breach
- ☠ Indwelling catheters
- ☠ Immunosuppressants
- ☠ Drug user

A96: Septic Shock

Septic Shock Main Signs

- Confirmed infection.
- Hypotension, to which fluid administration is ineffective, and vasopressors are needed to maintain MAP > 64 mmHg, in the absence of hypovolaemia, and lactate > 2 mmol/L (18 mg/dL).
- A serum lactate level greater than 2 mmol/litre.
- Altered mental state, slurred speech
- Diarrhoea
- Nausea/vomiting
- Cool, pale, clammy skin
- Dizziness
- Muscle pain
- Low urine output
- Unconsciousness

Note: A high serum lactate level, after fluid administration, suggests poor oxygenation to cells.

Immediate treatment: Assisted ventilation (if CPAP ineffective, intubation), vasopressors + Sepsis 6.

A97: Sequential Organ Failure Assessment

SOFA Organ System Scoring (0 = ok, 4 = most severe)

Respiration	0	1	2	3	4
PaO_2/FiO_2 [ie, P/F ratio]	≥ 400	< 400	< 300	< 200 with resp support	< 100 with resp support

Coagulation	0	1	2	3	4
Platelets 10^3/microlitre	>= 150	< 150	< 100	< 50	< 20

Liver	0	1	2	3	4
Bilirubin, mg/dL	< 1.2	1.2 – 1.9	2 – 5.9	6 – 11.9	12

Cardio-vascular	0	1	2	3	4
Mean Airway Pressure	> 69 mmHg (No vaso-pressors needed)	< 70 mmHg (No vaso-pressors needed)			
Vasopressors needed					
D = Dopamine A = Adrenaline Dt = Dobutamine N = Noradrenaline			**D** < 5 mcg/kg per min OR any dose **Dt**	**D** > 5 mcg/kg/min OR **A** <= 0.1 mcg/kg/min OR **N** <= 0.1 mcg/kg/min	**D** > 15 mcg/kg/min OR **A** > 0.1 mcg/kg/min OR **N** > 0.1 mcg/kg/min

CNS	0	1	2	3	4
GCS Score	15	13-14	10-12	6-9	< 6

Renal	0	1	2	3	4
Creatinine, mg/dL	< 1.2	1.2-1.9	2 - 3.4	3.5 - 4.9	> 5
Urine output/day				< 500 ml	< 200 ml

A98: Shock

Type	***Causes***
Hypovolaemic	Low blood volume: less than 80% of normal.
Cardiogenic (pump failure)	Myocardial infarction; arrhythmias.
Obstructive	Cardiac blood vessels flow impeded by pulmonary embolism, cardiac tamponade, or tension pneumothorax.
Distributive (sub-types below)	Excess vasodilation, as with SIRS, and septic, anaphylactic, insulin, and neurogenic shock.
Anaphylactic	Severe allergic reaction.
Neurogenic	CNS damage; spinal cord injury; sudden emotional distress.
Septic	Final phase of sepsis – large drop in BP.

Basic Observations

Shock Type	*HR*	*CVP*	*CO*	*Skin*
Hypovolaemic	↑	↓	↓	Cool clammy
Cardiogenic	↑	↑	↓↓	Pale
Obstructive	↑	↑	↓	Pale, cold, clammy
Anaphylactic	↑	↓	↓	Rash
Neurogenic	↓	↓	↓	Warm, then cool
Septic	↑	↓	↑ then ↓	Pale, cold, clammy

Key: **HR** Heart Rate, **CVP** Central Venous Pressure, **CO** Cardiac Output.

Symptoms common to all shock types

- Low systolic BP (< 90 mmHg)
- Hypovolaemia
- Tachypnoea
- Hypotension. Can be hypertension if anaphylactic shock
- Low urine output (oliguria) < 0.5 ml/kg/hour
- Metaboloc acidosis
- Reduced oxygen saturation

Other possible symptoms

- Reduced oxygen saturation
- Fever
- Capillary refill time: > 2 secs
- Peripheral shut down
- Thirst
- Dizziness, confusion, agitation, speech difficulty
- Diarrhoea
- Nausea/vomiting
- Muscle ache/weakness
- Chest pain

Treatment

Call for help, lay the patient down, elevate the legs, administer fluids, monitor for cardiac arrest.

A99: Spinal Block

A neuro-axial block, typically using Diamorphine and/or 0.5% Heavy Marcain, into the cerebrospinal fluid of the subarachnoid (aka intrathecal) space, below (inferior to) L2 (2nd lumbar), whilst avoiding piercing the spinal cord. This produces a temporary (2-3 hours) block of the sensory, motor, and autonomic nerves, which come into contact with the anaesthetic.

The sensory block gives the required analgesia, but the associated motor block causes weakness or paralysis, whilst the autonomic block causes vasodilation of blood vessels within the distribution of the block. Vasoconstrictors counter resultant hypotension.

Injection point

The level of the injection influences the rate of spread of the block, as does the amount of anaesthetic, and patient position. Injection is usually made below the 2nd Lumbar vertebra, where the spinal cord terminates, and there is less risk of nerve damage from the needle. Fine bore needles are used, with "pencil" point and smallest gauge being least likely to cause post-spinal headache, which is caused by CSF leakage through the hole in the dura mater, made by the needle.

Equipment

- Regional block trolley
- Stools for patient and Anaesthetist
- Basic Universal set (sterile gallipots, swabs etc)
- Extra drape (75*75)
- 0.5% Chlorhexadine Gluconate spray
- Syringes: 1 ml, 5 ml luer lock, 10 ml luer lock
- Saline: 10 ml
- 1% Lidocaine (10 ml syringe, blue/orange needle)
- 4 ml Heavy Marcain (5 ml syringe)
- Diamorphine 5 mg (powder, mix with normal saline)
- Whitacre/20g or 25g Abbocath/90mm (+ introducer) needle
- Opsite - post injection
- "Cryo" spray - to test effectiveness of spread

A100: Spinal (Quincke, Whitacre, Sprotte) & Epidural (Tuohy) Needles

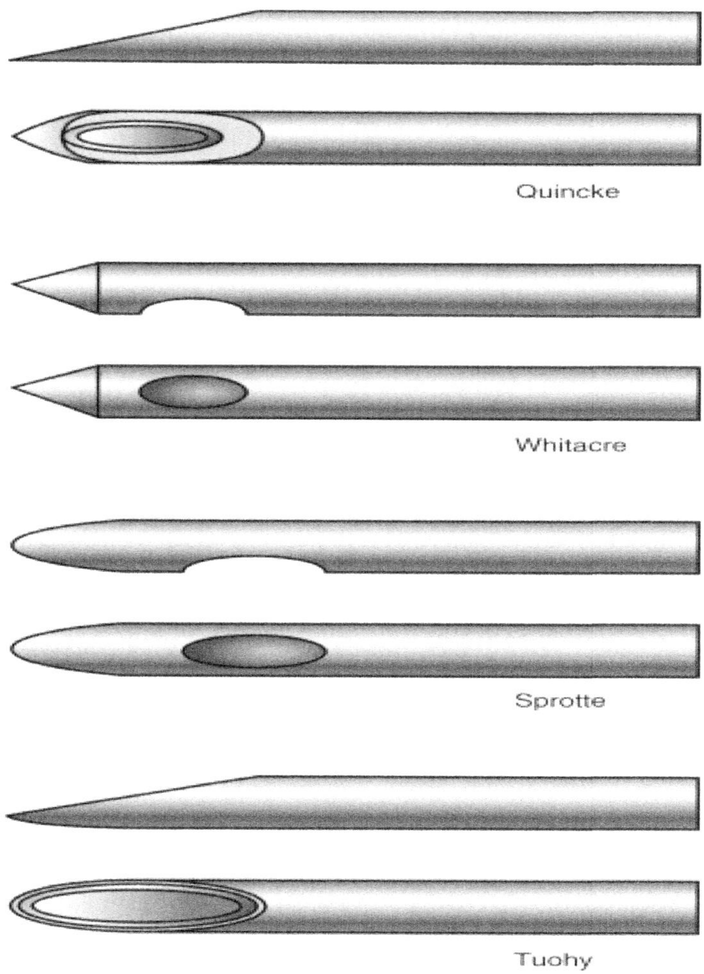

A101: Stroke

The brain needs the oxygen and nutrients provided by blood. If the supply of blood is restricted, brain cells begin to die, which may lead to brain damage and, possibly, death.

General Signs

- Drooping on one side of the face
- Cannot fully raise the arms
- Slurred speech/confusion
- Dysphagia

Two main types of Stroke

Ischaemic Stroke

Brain blood supply is stopped due to a clot, usually atherosclerosis.

Signs: Headache, numbness, one sided weakness, vision problems, imbalance, slurred speech, poor limb movement, confusion.

Treatments: Aspirin (antiplatelet), Acteplase to dissolve clots, Thrombectomy (surgery).

Haemorrhagic Stroke

A blood vessel supplying the brain bursts. Typical cause is hypertension.

Signs: Weakness, speech and walking problems, vomiting, irregular breathing, erratic eye movement, numbness or paralysis, coma.

Treatment: Surgical "clipping" to arrest bleeding.

ROSIER Score

Sign	***No***	***Yes***
Syncope	0	**-1**
Seizures	0	**-1**
Asymmetric facial weakness	0	1
Asymmetric arm weakness	0	1
Asymmetric leg weakness	0	1
Speech problems	0	1
Vision defects	0	1

Score Result

- Less than 1 (-2, -1, 0) means stroke is unlikely.
- Greater than 0 (1-5) means stroke is more likely.

A102: Subcutaneous Injection

General Description

A needle with a drug charged syringe, goes through the skin and into subcutaneous tissue. Subcut injections are not given if the skin is burnt, hardened, inflamed, swollen, or damaged by a previous injection.

If two inches (5 cm) of skin (not muscle) can be grasped between the thumb and index finger, the needle is inserted at right angles to the injection site. If only one inch (2.5 cm) of skin can be grasped, the angle is reduced to 45 degrees.

Injection Sites

- Outside of the upper arm
- Rear of the upper arm
- Upper thigh
- Abdomen - 1 inch from the navel

Method

- Clean injection site with an alcohol swab (spiral outwards).
- Allow to dry.

- Remove needle (12/15 mm length. 25/27/30 guage) cover.
- Hold the syringe like a dart.
- Grasp skin between thumb and index finger.
- Thrust the needle into the skin at an angle of 90°.
- Children and those with little subcutaneous fat – 45° angle.
- Once fully inserted, release the skin.
- Grasp the base of the syringe to stabilise it.
- Aspirate (pull the plunger) to ensure no blood is present.
- If blood is aspirated, discard the needle and start again.
- If no blood appears, inject medication over 10 seconds.
- After 10 secs, remove the needle, apply pressure (swab).
- Dispose of sharps.

A103: Submental Intubation

The patient undergoes a standard intubation with an armoured et (endotracheal) tube, ensuring that the circuit to tube connector can be removed and replaced.

On the operating table, the patient is preloaded with 100 % oxygen, before the surgical team perform the conversion to submental intubation:

Note: During this process, the ET tube must be stabilised, to avoid displacement.

► A local anaesthetic, with adrenaline (epinephrine), is injected into the midline of the submental region, to the floor of the mouth (oral cavity), and into the oral mucosa.

► The ET tube is held secure, to prevent displacement.

► A 1-2 cm (0.4 - 0.8 inch) lateral incision is made submentally.

► A blunt dissection is made, with curved artery forceps, through to the floor of the mouth, avoiding the lingual nerve, salivary duct, and salivary gland.

► A percutaneous tracheotomy dilator opens up the above passage, from the mouth, and out through the submental incision.

► The dilator is passed through again, from opposite direction.

► The ET tube pilot ballon is fed into the top (mouth) of the dilator.

► The dilator is pulled out, submentally, taking the secured pilot balloon with it.

► The dilator is fed back up through the incision to the mouth.

► The ET tube is disconnected from the circuit, and its connector.

► Circuit end of the ET tube is railroaded over the tip of the dilator, then the dilator leads the tube out through the submental opening.

► The connector and circuit are reconnected to the ET tube.

► The ET tube is secured/sutured in place.

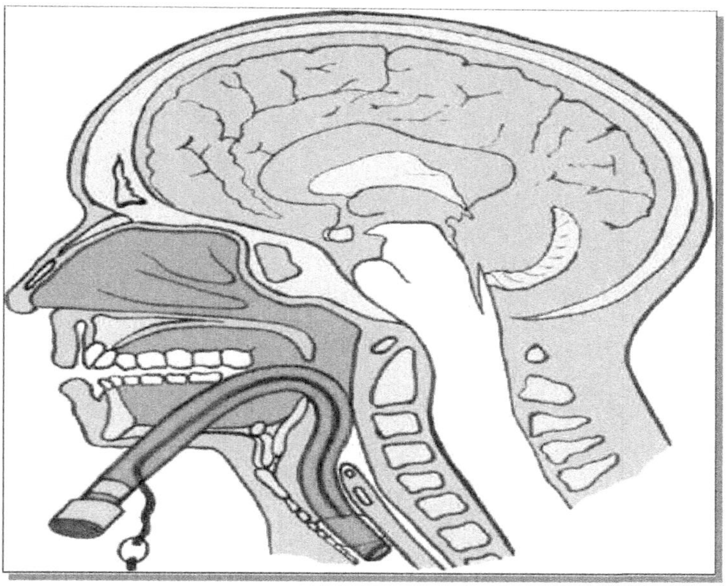

When submental intubation is completed, the ET tube is seen leading up through the mentum (chin), and no part of the tube is in the nasal or oral cavities. (Image courtesy of *Trauma Pro*)

A104: Tension Pneumothorax

Pneumothorax due to air escaping into the pleural cavity, typically as a consequence of a penetrating injury. Increasing air pressure in the pleural cavity progressively collapses the lung. Intrapleural pressure can increase to the point where it compresses the vena cava, and interferes with venous return (cardiac preload), resulting in blood pooling in capacitance vessels, and reduced cardiac output, with ensuing cardiovascular collapse and shock.

Signs

- Respiratory distress
- Tachypnoea
- **Hypotension**
- **Hypoxia**
- Muffled lung sounds
- Hyper-expanded chest
- Distended jugular veins (JVD)
- Sudden onset sharp chest pain
- Mediastinal shift to opposite side
- Tracheal deviation opposite to the tension side

Treatment

Emergency decompression, to alleviate intrapleural pressure, by thoracocentesis with a 12-16 g needle in the 2nd intercostal space. If pneumothorax recurs, a tube thoracostomy may be performed.

A105: Target Controlled Infusion

Software governed infusion device to control drug dosages, according to parameters such as gender, age, and weight. The object is to produce an optimal target concentration of the drug in the brain, and so provide the required anaesthetic effect, rather than the patient experiencing the highs and falls in concentration when given boluses. Other advantages are reduced nausea/vomiting, and an increased blood flow in the brain.

Equipment

- TCI Pump and power cable
- 2 * 50 ml luer lock syringes
- 2 * Electro-cath tubing + Electro-cath union connector
- 2% propofol and mini spikes
- Remifentanil
- Normal saline

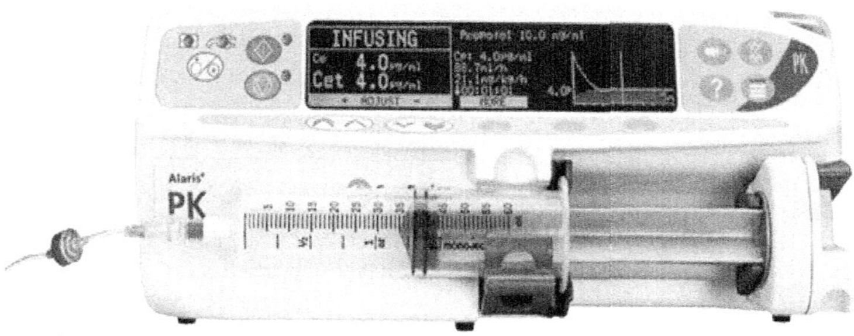

A106: Thiopentone

The following points govern the use of Thiopentone:

- Airway reflexes are maintained
- Not suitable with LMA use – laryngospasm, because of above
- Does not cause significant hypotension
- Reduces intracranial pressure
- Prompt return of protective airway reflexes
- Decreases cerebral metabolism and cerebral blood flow
- Safe for induction of obstetric cases (but crosses the placenta)
- Contraindicated in hypovolaemic patients
- May cause bronchospasm in asthmatics
- Increases heart rate
- Reduces cardiac output & blood pressure

A107: Two Bag Test

Stages:

- Attach a reservoir bag (test lung) to the patient end of the circuit, include the HME filter and angle piece (if used).
- Set a gas flow of 5 litre/minute.
- Set the APL valve to 30 cmH_2O.
- Manually ventilate the test lung.
- Ensure there is no loss of pressure.
- Observe the 1-way valves are functioning.
- Squeeze both bags to verify the APL valve pressure release.
- Switch to “ventilator” mode, and verify there are no leaks.
- Turn off gas flow and check there are no leaks.
- For each vaporiser; turn on and ensure no leaks; turn off.

A108: Universal/Standard Precautions

Specific aspects to manage include:

- Hand wash (WHO 5 moments)
- Staff immunity
- Safe use/disposal of sharps
- Clinical waste disposal
- Management of body fluids
- Isolation policy
- Environmental cleaning
- Use of indwelling devices
- Communication skills
- Aseptic non-touch technique
- Waste management
- Safe handling of linen
- Personal protective equipment
- Respiratory hygiene and coughing control
- Decontamination of reusable medical equipment

A109: Vasopressors

Perioperatively, Ephedrine and Metaraminol should always be immediately available. Ephedrine has a faster onset than Metaraminol, but only lasts for about 10 minutes; whereas Metaraminol lasts 20-60 minutes.

Vasoconstriction routes

- Exogenous (external source)
- Adrenaline and Noradrenaline (internally secreted)
- Angiotensin
- Antidiuretic hormone (ADH)
- Alpha-adrenergic sympathomimetic drugs

Exogenous causes of vasoconstriction

- Cold
- Fear/Stress
- Nicotine

Alpha-adrenergic sympathomimetics

Vasopressors that are used to maintain blood pressure during anaesthesia, and in treating hypotension.

♦ Metaraminol ♦ Ephedrine ♦ Noradrenaline ♦ Phenylephrine

A110: Ventilation/Perfusion (V/Q)

V (ventilation) is the air breathed in through the nose and mouth, down the trachea, into the bronchi, and then through smaller airways to the alveoli, where the exchange of oxygen and carbon dioxide takes place.

Q (perfusion) is the flow of oxygenated blood to the capillary bed, in order to conduct nutrient and gas exchange.

V/Q (ventilation/perfusion): The ratio which illustrates the relationship between the volume of air (V) which reaches the alveoli, and the volume of blood (Q) which flows through the lung capillaries. V/Q is used to assess the efficiency of how ventilation and perfusion are matched.

Normal ventilation is 4 litre/minute. Normal perfusion is 5 litre/minute. This gives a V/Q ratio of 0.8. Anything other than 0.8 is a V/Q mismatch - a feature of COPD.

In right to left pulmonary shunt, V/Q is 0.

Note: Ventilation and perfusion volumes are higher in the lower parts of the lung, but the V/Q ratio is higher in the upper parts.

A111: Ventilator Settings (example)

Setting	*Value*
FiO_2	1
PEEP	5-10 cmH_2O
Mode	SIMV
Inspiratory pressure	25 cmH_2O
I:E ratio	1:2
Respiratory rate	12/minute

A112: VF and VT ECG Traces

Ventricular Fibrillation

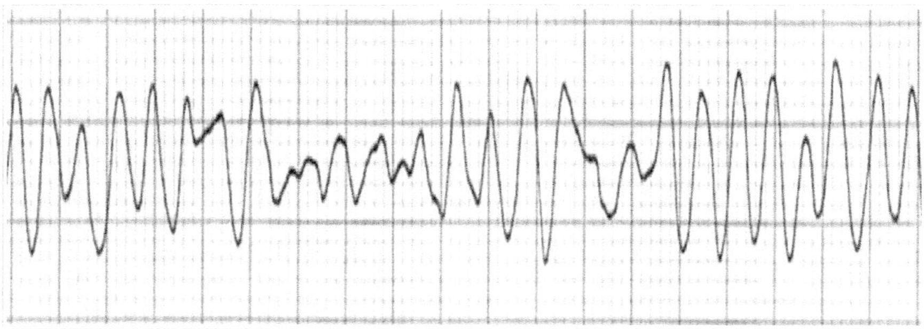

Ventricular Tachycardia

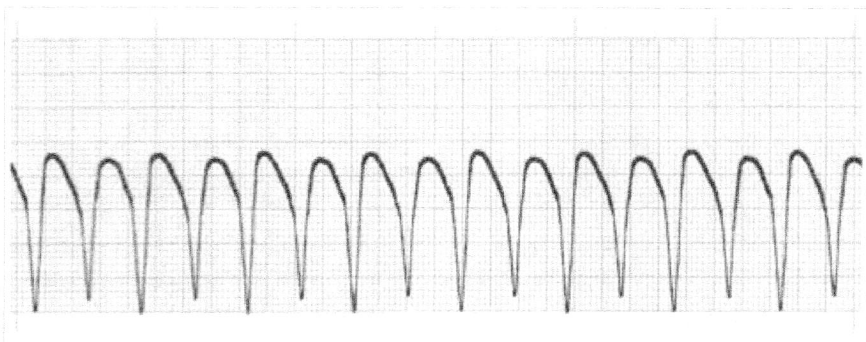

A113: VivaSight D-L

A camera guided double lumen endotracheal/bronchial tube, to isolate one lung - with or without a laryngoscope. The distal (blue) part of the tube is passed into the left main bronchus, and the lung is isolated with an inflation cuff (max pressure 25 cmH_2O). The more proximal part of the tube (white) sits in the trachea, which is sealed by another cuff. Between the two cuffs is the camera and LED light source. Placement is made easier with a dedicated VivaSight stylet. A small cable (white) connects the camera with an external monitor, and an injection port (brown) is used for flushing the camera lens with air or normal saline, but not for suctioning the airway. Fr type sizes are 35, 37, 39, 41.

Setting up

- Test and deflate the cuffs.
- Connect camera and monitor.
- Lightly lubricate the tube with water based gel.
- Suction the airway.

Technique

- Pass bronchial tip (blue) through vocal cords – bevel up.
- Remove the stylet.
- Rotate tube 90° anti-clockwise, so camera pointing up.
- Advance tracheal lumen (white) until passed vocal cords.

- Advance until tip (blue) in left bronchus, and carina in view.
- Inflate cuffs.

Note: For gas to flow through a lumen, the arrow on the rotator must be in line with the arrow on the Y-connector.

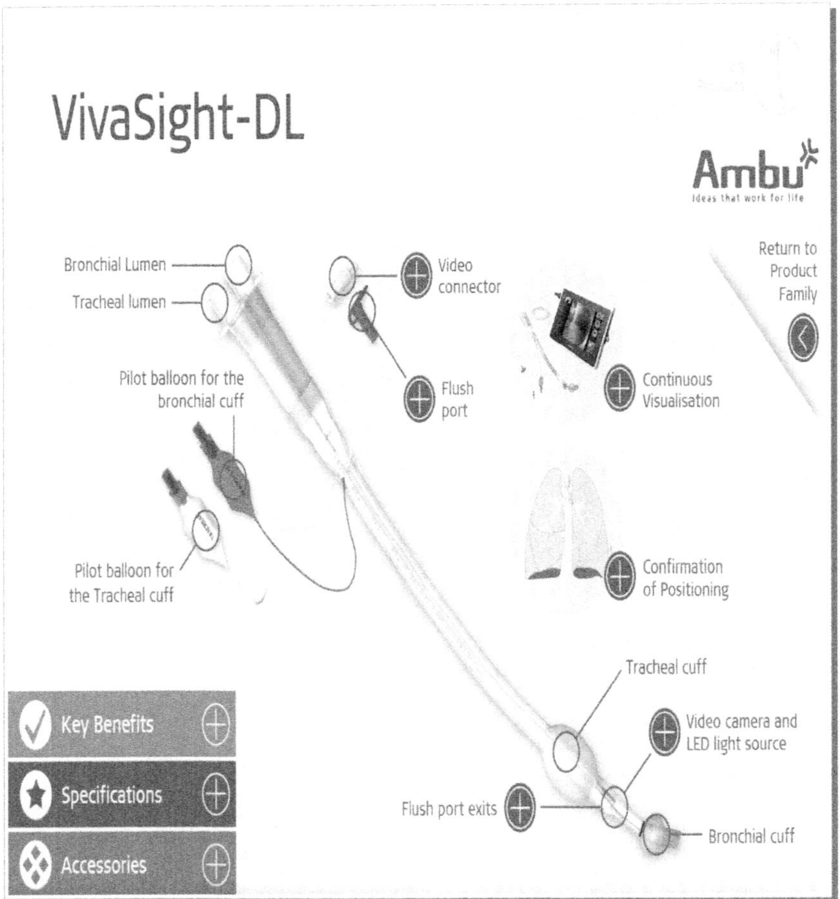

A114: British Thoracic Society Oxygen Codes

Code	Description
A	Breathing ambient (room) air
CP	CPAP device
H	Humidified oxygen and % eg, H40
N	Nasal cannula
NIV	Non-invasive device: BiPAP, NPV.
RM	Reservoir mask
SM	Simple mask
TM	Tracheostomy mask
V	Venturi mask and % eg, V24
OTH	Other, specify:

Books by John England

📖 **Blood Gases**
https://www.amazon.co.uk/dp/B09755Pd1F/ref

📖 **Q & A: Anaesthetic Principles, Volume 1**
http://amzn.eu/iIbr8eK

📖 **Q & A: Anaesthetic Principles, Volume 2**
http://amzn.eu/4eKMyRe

📖 **Q & A: Anaesthetic Principles, Volume 3**
http://www.amazon.co.uk/dp/B0876F7V6S

📖 **Q & A: Anaesthetic Principles, Volumes 1-3**
https://www.amazon.co.uk/dp/B087BJ7YXW

📖 **Perioperative Topics: Test and Learn**
http://amzn.eu/gMhiDvm

📖 **Q & A: Basic Life Support**
http://amzn.eu/acoxDel

📖 **Science Glossary**
https://www.amazon.co.uk/dp/B08DMV7GM/ref

📖 **Pass Your Drug Calculation Test**
http://amzn.eu/duk6uT7

📖 **Basic Drug Calculations**
http://amzn.eu/d0SWt0c

📖 **Drug Calculation Workbook**
http://amzn.eu/d39gtl3

📖 **Drug Calculation Examples**
http://amzn.eu/76zGfkJ

📖 **Drug Calculations By Formula**
http://amzn.eu/eW9SEg3

📖 **Advanced Drug Calculation Workbook**
http://amzn.eu/7zDyFQh

📖 **Nurse Q & A: Anatomy and Physiology**
http://amzn.eu/f6nRC6G

📖 **Q & A: Respiratory System**
http://amzn.eu/7RqNNxa

Printed in Great Britain
by Amazon

86857379R00312